# Psychiatry

SECOND EDITION

## AN ILLUSTRATED COLOUR TEXT

*Commissioning Editor:* Timothy Horne
*Development Editor:* Sheila Black
*Project Manager:* Frances Affleck
*Designer:* Kirsteen Wright
*Illustration Manager:* Merlyn Harvey
*Illustrators:* Evi Antioniou-Tibbits, Cactus Design & Illustration Ltd

# Psychiatry

SECOND EDITION

## AN ILLUSTRATED COLOUR TEXT

**Lesley Stevens** MB BS FRCPsych
Consultant Psychiatrist,
Hampshire Partnership NHS Foundation Trust,
Winchester, UK

**Ian Rodin** BM MRCPsych
Consultant Psychiatrist,
Dorset Community Health Services,
NHS Dorset, UK

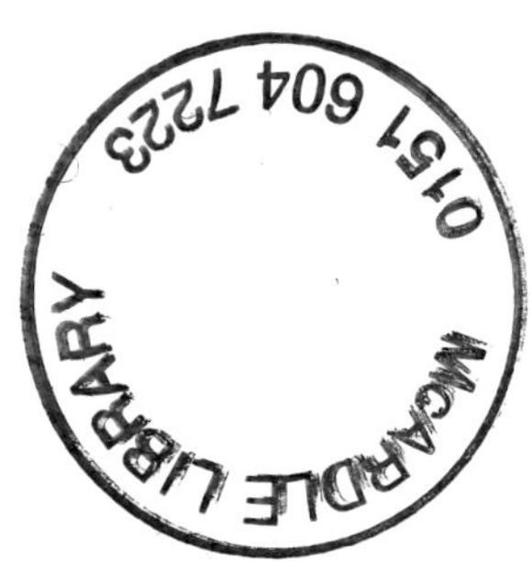


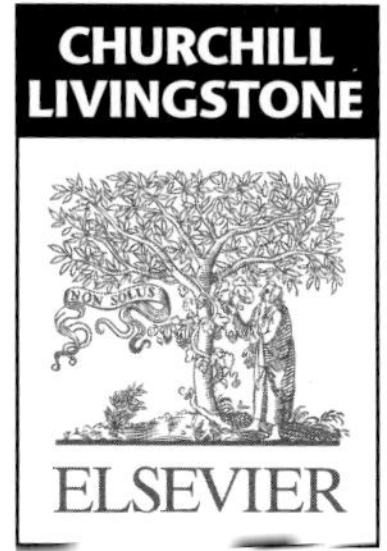


EDINBURGH LONDON NEW YORK OXFORD PHILADELPHIA ST LOUIS SYDNEY TORONTO 2011

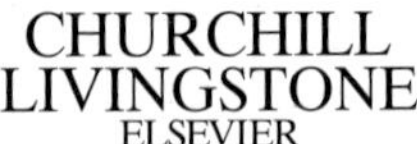



ISBN 978-0-7020-3396-4

**British Library Cataloguing in Publication Data**
A catalogue record for this book is available from the British Library

**Library of Congress Cataloging in Publication Data**
A catalog record for this book is available from the Library of Congress

**Notices**

Knowledge and best practice in this field are constantly changing. As new research and experience broaden our understanding, changes in research methods, professional practices, or medical treatment may become necessary.

Practitioners and researchers must always rely on their own experience and knowledge in evaluating and using any information, methods, compounds, or experiments described herein. In using such information or methods they should be mindful of their own safety and the safety of others, including parties for whom they have a professional responsibility.

With respect to any drug or pharmaceutical products identified, readers are advised to check the most current information provided (i) on procedures featured or (ii) by the manufacturer of each product to be administered, to verify the recommended dose or formula, the method and duration of administration, and contraindications. It is the responsibility of practitioners, relying on their own experience and knowledge of their patients, to make diagnoses, to determine dosages and the best treatment for each individual patient, and to take all appropriate safety precautions.

To the fullest extent of the law, neither the Publisher nor the authors, contributors, or editors, assume any liability for any injury and/or damage to persons or property as a matter of products liability, negligence or otherwise, or from any use or operation of any methods, products, instructions, or ideas contained in the material herein.



The publisher's policy is to use **paper manufactured from sustainable forests**

Printed in China

# Preface

This book is aimed at medical students, but should be suitable for anyone learning about psychiatry for the first time, or needing to refresh their knowledge. What makes it different from other introductory psychiatry texts is its format, which will be familiar to readers of other books from the Illustrated Colour Text series. There are illustrations and clinical examples throughout, and each topic is covered in two facing pages. This has allowed us to keep the book relatively brief and still cover a wide range of information. There are summary boxes, questions and answers about clinical problems, and a new self-assessment section, all of which should help you monitor and revise your learning. We have tried to produce a book that is stimulating and easy to read. Psychiatry is a fascinating and highly rewarding field and we hope this book will help you make the most of it. If we encourage you to meet and work with psychiatric patients and their families, and give you the knowledge you need to do this effectively, then we will have succeeded.

Lesley Stevens
Ian Rodin
2011

# Acknowledgements

We wrote the first edition of the book when we were lecturers in psychiatry at the University of Southampton and continue to teach students from the School of Medicine. This experience, and the encouragement and guidance given to us by Chris Thompson, Robert Peveler and David Baldwin, has been invaluable. We couldn't have written this second edition without the advice of Alison Taylor and Sheila Black at Elsevier and, once again, the tolerance and support of our partners, Joe and Deborah.

# Contents

# Mental health services I

## Case history 1

John is a 23-year-old unemployed, single man who lives with his parents. He has chronic schizophrenia. When he is acutely unwell he becomes distressed because he hears threatening voices, and is suspicious and frightened of his parents. He has threatened his mother in the past, and she is frightened of him, although he has never hurt her physically. Medication is effective in controlling these episodes, but he does not like taking it and often 'forgets'. Between these episodes he is withdrawn, spending most of his time lying on his bed, with little contact with his family and no friends. His father is angry that he is 'lazy' and would like him to move out, but John shows no signs of going.

a. Which members of the psychiatric multidisciplinary team should be involved in John's care, and what are their roles?
b. Which team member would be the most appropriate care co-ordinator, and why?

Most mental illnesses are caused by a combination of biological, psychological and social factors. Some patients have complex needs that cannot be met by a single mental health professional. When ill, patients are often unable to fulfil their usual role at home, work and elsewhere, and may neglect or harm themselves. Their behaviour may be odd, impulsive, disinhibited or violent, and this may damage relationships or lead to others being harmed. Social factors such as homelessness and unemployment may act as precipitating or maintaining factors in the illness, and clearly cannot be ignored in treatment. It is essential, therefore, that a mental health service should include psychiatric services, social services, housing agencies, voluntary agencies and others working closely together (Fig. 1). This style of inter-agency working is characteristic of psychiatry and distinguishes it from many other branches of medicine. Psychiatrists usually work in multidisciplinary teams, in a variety of settings, including hospitals and the community.

## The changing face of psychiatry

The majority of old psychiatric hospitals were built as a result of the Lunatics Act of 1845. They were generally large, imposing buildings in isolated rural locations, cut off from the outside world. The hospitals were rapidly filled, and bed numbers over the following 100 years rose at an alarming rate. In the absence of adequate systems for assessment and diagnosis, many patients were admitted inappropriately and lack of effective treatments meant that management was largely custodial. Patients were generally held against their will and for long periods. Wards were locked, with patients allowed outside only under supervision from staff.

In the late 1930s, electroconvulsive therapy (ECT) was introduced, and there was a slow move towards unlocking wards, voluntary treatment and provision of outpatient services. The number of psychiatric beds began to reduce and this process was accelerated by the discovery of the first effective drug treatment for schizophrenia, chlorpromazine, in 1952. Patients who had previously been very disturbed and difficult to manage improved on this drug, allowing more wards to be unlocked and patients to be discharged. Rehabilitation techniques accelerated the discharge process by tackling the effects of institutional living that in itself left many patients disabled and unable to live independently.

Since then there has been a steady move towards providing psychiatric treatment in the community. Psychiatric inpatient beds have been closed in large numbers (Fig. 2), and long stay residents of the old institutions have been rehoused, some to independent living and others to wards in the community, staffed hostels or supported lodgings. Where possible, patients are now treated in their own homes, outpatient clinics or day hospitals. Inpatient treatment will always be necessary for some and, ideally, should be provided in purpose-built units close to the community that the patient comes from, allowing regular contact with family and friends and a smooth transition from hospital to home when well.

## Psychiatric treatment settings

### *Inpatient treatment*

In general, very thorough psychiatric assessments and treatments can be provided in the community, and few patients need admission. When it is necessary, psychiatric wards can provide a safe, supportive environment for the most unwell patients. Urgent admission may be needed if the patient is at risk of neglect, deliberate self harm or suicide, or is violent. Some treatments, such as electroconvulsive therapy (ECT) or initiation

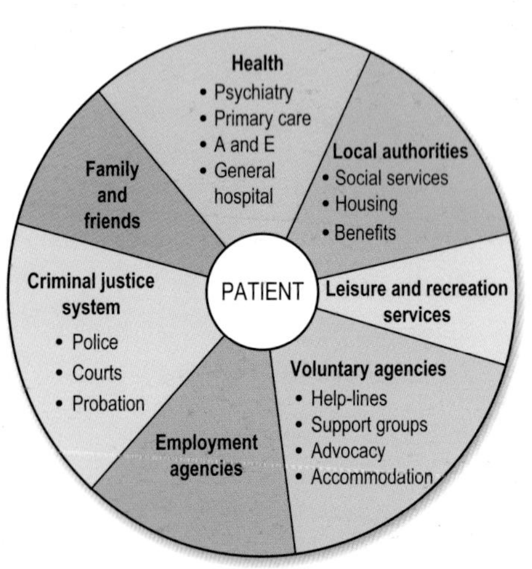


Fig. 1 **Agencies involved in mental health services.**

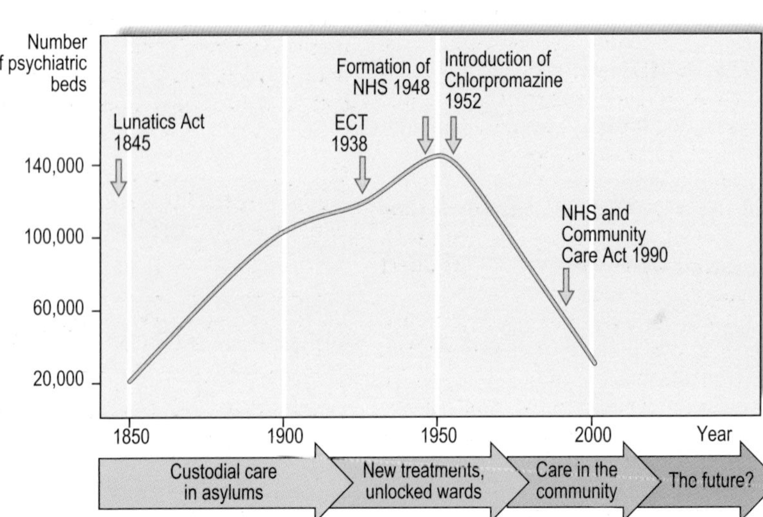


Fig. 2 **Changes in psychiatric services.**

of clozapine, will often require a period of admission, although services are increasingly flexible in delivering even the most complex treatments outside hospital.

### *Outpatient clinics*

Outpatient clinics tend to be run in community settings, such as GP surgeries and community mental health centres, rather than in hospitals. Most non-urgent referrals to psychiatrists are assessed and treated in these clinics. Some offer specialist services (e.g. lithium or clozapine clinics or depot injection clinics). Often these clinics are run by other mental health practitioners.

### *Day hospitals*

Day hospitals are staffed by multidisciplinary teams and can provide a comprehensive service. They may be used as an alternative to admission for patients requiring a high level of support and monitoring but considered to be well enough to go home for evenings and weekends. This is often made possible through the support of relatives and carers. Their use has declined in adult services, but they are still often used in Older Persons' Mental Health services.

### *Community Mental Health Teams (CMHTs)*

CMHTs consist of psychiatrists, community mental health nurses, social workers, psychologists, occupational therapists and support workers who work together to provide a community service. They are based in centres away from the hospital and convenient for the community they serve. They see patients in their own homes and in clinics. This model has been adapted to develop specialist teams, described overleaf.

## The Multidisciplinary Team (MDT)

Psychiatrists routinely work as part of an MDT, in order to be able to offer patients comprehensive care that addresses their medical, social and psychological needs. Ideally, an MDT works closely together, with regular meetings to discuss patients in their care. Referrals are discussed and allocated to the most appropriate team member for assessment. Some patients will only require contact with one member of the team, while others with more complicated needs may have direct contact with several.

Teams work most efficiently if they share a common goal, communicate well with each other and have clear leadership. In most cases, the consultant psychiatrist has a leadership role in the team. There is unlikely to be a clear hierarchy across the professional groups involved and there may be some conflict about leadership. It is vital that the members are comfortable with the leadership arrangements. Open discussion of the issues by all members of the team is important.

The role of each team member and the skills they can contribute must be clearly understood by all. There is likely to be some overlapping of roles, and it is essential that the responsibilities of each individual in caring for a particular patient are made clear to all concerned.

## Who is in the MDT?

**Psychiatrists** are doctors who have undertaken a specialist training in mental health that is accredited by the Royal College of Psychiatrists. They are responsible for the medical care of mentally ill patients, including assessment, diagnosis and management, and are the only member of the team able to prescribe drugs. They also have responsibilities under the Mental Health Act, 1983 (see p. 18).

**Psychiatric nurses** are Registered Mental Nurses (RMNs) who have completed a 3-year training in mental health. Their roles are varied, and they may work in many different settings, including wards, day hospitals, outpatient clinics and the community. In hospitals they have responsibility for ensuring the environment is therapeutic and safe, and for observing and monitoring patients.

**Community psychiatric nurses (CPNs)** are RMNs who have been trained in community nursing. They usually work in CMHTs. Their role includes provision of psychological therapies, long-term support for the chronically mentally ill, counselling and administration of injected depot medication.

**Clinical psychologists** have a degree in psychology and a postgraduate qualification in clinical work, usually an MSc. Their role is in assessment of patients and provision and supervision of psychological therapies. Special skills enable them to test intelligence, personality and neuropsychological functioning of patients with suspected brain damage or dementia.

**Occupational therapists (OTs)** have a 3-year specialist training in occupational therapy. They work in hospital and increasingly in the community assisting mentally ill patients to develop confidence and skills in social and occupational environments using a wide range of activities.

**Social workers** have a general qualification in social work and may specialise in mental health. Social workers in mental health teams often act as Approved Mental Health Practitioners, exercising responsibilities under the Mental Health Act, 2007. They have a wide ranging role, applying a social perspective to the problems they encounter.

**Support, Time and Recovery (STR) Workers** are so called because their role is to offer support and give time to the patient on their journey to recovery. They work under the supervision of the care co-ordinator.

## Care Programme Approach

The Care Programme Approach (CPA) is an important part of mental health policy in the UK. It was first implemented in 1991 following concerns that some patients were falling through the network of services. It is designed to ensure that the various agencies and professionals involved in the care of the vulnerable mentally ill work with the patient and their family to develop co-ordinated management plans (Fig. 3). A 'Care Co-ordinator' is appointed from the multidisciplinary team to ensure the plans are put into action. In 2008 the CPA policy was modified so that only those with more complex needs come under CPA. All other patients must have their care planned and documented by a 'Lead Professional'.

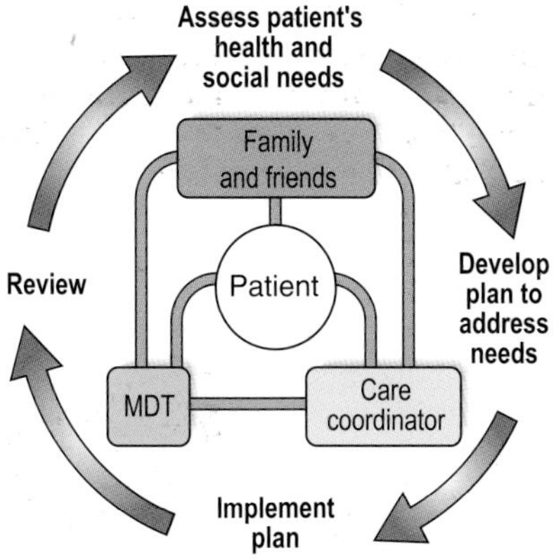


Fig. 3 **The Care Programme Approach.**

### Mental Health Services

- The medical, psychological and social needs of mentally ill patients must be considered
- Psychiatric services work with other agencies to provide for their patient's needs, including social services, housing departments and voluntary agencies
- Psychiatrists work in multidisciplinary teams including nurses, social workers, psychologists and OTs

# Mental health services II

## *Case history 2*

Jess has been treated in an inpatient unit under section 3 of the Mental Health Act. She was admitted with an acute manic episode. She had stopped taking her lithium a few weeks before admission, and had not kept any appointments with her care co-ordinator or psychiatrist from the Community Mental Health Team. She has responded well to treatment in hospital, and has had some successful home leave. However, she still has little insight into her illness, and is ambivalent about taking lithium when out of hospital. The ward has requested a Care Programme Approach (CPA) meeting to plan her discharge.

a. Who should be invited to attend the CPA meeting?
b. What might be included in the plan?

In recent years the way mental health services are organised has changed dramatically, with the emergence of new teams, with a focus on caring for people in their own homes as far as possible. These teams specialise in a particular area of health care, and patients will often move between teams as their illness or circumstances change. They may also have input from several teams at the same time. In these circumstances the care co-ordinator plays a key role in providing a consistent point of contact for the patient, and all teams have to work hard on their communication with other teams. This section describes three specialist teams – Crisis Resolution and Home Treatment teams (CRHT), Early Intervention in Psychosis teams (EIP) and Assertive Outreach teams (AOT). There are many other types of specialist teams such as perinatal services, liaison services, memory clinics, drug and alcohol services, which will be described in the appropriate chapters later in the book.

Figure 1 illustrates the pathway through four different mental health teams taken by Sam, a 19-year-old man. Sam presents to his GP for the first time, at the insistence of his mother who is concerned that he is spending all of his time in his bedroom, not seeing his friends, and tending to sleep all day, and stay awake all night. The GP is concerned that he may be depressed and refers him to the Community Mental Health Team (CMHT). He is seen initially by a social worker from the team, who visits him at home. He tells the social worker that he is spending most of his time on his computer because he has discovered a conspiracy that involves police forces in several countries working together to support terrorist activity. He is concerned that as he knows about it he will himself become a terrorist target, and feels he needs to lie low. He is very frightened and distressed by these beliefs, but has not discussed them with anyone else. The social worker is concerned that he is psychotic, and takes him in to the CMHT team base to see the psychiatrist in clinic for an urgent assessment.

The psychiatrist agrees that Sam has a psychotic illness, and prescribes antipsychotic medication. As he is young, and presenting with psychotic symptoms for the first time they agree to refer him to the Early Intervention in Psychosis service (EIP). A nurse from this team meets with Sam and his mother at home the next day, and agrees to become his care co-ordinator, and to visit him daily initially, to complete an assessment, monitor his progress, and offer support to his mother. However, Sam's mental state deteriorates. He is very suspicious of the medication, fearing that it may poison him, and becomes increasingly suspicious of staff, and regretful that he has talked about his fears, as he thinks this will put him in danger. The EIP team decides that as things are deteriorating he may need admission to hospital. They therefore refer him to the Crisis Resolution and Home Treatment Team (CRHT). Their role is to assess whether it is possible to safely treat him at home with more intensive support from their team.

The CRHT consultant and nurse see Sam at home, and decide that it is not going to be possible to treat him at home because of the level of distress he is experiencing and his adamant refusal to take any medication. He is therefore admitted to the local inpatient unit under a section of the Mental Health Act. He is assessed and treated by the inpatient medical and nursing staff, and responds well to antipsychotic medication, which he agrees to take in hospital, and following his discharge. During his stay his care co-ordinator from EIP visits him regularly, and as his mental state improves takes him out for visits home. Prior to his discharge a CPA meeting is held, involving the inpatient team, EIP and CRHT, and they agree that as he now has a good relationship with his care co-ordinator he can be discharged without CRHT support.

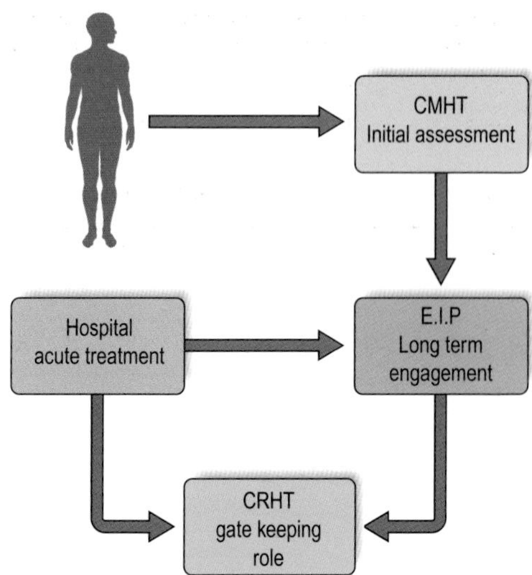


Fig. 1 **Sam's pathway through mental health services.**

### Crisis Resolution and Home Treatment teams (CRHT)

These teams are sometimes known as Crisis Intervention, Crisis Response, or Rapid Response Teams. They are community teams, but their role is closely allied to that of the inpatient unit. They treat patients who would, in the past, have been treated in hospital. They are often based in inpatient units, and function 24 hours a day, 7 days a week. Their role includes:

- Gatekeeping inpatient beds – this means that they are the final arbiters of whether a patient can be admitted to an acute inpatient bed. They will consider whether the treatment required can be delivered at home instead of in hospital, and if so will provide the necessary care.
- Home Treatment – CRHT teams care for people in their own homes who, without this intervention, would need an admission to hospital. They are able to prevent admission, by providing intensive and flexible support to acutely unwell people, visiting several times a day if necessary, supervising medication, and supporting the family. They also work with inpatient units to ensure that inpatients are discharged at the earliest opportunity, and continue their acute care at home. There ought to be a seamless transition from inpatient treatment to home treatment.
- Crisis Resolution – CRHTs are able to respond to psychiatric emergencies in the community at any time of the day or night, and any day of the week. During office hours CMHTs usually do this work, but out of hours it will come to the CRHT. They can take referrals from GPs, directly from known patients, and from general hospitals. They can also attend Mental Health Act assessments, in order to look for alternatives to admission.

CRHTs do not usually take the role of care co-ordinator, but instead work alongside a care co-ordinator from another community team. Their input is intensive, but short term. The teams are multidisciplinary, and include consultant psychiatrists. The staff within the team work closely together to ensure they are providing a consistent approach to treatment even when several different members of staff are involved.

## Early Intervention in Psychosis teams (EIP)

These teams are founded on the principle that the earlier and more effectively psychotic illnesses such as schizophrenia are treated the better the long-term outcome for the patient. Engagement at an early stage in the illness can avoid a later traumatic first contact with mental health services (i.e. admission under a section of the Mental Health Act), and increases the likelihood of the patient continuing to take treatment and stay engaged with services in the long term. EIP teams generally work with people between the ages of 14 and 35 years who are experiencing their first psychotic episode, therefore crossing traditional barriers between Child and Adolescent services and Adult services. The teams include consultant psychiatrists who may be trained as either adolescent or adult specialists. The team members act as care co-ordinators for their patients, and tend to have much smaller case loads than CMHT workers, so that they can provide a more intensive input. They usually work with patients for about 3 years before handing over to CMHTs or AOTs.

## Assertive Outreach teams (AOT)

AOTs work with patients who have a serious mental illness, usually schizophrenia, and are at high risk of causing harm to themselves or others, and do not want to engage with mental health services. Typically their patients will have schizophrenia, complicated by substance abuse, and have a history of aggressive behaviour when unwell, and will have had repeated admissions to hospital under a section of the Mental Health Act. They often have no insight into their illness, do not believe that they have a mental illness, and therefore do not want to take medication or see mental health staff. AOT overcome these difficulties by working intensively with small case loads. They focus on engaging with the patient in order to be able to deliver effective treatment (Fig. 2). This is often achieved by taking the focus away from talking about mental health issues, and providing practical help with finance, housing or other difficulties, or helping with providing day to day needs and befriending. AOTs act as care co-ordinators for their patients, and will often work with them for several years before transferring back to the CMHTs.

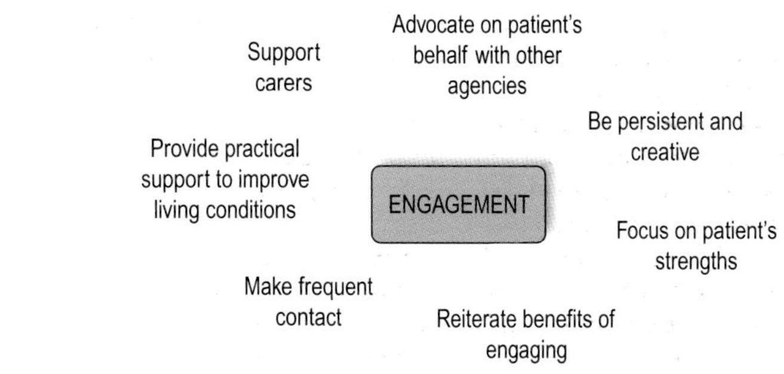


Fig. 2 **AOT techniques in engagement.**

## Mental Health Services

- Mental health services are organised with a focus on caring for people in their own homes as far as is safely possible
- CRHT teams care for people who, without this intervention, would need an admission to hospital, and support inpatients to be discharged home at the earliest opportunity
- EIP teams generally work with young people who are experiencing their first psychotic episode, with the aim of improving their long-term prognosis
- AOTs work with patients who have a serious mental illness, are at high risk of causing harm to themselves or others, and do not want to engage with mental health services

# Classification in psychiatry

> ### *Case history 3*
>
> From the age of 18 years, Emily has always manipulated situations so that other people sort things out for her. If they refuse to do this she becomes angry and tearful. From the age of 30, she has experienced panic attacks when in crowds or shops. When 45, she had an episode of depression and obsessional symptoms occurring and remitting at the same time. She had a further episode of depression when given steroids for treatment of COAD when 54.
>
> a. What psychiatric disorders do you think Emily has experienced?

Before the 1970s, it was thought that schizophrenia was more common in the US than the UK. However, when this was properly researched, it turned out that there was no real difference in prevalence. The reason for the previously observed difference was that psychiatrists in the two countries had different views about the nature of the condition: American psychiatrists were more likely to diagnose schizophrenia and British psychiatrists more likely to diagnose manic-depression.

The development of standardised methods of classifying psychiatric disorders has improved communication between clinicians and has made it possible to research the aetiology, management and prognosis of a particular diagnosis, thereby providing an empirical basis for clinical practice. As a result, diagnosis becomes a useful procedure rather than just a way of labelling people (Fig. 1).

## Classification systems

There are two major classification systems used in psychiatry. The first is the International Classification of Disease, 10th version (ICD10), devised by the World Health Organization in 1993. The second classification system is the Diagnostic Systems Manual, currently in its 4th version (DSM IV), which has been produced by the American Psychiatric Association. The two systems are broadly similar and in this book we have mostly followed ICD10. Table 1 outlines the ICD10 classification of psychiatric disorders.

DSM V is due in 2012 and ICD11 in 2014. The greatest change is likely to be the introduction of dimensional measures for some conditions, in contrast to the sole use until now of categorical diagnoses. In general medicine, blood pressure is a dimensional measure, hypertension a category. Metabolic syndrome is a categorical construct that is based on a number of dimensional measures, such as waist circumference, blood pressure and serum glucose and lipids. In psychiatry, there are scales that can be used, for example, to give dimensional measures of psychosis, mood, anxiety and traits of personality, and these can be used as an alternative or, perhaps more pragmatically, as an adjunct to categorical diagnosis.

## Psychiatric diagnosis

It is important not to confuse symptoms with diagnosis in psychiatry. This is often done in the case of symptoms, such as depression or anxiety, which also give their name to a diagnosis (depressive disorder, anxiety disorder). To make these diagnoses, other symptoms have to be present. In addition, a minimum duration of symptoms is usually specified. In other words, most psychiatric diagnoses are made on the basis of a particular collection of symptoms, or syndrome, being present for a minimum period of time. These principles are represented in Figure 2.

### *Diagnostic categories*

The standard categories of psychiatric diagnosis are shown in Figure 3. When you are making a differential diagnosis it is helpful to run through these categories one by one to check you haven't forgotten any relevant disorders. You may be familiar with the 'surgical sieve' (inflammatory, infective, neoplastic, etc.) which provides a similar structure for



Fig. 1 **If a diagnosis is used to inform clinical practice, it becomes more than just a label.**

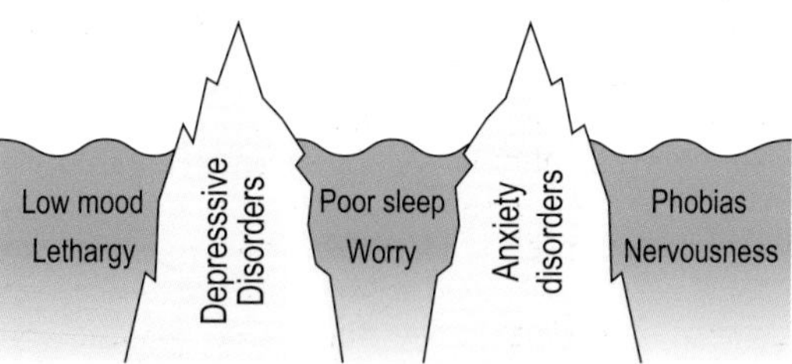


Fig. 2 **Symptoms versus diagnosis.** The 'sea' of symptoms represents the high prevalence of symptoms in a normal population. Disorders occur when particular symptoms occur at the same time.

Table 1 **Outline of ICD10 classification of psychiatric disorders**

| | |
|---|---|
| **Organic** | Organic disorders: includes dementia, delirium, other organic disorders |
| | Mental and behavioural disorders due to psychoactive substance use |
| **Functional** | Schizophrenia, schizotypal and delusional disorders |
| | Mood disorders: includes bipolar disorder, depressive illness, cyclothymia, dysthymia |
| | Neurotic, stress-related and somatoform disorders: includes anxiety disorders, obsessive-compulsive disorders, reactions to stress, dissociative and somatoform disorders |
| | Behavioural syndromes associated with physiological disturbances and physical factors: includes eating disorders, sleep disorders, sexual dysfunction |
| | Disorders of adult personality and behaviour: includes personality disorders, factitious disorders |
| | Mental retardation |
| | Disorders of psychological development |
| | Behavioural and emotional disorders with onset usually occurring in childhood and adolescence |
| | Unspecified mental disorder |

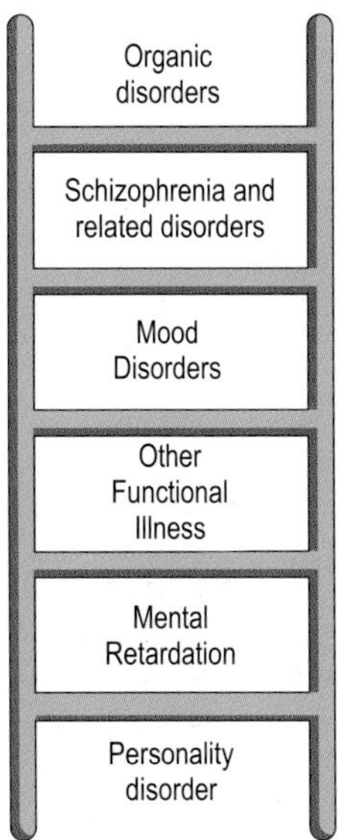


Fig. 3 **The psychiatric diagnostic hierarchy.** Diagnoses further up the ladder take precedence.

thinking about the diagnosis of organic disease. Diagnoses from categories higher up the list in Figure 3 take precedence over those lower down. For example, if a patient has panic attacks because they are in an acute state of fear as a result of persecutory delusions, then a diagnosis of paranoid schizophrenia would be made and not one of panic disorder. Similarly, if a patient develops typical symptoms of schizophrenia while taking illicit drugs, the diagnosis would be drug-induced psychosis, not schizophrenia. Often though, people will have more than one diagnosis, reflecting the fact that they have had different abnormalities of mental state occurring at different times, or with different times of onset. Such comorbidity is common, as having one form of mental disorder often increases the chance of developing another. For example, someone with social phobia is at raised risk of developing a depressive disorder and alcohol dependence.

### *Psychotic and neurotic disorders*

In the past, a distinction was made between psychotic and neurotic disorders, but this is no longer so. The term psychotic is still used to describe symptoms characterised by loss of contact with reality, such as hallucinations and delusions. In other words, it describes those symptoms that in lay terms would be described as madness. Neurotic is a less precise term that in the past described all non-psychotic illnesses. In ICD10 it is only used to describe what are called anxiety disorders in DSM IV. DSM IV does not use the term at all.

### *Organic disorder*

Organic disorder is a broad term which can crudely be defined as 'physical' disorders which cause psychiatric symptoms. Many organic disorders involve structural damage to the brain with consequent psychiatric symptoms. Examples of these include tumours, injury, infection and degenerative processes such as dementia. Organic disorder also includes metabolic disturbance and endocrine disease which causes psychiatric symptoms, along with any toxic effect of medication, alcohol or drugs on the brain.

### *Functional illness*

Functional illness is the term given to all psychiatric illness other than organic disorder. In this case, a crude definition would be that functional illness is psychiatric illness without a 'physical' cause. The distinction between organic and functional conditions was made at a time when body and mind were considered separate entities and, in that context, it was perfectly valid. It remains a useful way of classifying psychiatric disorders. The danger of making such a distinction is that it encourages the belief that functional illness is the result only of psychological and social factors. In fact, there is increasing evidence that structural, neurochemical and neuroendocrine abnormalities of the brain are important factors in some functional illnesses. Therefore, while the terms organic and functional are useful for classification, they can be misleading about aetiology, as the following example shows.

Cardiac failure is a syndrome, the causes of which are known. Imagine, though, if it had never been possible to investigate the internal workings of the human body. Cardiac failure would remain a common clinical problem but its aetiology would be unknown. The presence of oedema in some cases would suggest that excess water was a problem and so treatment with venesection (drainage of blood) or diuretics might be developed. The association with symptoms such as chest pain and signs such as heart murmurs would give clues to the aetiology but it would be impossible to determine it for sure. Therefore, cardiac failure would be an illness defined in syndromal terms but the underlying tissue pathology would not be known. In other words, it would be equivalent to functional psychiatric illness.

The main difference from organic disorder is that the underlying cause of functional psychiatric illness has not yet been determined, largely because it is so difficult to investigate brain function during life. This is not to underestimate the importance of psychological and social factors but should serve as a reminder that biological processes are also important in functional illness.

The other important thing to note about functional illnesses is that they *are* illnesses; that is, they represent a change from what is normal for the patient. This differentiates them from the final broad categories of psychiatric disorder, personality disorder and mental retardation.

### *Mental retardation (learning disability)*

Mental retardation, referred to as learning disability in the UK, is a general impairment in intellectual function that usually presents early in life. An intelligence quotient of less than 70 is usually required to make the diagnosis.

### *Personality disorders*

The way people react to different circumstances depends on their personality. If their personality repeatedly results in excessive distress or abnormal behaviour in situations most people would cope with, then they are considered to have a personality disorder. In severe cases of personality disorder, behaviour or levels of distress are abnormal most of the time.

There are three essential features that must be established before a diagnosis of personality disorder is made. First it is important to establish that the abnormalities of personality cause distress either to the patient or to others. Secondly, the problems the disorder causes must have been present since late adolescence, as personality is usually well established by this stage of development. Thirdly, personality disorder is persistent and long-standing, so while it may be worse at times of stress, there will never be periods of complete remission as there often is with illness.

### Classification in psychiatry

- Most psychiatric diagnoses are syndromes, i.e. they are based on symptoms rather than tissue abnormalities. It is important, therefore, to have a clear idea of the symptoms needed to make a particular diagnosis.
- Making a diagnosis means that research evidence about aetiology, treatment and prognosis of that condition can be used in individual patients' care.

# History and aetiology

The standard sections covered by the psychiatric history are shown in Figure 1. An important thing to note is how similar these are to those covered by the standard medical history. As you are probably already familiar with medical history-taking, you will already have many of the skills necessary for taking a psychiatric history.

The most important difference with the psychiatric history is the amount of background information you need to collect. This is because it is meaningless to consider psychiatric disorders outside the context in which they occur, as exemplified in Figure 2. Because of this, the psychiatric history includes two sections (personal history and premorbid personality) which are not used in other medical specialities. For the same reason, social circumstances are particularly important in psychiatry and should be recorded in detail. As well as giving you a better understanding of the patient and their problems, this background information will help you understand the aetiology of the patient's problems.

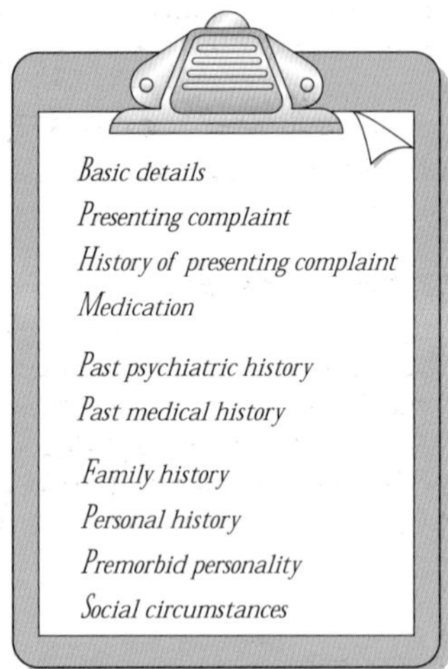


Fig. 1 **The psychiatric history.**

## Aetiology of psychiatric disorders

Psychiatric aetiology should be split into three components:

- predisposing factors
- precipitating factors
- maintaining factors.

In other words: why is this patient vulnerable to developing this disorder, what caused them to develop it now, and what is stopping them getting better? Possible aetiological factors are shown in Figure 3. Identifying these factors is important for several reasons.

If you can explain why a particular patient has developed a particular disorder, then you will feel much more confident about the diagnosis. For instance, a diagnosis of angina is much more likely in a 60-year-old male smoker than in a 30-year-old healthy female non-smoker. A knowledge of the aetiology of ischaemic heart disease, therefore, helps you make a diagnosis. This process is important in all areas of medicine but particularly so in psychiatry. This is because there are no tests available to confirm most psychiatric diagnoses and so aetiology provides a useful way of assessing the likelihood of the diagnoses you are considering for a particular patient.

Aetiology is important for other reasons. Firstly, many patients find it helpful to know why they have developed an illness. Secondly, identifying what has precipitated a disorder, or what is preventing recovery, will influence the treatment a patient receives. Finally, it is often necessary to understand the aetiology of a patient's problems in order to make accurate predictions about their prognosis.

## The psychiatric history

### Presenting complaint

This part of the psychiatric history is very similar to that in other medical specialities. The basic principles are laid out in Figure 4. The reasons for presentation are determined and then clarified by further questioning. Questions are then asked about other symptoms that will help clarify the diagnosis.

An example of this process in general medicine is when a patient complains of chest pain. The nature and duration of the pain is determined and then enquiry is made about symptoms of cardiovascular, pulmonary and gastro-oesophageal disease. Possible precipitants of the complaint are identified, along with exacerbating and relieving factors.

The same process is used in psychiatry. For instance, if a patient complains of auditory hallucinations, first deter-

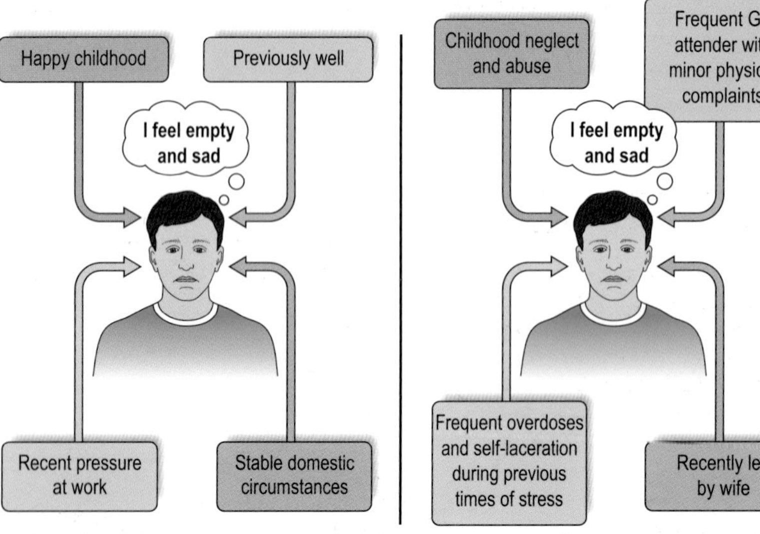


Fig. 2 **The symptoms are the same but the clinical picture is completely different.**

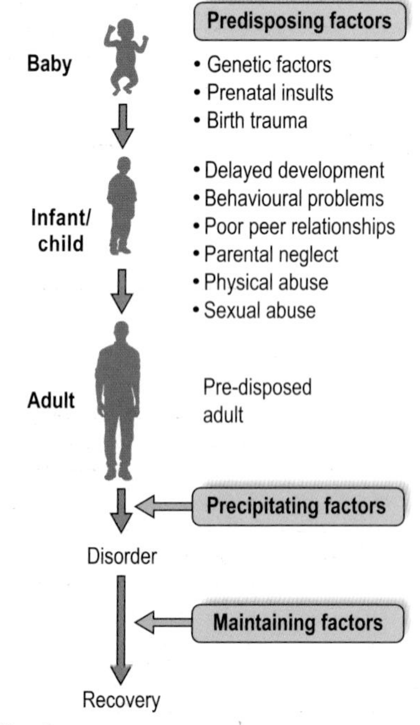


Fig. 3 **Aetiological factors in psychiatric illness.**

mine their nature and duration. Find out if anything makes them better or worse and ask about possible precipitants such as stressful life events or poor compliance with medication. Once you have a clear picture of these symptoms, try to think of all the conditions which could give rise to them. If you cannot remember many causes, try to jog your memory by running through the diagnostic categories listed in the previous chapter. This process should lead you to enquire about symptoms of schizophrenia, depressive illness and drug and alcohol problems. Once you have asked all these questions, you will hopefully have a good idea of likely diagnoses. The rest of the history will help you put this information in context.

## Medication

Enquire about the type and dose of all medication. Find out how long the patient has been taking each drug, as most psychiatric medication takes at least two weeks to start working. Do not forget to ask about medication being prescribed for non-psychiatric problems, as it may have important interactions with psychiatric treatments or may even be the cause of psychiatric symptoms.

## Past psychiatric history

Find out about the date, duration and nature of all previous episodes of illness. Episodes serious enough to require treatment are of particular interest, although it is worth remembering that doctors often fail to recognise or adequately treat mental illness. If treatment was given, find out what it was and whether it helped as this may clarify the diagnosis and also may indicate whether similar treatments are likely to be effective for the current episode. If the patient has difficulty remembering previous treatment, try to jog their memory by asking direct questions like:

- Have you ever been given regular injections?
- Have you ever needed to have blood tests to check on the tablets you were taking?
- Have you ever had ECT?

Always ask whether the patient has seen a psychiatrist before or has required psychiatric admission. Also ask directly about any history of self-harm and try to get an idea of the seriousness of any suicide attempts. In some cases, it may be appropriate to ask direct questions to find out whether particular symptoms have occurred in the past, such as a history of mania in someone presenting with depression, or psychotic symptoms if a psychotic illness is suspected.

## Past medical history

Organic disease, especially if it causes disability or pain, may precipitate or maintain psychiatric illness. Some organic diseases cause psychiatric as well as physical symptoms. Alternatively, psychiatric illness, such as somatoform disorders, may masquerade as organic disease. Finally, it is important to identify organic disease as it may be exacerbated by some psychiatric treatments. For example, tricyclic antidepressants should be used with caution in patients with prostatism because of antimuscarinic effects on the urinary tract.

## Family history

Many psychiatric illnesses have a genetic basis, so family history of mental illness should be determined in as much detail as possible. Early relationships within the family are considered important in the aetiology of some psychiatric illnesses, especially in depressive illness where strong associations with parental neglect and abuse have been demonstrated.

## Personal history

The personal history is the main difference between history taking in psychiatry and in other medical specialities. It aims to trace the patient's development and achievements from conception to the present. The main areas to cover are listed in Table 1. Compare these with Figure 2 and it will be obvious that one of the aims of the personal history is to identify predisposing factors for psychiatric illness. The personal history also gives a baseline level of function so that the effect of illness can be assessed. For example, losing a job because of lethargy and apathy is of greater significance if the previous work record has been flawless.

## Premorbid personality

This is conventionally divided into character, habits and interests. It is very important to know what the patient's character was like before the onset of illness as it helps assess the severity of symptoms. For instance, anxiety symptoms in a usually outgoing, self-confident patient should be viewed differently to identical symptoms in a patient who admits to lifelong nervousness. Assessment of character should include a forensic history (history of criminal behaviour). A history of violence is particularly important as it increases the risk of violence in the future. Enquiry about habits should include alcohol and illicit drugs.

## Social circumstances

You may have covered many of these in earlier sections of the history but make sure you know the type of accommodation the patient lives in, who they live with, what kind of support they have and whether they have any financial problems.

| Table 1 **Personal history** |
|---|
| Gestation and delivery |
| Childhood milestones |
| Family relationships and upbringing |
| Peer relationships |
| Schooling and academic achievements |
| Occupational history |
| Marital and sexual history |

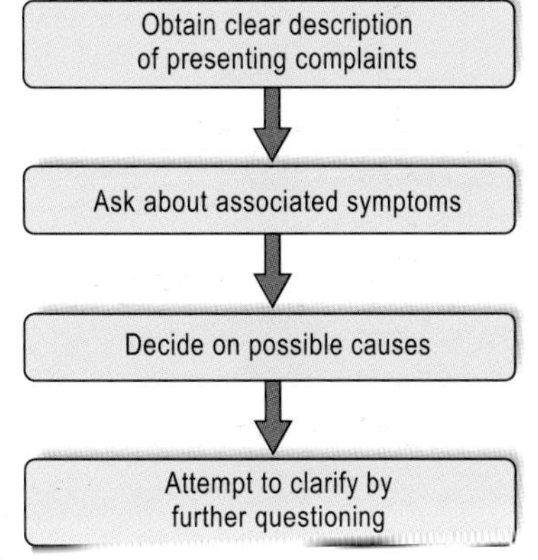

Fig. 4 **Taking the history of presenting complaint.**

## History and aetiology

- The psychiatric history is similar to other medical histories but aims to collect much more background information
- The information gathered should tell you who, what and why. In other words, it should give you an understanding of:
  - the patient's personality
  - the patient's background
  - the patient's current circumstances
  - the nature of the problems
  - the reasons these problems have developed

# Mental state examination

In psychiatry we are largely dependent upon the patient's subjective account of symptoms in order to reach a diagnosis, with few opportunities to do objective diagnostic tests. This can be a difficult task for the patient, struggling to put complex feelings and experiences into words, and for the interviewer, looking for diagnostic signs among all the information given. The mental state examination helps to overcome these difficulties by providing a structure for a detailed, systematic description of the patient's symptoms and behaviour.

The mental state examination is divided into seven sections (Fig. 1) which are described below.

## Appearance and behaviour

Self neglect, often characterised by a dirty, unkempt appearance, may be associated with a number of psychiatric disorders, including depression, schizophrenia and alcohol dependence. Odd or inappropriate dress can be a useful clue to the presence of mania, when bright colours or excessive make-up may reflect the patient's elated mood, or schizophrenia, when it may be associated with psychotic symptoms (e.g. wearing a motorcycle helmet indoors in the belief that it will protect against 'voices').

Facial expression and posture can give an indication of mood. Does the patient look sad, worried, frightened, angry, happy, or does the face betray no emotion? Movement and behaviour during the interview should also be described. Is there restlessness or agitation? Agitation often indicates distress, and can occur with most psychiatric disorders. Reduced movement or motor retardation is commonly associated with depression, but also occurs in schizophrenia and can be induced by sedative and antipsychotic drugs.

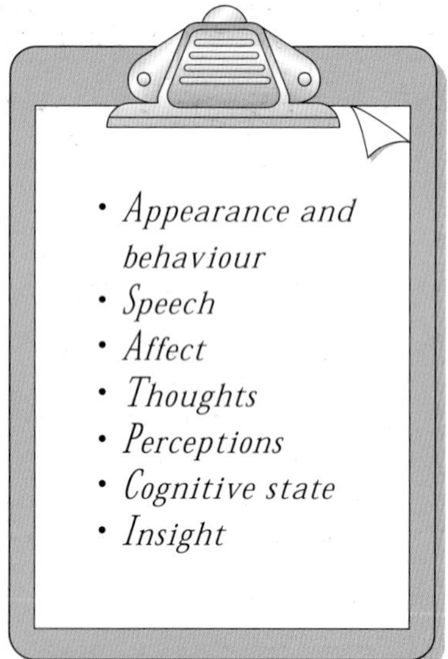


Fig. 1 **Mental state examination** – a detailed description should be entered under each heading.

The patient's co-operation with the assessment and interaction with the interviewer should be described. Is their behaviour disinhibited or aggressive? Do they seem to be responding to psychotic phenomena such as hallucinations?

## Speech

The way in which speech is delivered is described in this section of the examination. For example, the rate of speech may be reduced in depression or increased in mania. A particularly marked increase in rate, where the words seem to fall on top of each other, is described as 'pressure of speech'. Abnormalities in the volume of speech, such as whispering or shouting, should also be recorded. The content of the speech is considered under the heading 'Thoughts'.

## Affect

The term 'affect' refers to the emotional state in the short term, such as during the course of an interview. 'Mood' is the prevailing emotional state over a longer period. Abnormalities of affect include depression, elation, anxiety or anger, all of which are normal emotions in the right circumstances. Affect should be considered both objectively (based on appearance, behaviour and content of speech during the interview) and subjectively by asking the patient 'how are you feeling in yourself?'.

You should consider the predominant affect during the interview, and the degree of variation. Normally, the affect is appropriate to the circumstances of the individual and is reactive to events, so it is likely to vary during the course of an interview depending on the topic discussed. Reduced reactivity (variation) of affect is typical of depression and increased reactivity, known also as emotional lability, occurs in mania and some organic disorders. In schizophrenia, the person can seem emotionally empty (blunting of affect) or their affect can be out of keeping with the circumstances (incongruity of affect).

It is appropriate to ask about suicidal thoughts alongside affect (see p. 13).

## Thoughts

We gain access to the patient's thoughts via their speech, and it is important to listen carefully to the way our patients speak to us (form), as well as what they tell us (content). Abnormalities of the rhythm and flow of thought are known as 'formal thought disorder' and are most commonly associated with schizophrenia, but can occur in mania and organic brain disorders (Fig. 2). Changes can be subtle, and you should be alerted to the possibility of formal thought disorder if you find yourself losing the thread of the conversation.

The abnormalities of thought content to look for include delusions and obsessional thoughts.

### *Delusions*

Delusions are false beliefs that are firmly held by the patient, even in the face of clear evidence that they are not true. It is important to consider the patient's cultural background in deciding whether a belief is delusional.

For example, unusual religious beliefs that are shared by many others in a sect are not considered to be delusions, whereas idiosyncratic religious beliefs not shared by others (such as 'I am the Messiah') are. Delusions are symptoms of psychotic illness and can occur in schizophrenia and severe mood disorders. Some commonly encountered delusions are illustrated in Table 1. Direct questions are useful in revealing delusions, but should be prefixed with a reassurance that they are routine as they may sound odd to the non-psychotic patient. For example:

- Do you feel as though you are in danger? (persecutory delusions)
- Do people watch you, or talk about you? (delusions of reference)
- Do you feel as though you have special powers that other people do not have? (grandiose delusions).

### *Obsessional thoughts*

Obsessional thoughts are repetitive and intrusive thoughts. The patient recognises that they are their own thoughts, but feels unable to stop them, despite efforts to do so. They tend to be unpleasant, and patients often feel ashamed of them, and may not talk about them unless asked directly.

## Perceptions

A perception is a sensation of an external object, and may be experienced in any of the five senses. There are two types of abnormal perception: illusions and hallucinations (Fig. 3).

### *Illusions*

Illusions are distorted perceptions in which a real external object is perceived inaccurately. Illusions are more likely to occur if perception is difficult, such as

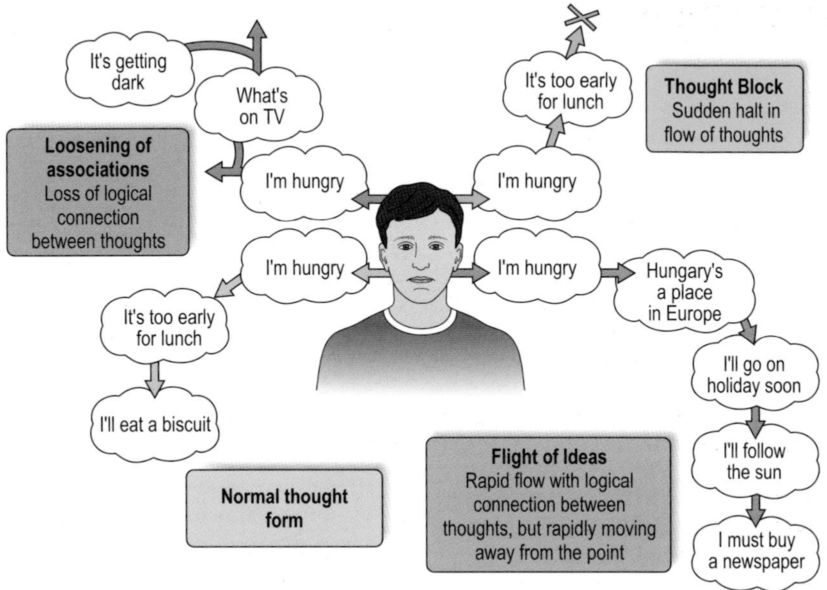


Fig. 2 **Abnormalities of thought form.**

| Table 1 **Commonly encountered delusions** | |
|---|---|
| Persecutory | 'They're going to get me' |
| Reference | 'Everyone is looking at me'<br>'They are talking about me on TV' |
| Grandiose | 'I'm the richest person in the world' |
| Guilt | 'It's my fault there are so many people unemployed' |
| Nihilism | 'I'm dead' |

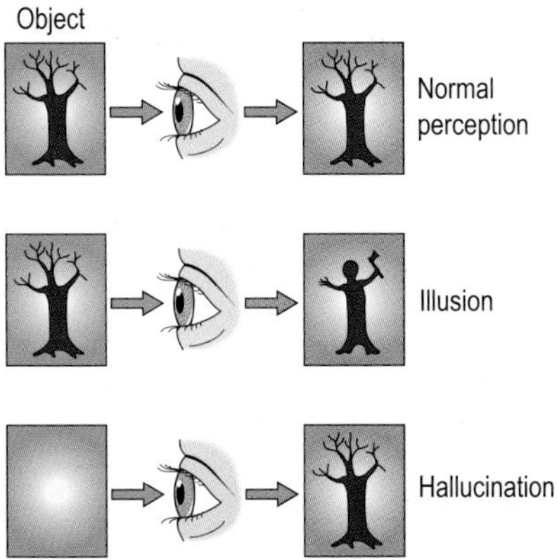


Fig. 3 **Perception, illusion and hallucination.**

with dim lighting, reduced vision or hearing, or heightened anxiety. Illusions can be normal phenomena, but are more likely to occur in the presence of some forms of mental illness, such as anxiety disorders and delirium.

### *Hallucinations*

Hallucinations are perceptions occurring in the absence of an external stimulus. An hallucination has all the qualities of a normal perception. They are psychotic symptoms and always abnormal. Types include:

- **Auditory hallucinations** (of sound). These are the most common type encountered in psychiatry. In schizophrenia, auditory hallucinations are typically of one or more voices speaking about the patient (third person hallucinations). In psychotic mood disorders they tend to be simpler, with a voice repeating a few words or phrases, and speaking directly to the patient (second person hallucinations). The content is in keeping with the mood ('mood congruent'). In depression the voice will say negative things ('you're useless') and in mania will conform to the elated mood ('you're wonderful').
- **Visual hallucinations**. These are usually associated with organic brain disorders. They occur in states of drug intoxication (e.g. with LSD, drug and alcohol withdrawal), delirium and neurological conditions, such as epilepsy.
- **Olfactory hallucinations** (of smell). These occur in organic disorders and occasionally in severe depression, when they are mood congruent. For example, the patient may perceive a rotting smell and believe they are dying and rotting away.
- **Gustatory hallucinations** (of taste). These are rare and may occur in organic disorders.
- **Tactile hallucinations** (of touch). These may occur in organic disorders. For example, in withdrawal states there may be a sensation of something crawling under the skin (formication).

Some patients will volunteer information about their hallucinations during the interview, others will need to be asked directly, for example, 'have you ever heard a voice when there has been no-one or nothing there to account for it?'.

## Cognitive state

Orientation, attention, concentration and memory are assessed in this section. Abnormalities are suggestive of organic brain disorders.

Orientation is the awareness of time, place and person. The patient should be asked the day, date and time, where they are, and who they are. It is important to take account of the patient's circumstances. If they have just been admitted to hospital they may be unsure of the ward name, and it is common for healthy people to not know the exact date.

Tests of attention and concentration include 'serial sevens', where the patient is asked to subtract 7 from 100, and 7 from the resulting number, etc., and months of the year in reverse, for those who find arithmetic too difficult.

Immediate recall is tested with 'digit span' in which the patient is asked to repeat a series of numbers. Normally, 7 digits can be repeated accurately, and 4 or less is abnormal. Short-term memory is tested with a name and address (e.g. 'Patricia Jones, 23 Brook St, Grimsby'). Check they have registered it by asking them to repeat it back immediately, then again after 5 minutes.

## Insight

This is an assessment of how aware the patient is of their own mental state. Does the patient believe himself to be mentally ill and in need of treatment? What is the patient's understanding of the abnormal signs and symptoms that you have observed in the interview? Insight is not simply present or absent. For example, in schizophrenia, the patient may have no insight into his delusions yet be aware that he is ill and prepared to co-operate with treatment.

### Mental state examination

- The mental state examination is a structured description of diagnostic signs and symptoms exhibited by the patient during a consultation
- It is important to be aware of the non-verbal communications, and to consider how things are said in addition to what is said

# Assessment of risk

Assessment of patients with mental illness is not complete without an assessment of risk. The following risks should be considered in every case:

- suicide
- deliberate self harm
- aggressive behaviour
- neglect or exploitation by others
- self neglect.

Assessing risk needs a systematic and holistic approach. There are questionnaires available to help in the assessment, but they are no substitute for taking a thorough history and detailed mental state examination, and carefully weighing up the various risk and protective factors that are present. The physical, psychological and social influences on the individual should be considered, along with the likelihood of them changing. Past history of high-risk behaviour is important, and if present the current risk should be considered to be greater. Assessing risk can be a difficult and highly skilled task. If you ever find yourself in doubt about the risk faced by a patient it is essential to seek advice from an experienced psychiatrist.

The emphasis here will be on assessing and managing risk of suicide and deliberate self harm. The principles of this form of risk assessment can be applied to assessing other risks. In particular, it is important to ask the patient directly about the risk faced by themselves or others, and to ask in detail about any incidents that have occurred.

## Suicide and deliberate self harm

Suicide is deliberate self murder, and the cause of at least 1% of all deaths in the UK. The annual rate has steadily fallen to around 8.5 per 100,000 and is highest in men and the elderly. In the 1980s and 1990s there was a dramatic increase in the suicide rate in young men, however this trend is now reversing, and the suicide rates in this group are falling year on year. But suicide remains the second most common cause of death in 15- to 44-year-old men (accidental death is the most common cause). Over all ages men are three times more likely to die by suicide than women, and for the 20 to 24 years age group men are four times more likely than women to die in this way. Young Asian women have been identified as particularly vulnerable, with a suicide rate that is twice the national average. The method for committing suicide is determined to some extent by the availability of means. In the UK the commonest methods are hanging, self poisoning (most often painkillers or antidepressants), jumping and drowning. In the USA, firearms are the commonest means of suicide.

Deliberate self harm (DSH) is much more common than suicide. The annual rate is about 3 per 1000. In contrast with suicide, DSH is most common in young women, and drug overdose is the most frequently used method. A significant number of people who harm themselves go on to commit suicide, with 1% of those presenting to hospital following a suicide attempt dying by suicide in the following year, and 5% over the following 10 years.

### Aetiology

Mental illness is by far the most important cause of suicide, present in about 90% of cases. In 70% of suicides the mental illness is depressive disorder. It is important to be aware that the early stage of recovery from depression is a vulnerable time as energy and motivation may return before the mood lifts, so the person is more able to act on continuing suicidal ideas. Up to 15% of people with severe mood disorders will kill themselves. About 20% of those dying by suicide are alcoholics, and alcoholics have a suicide rate of 10%. As schizophrenia is relatively uncommon it is present in only 2–3% of suicides but, of those suffering from schizophrenia, 10% die by suicide, with the greatest risk in the earlier stages of the illness when the patient is struggling to come to terms with the potentially devastating effects of the condition.

A number of social and medical factors are associated with suicide. These are listed in Table 1. They are not necessarily causes of suicide and are not present in all cases, but it is useful to bear them in mind when assessing a patient who may be at risk of committing suicide.

The causes and motivations for DSH vary enormously. Three groups may be identified, although there is considerable overlap:

- *Failed suicide attempt.* These individuals are likely to be similar to those who succeed in completing suicide (see Table 1) and are at high risk of repeating the attempt, with fatal results. They are likely to have a mental illness.
- *Impulsive self harm, with ambivalence about the wish to die.* Often an overdose is taken immediately after a stressful event, with no advance planning and help is sought quickly. There may be a genuine wish to die at the time of the act or lack of concern about the outcome. Often there is no real suicidal intent, but instead an attempt to cope with a difficult situation by gaining attention, self-punishment or manipulation of others. The characteristics of such individuals are quite different from those with serious suicide intent. They are unlikely to be mentally ill, and tend to be young and female (Fig. 1).
- *Repeated self harm with no suicide intent.* There are a small group of individuals who repeatedly act on impulses to harm themselves, most often by cutting their arms superficially or taking small overdoses. This behaviour is usually due to a severe personality disorder.

### Assessing suicide risk

Suicide risk is not easily quantifiable and can fluctuate. Some patients will describe suicidal thoughts, accompanied by a plan to put the thoughts into action, and a definite intention to act on the plan. They clearly have a very high risk of committing suicide and urgent action is required. However, it is not usually this clear cut. For most patients there are protective factors that make it less likely that they will act on suicidal thoughts. The protective factors will vary from one individual to another, but often include

| Table 1 **Factors associated with suicide** |
|---|
| ■ Male |
| ■ Older age – the greatest risk is in men over 75 |
| ■ Previous attempts – up to 30% of people who commit suicide have attempted suicide previously |
| ■ Mental illness – present in 90%, mainly depressive disorder |
| ■ Divorced, single, or widowed |
| ■ Bereavement – in particular loss of a spouse |
| ■ Social isolation |
| ■ Living in urban environment |
| ■ Physical ill-health – chronic, painful and life-threatening illnesses |
| ■ Unemployment – the rate increases with duration of unemployment and is also raised in the wives of unemployed men |

| DSH | Suicide |
|---|---|
| Young | Older (age > 40 years) |
| Female | Male |
| Overdose | Violent method |
| Impulsive | Planned |
| Rarely serious mental illness | 90% mentally ill |

Fig. 1 **Comparison of characteristics of those who deliberately harm themselves and those who complete suicide.**

*'It sounds as though things have been very difficult for you recently, have they ever been so bad that.......'*

*'......life is not worth living?'*
*'......life seems hopeless or pointless?'*
*'Do you have any plans for the future?'*

*'Do you feel suicidal?'*
*'Have you thought of ending it all?'*

*'Can you tell me about the suicidal thoughts?'*
*'What methods have you considered?'*
*'Have you made a plan?'*

Fig. 2 **Asking about suicide.**

concern about the impact of suicide on family, a religious belief that suicide is sinful, or fears about dying painfully or being left in a worse situation as a consequence of the suicide attempt. These protective factors will vary with changes in social circumstances and the severity of mental illness. For example, with a worsening of a depressive disorder a mother may move from resisting suicide for the sake of her children to feeling that they would be better off without her. It is therefore important to reassess suicide risk in vulnerable patients at frequent intervals, and look for and promote protective factors. Assessment must include an exploration of the suicidal ideas and DSH if present. It is also important to complete a full psychiatric history and mental state examination, looking for factors associated with suicide (Table 1).

### *Asking about suicide*

Asking about suicidal thoughts is a skill that requires practice and can raise anxiety initially. It is vital that you put your anxieties aside and ask these questions of all psychiatric patients and any other patients who appear to be low in mood or have harmed themselves. Asking about suicide in a sensitive way is very unlikely to cause offence, and may give a distressed patient their first opportunity to voice thoughts about which they have felt guilty, ashamed or afraid. This can be a great relief for some patients and those with no suicidal ideas will not become suicidal simply because you have raised the subject with them.

There are many ways of asking about suicide, and you should find a form of questioning that you feel comfortable with and then use it routinely. Examples are given in Figure 2.

### *Assessment following DSH*

The aims of a psychiatric assessment following DSH are to evaluate the suicide risk, determine whether a mental illness is present and develop a management plan that will ensure the patient's safety. All doctors should be able to assess suicide risk in order to take the necessary precautions to prevent a high-risk patient from harming themselves.

The following questions are useful in considering whether the DSH was a serious attempt at suicide:

- *Events preceding the act.* Why did they harm themselves? Was there a single specific incident or a build up of stressors over time and, if so, what was the 'final straw'? Was the attempt planned and, if so, how detailed were the plans and how long ago were they made? A planned episode of DSH is likely to have been a serious suicide attempt.
- *The act itself.* What method was used? Consider the potential fatality of the method objectively and from the patient's view. The attempt is serious if the patient believed the method used to be highly dangerous, even if in reality it was unlikely to be so. For example, benzodiazepines are relatively safe in overdose but are frequently perceived as dangerous by patients, while many believe that the potentially lethal paracetamol is safe. What were the circumstances of the act? Did they intend to die? If not, what was their intention? Did they write a suicide note? How did they reach medical care? Did they try to avoid being found?
- *Current thoughts about suicide.* What is their view about the self harm now? Do they wish they had succeeded or are they relieved to still be alive, or are they not sure? What has been the reaction of friends and family? Has anything changed as a consequence of the self harm? Discharging a patient back into the stressful environment that prompted the self harm may be risky. Do they think they might repeat the act?

## Management

When the suicide risk assessment has been completed, a management plan can be developed. The priority must be to ensure the patient's safety.

Medical treatment for the effects of the self harm may be needed before starting psychiatric treatment. The place of treatment should be carefully considered. Patients with high risk are likely to need admission to the safe environment of a psychiatric inpatient unit. In some cases compulsory admission under the Mental Health Act 1983 (see p. 18) will be needed. General medical wards are not safe places for patients at high risk of suicide. If it is essential to care for them in this environment then constant nursing attendance must be arranged.

It is possible to manage a patient with moderate suicide risk in the community if they are prepared to accept treatment, rapid follow-up can be arranged and they have support at home. Involvement of the Crisis Resolution and Home Treatment team to provide support immediately following discharge can be invaluable, and some patients need ongoing support from mental health services.

Once safety has been ensured any underlying mental illness may be treated in the usual way.

**Assessment of risk**

- 90% of all those who die by suicide are mentally ill
- Those who deliberately harm themselves are 100 times more likely to die by suicide in the next year than the general population
- It is important to routinely ask all psychiatric patients, and all other patients who are low in mood, about suicide

# Management plan and formulation

## Management plan

The management plan is a comprehensive plan of action that starts with the differential diagnosis and investigations necessary to reach a firm diagnosis, and progresses through immediate, short- and long-term treatments. Physical, psychological and social interventions should be considered in every case.

### Differential diagnosis

The differential diagnosis is a list of possible diagnoses drawn up after taking a full history and performing both mental state and physical examinations. It is helpful to consider each of the following categories for patients presenting with psychiatric symptoms:

- **Functional mental illness**. These are psychiatric illnesses occurring without a physical cause (p. 7).
- **Organic mental illness**. These are physical disorders causing psychiatric symptoms and include neurological disorders, metabolic disturbance, endocrine disorders and toxic effects of medication, alcohol or drugs.
- **Personality disorder**. This may be the primary diagnosis, or occur concurrently with another disorder.
- **Mental retardation**. This may result in presentation with emotional or behavioural abnormalities. Both functional and organic mental illnesses occur more frequently in people with mental retardation.
- **Medical disorder**. There may be a coincident medical disorder which, although not directly causing the mental illness, may have an impact on its presentation and response to treatment.

The correct diagnosis may be glaringly obvious, but in most cases there will be three or four realistic alternative differential diagnoses, with one favourite. There will often be more than one correct diagnosis present at the same time (Fig. 1).

### Investigations

The purpose of investigations is to reach a firm diagnosis by confirming or excluding each differential diagnosis in turn. It is not acceptable to do 'routine investigations' without adequate justification for each. All investigations have a cost, either financial or in terms of discomfort or side-effects for the patient, or clinicians' time.

Investigations should start with information gathering from psychiatric and medical case notes and the GP. Relatives or friends may be interviewed with the patient's consent. If possible, the patient should not be present at these interviews in order to give the informant an opportunity to speak freely. They should be asked for their view of the patient's problems, and may be able to clarify or confirm aspects of the history you are uncertain about. It is helpful to engage the family at an early stage as they may have an important role in the later management of the patient. Psychological and physical investigations may be helpful if abnormalities are found in routine cognitive testing or physical examination (Fig. 2).

### Treatment

Treatment should be a comprehensive package of care designed to meet the patient's physical, psychological and social needs. The patient must be involved in the planning of treatment, and it is up to the doctor to ensure the patient is sufficiently informed about the diagnosis and the options available to be able to do so.

There are generally three phases of treatment:

- **Immediate care**. It is important to think about where the patient should be treated. Admission to an inpatient unit or day hospital may be required (Fig. 3), although the majority are treated in the community – either in their own homes or in outpatient clinics. In general, treatment should not be started until a firm diagnosis is made, but if the patient is distressed it may be possible to provide some immediate symptomatic relief. This may take the form of a physical treatment, such as an antipsychotic drug to relieve severe agitation, or a psychological treatment, such as arranging for a CPN to provide support while investigations are underway, or a social intervention, such as provision of information about hostels for a homeless patient.
- **Short-term treatment**. Once a diagnosis has been made, appropriate physical, psychological and social treatments should be started, and progress carefully monitored until the acute episode has fully resolved.

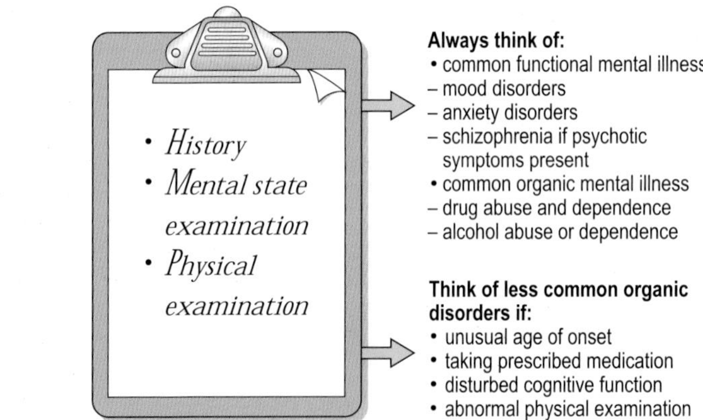


Fig. 1 **Differential diagnosis.**

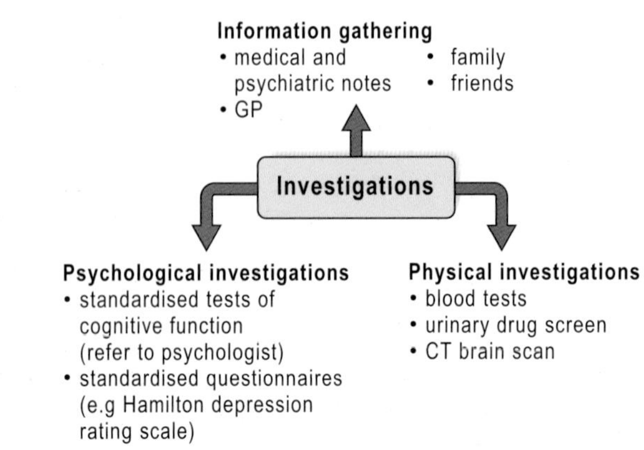


Fig. 2 **Investigations.**

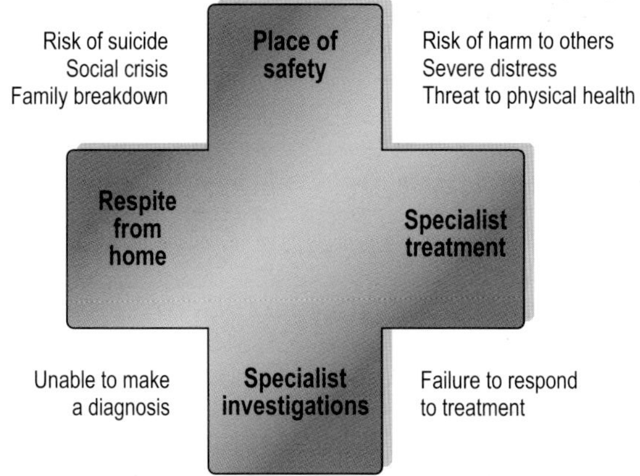


Fig. 3 **Reasons for admission to hospital.**

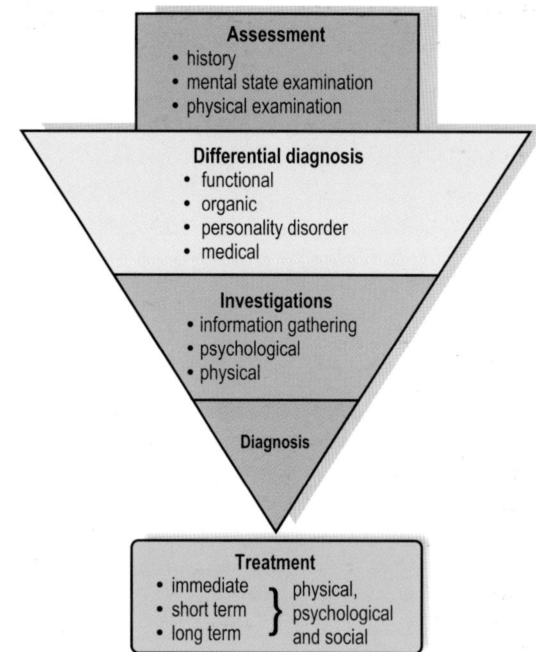


Fig. 4 **Formulation.**

- **Long-term treatment**. Treatment may be continued long term for two reasons:
  1. continued treatment of a chronic illness, such as schizophrenia
  2. prevention of recurrence (prophylaxis) in illnesses such as bipolar disorder.

## Formulation

The formulation is a concise summary of your assessment of the patient. It is used to communicate information in clinical notes, letters, and when presenting a case in ward rounds or exams. It begins with a brief description of the patient, for example: '*Mrs Smith is a 38-year-old married housewife with three children, presenting with a 6 month history of panic attacks*'. It then progresses through the history, mental state examination and physical examination, summarising the important aspects of the case. It is not necessary to repeat every detail of history if not directly relevant, but important negative findings must be included, such as no family history of mental illness, no suicidal ideation, no psychotic symptoms, etc. The formulation ends with a discussion of the differential diagnosis, including the arguments for and against the various possibilities raised, the relevant aetiological factors, investigations, and immediate short and long-term treatment plans (Fig. 4).

### Clinical exam technique

All clinical exams are forbidding experiences, but many students particularly dread the psychiatric variety, complaining that there are too many history questions to remember, chaotic stories to make sense of, and the risk of having a patient who is unco-operative, thought disordered, agitated or sedated. The secret of success is to stay calm, approach the task in a logical, structured way and practise. The following hints may be helpful.

#### *Before the exam*

- Have a clear structure for the history, mental state and formulation worked out. Some centres will allow you to take in a crib sheet listing the major headings.

#### *With the patient*

- Take time to put the patient at ease. Explain that you are being tested, not them.
- Make notes as you go along, ordering the information under appropriate headings.
- Control the interview. If the patient is too verbose then politely explain that you have a lot of questions to ask in a short time, and you may need to interrupt occasionally to complete the task.
- Do not worry about missing things. It often takes several interviews to complete a full psychiatric assessment. Concentrate on the key facts and tell the examiner what further information you would like to collect, given enough time.
- Do not panic if the patient is unco-operative. Think about why they are being difficult – is it a symptom of their illness? Do as thorough a mental state examination as possible, and use the time to work out a comprehensive management plan. Explain the problems to the examiner, who will make allowances.
- Allow time (about 10 minutes) at the end to gather your thoughts and write notes on:
  - *differential diagnosis*: consider both functional and organic diagnoses
  - *aetiology*: include predisposing, precipitating and perpetuating factors
  - *investigations*: must include looking at the case notes, and speaking to informants (GP and nearest relative usually)
  - *management plan*: consider physical, psychological and social treatments required immediately, and over the short and long term.

#### *With the examiner*

- Present yourself in an appropriate, professional manner. Try to appear confident without being cocky, be polite and pleasant, make eye contact and speak clearly.
- Make the presentation interesting. Summarise the relevant information, including important negatives, and avoid repetition.

### Management plan and formulation

- A management plan must include consideration of differential diagnoses, investigations and treatment
- Treatment plans should consider physical, psychological and social interventions in the immediate, short and long term
- A formulation is a concise summary of your assessment

# Mental capacity

> ### *Case history 4*
> Sarah, a 75-year-old widowed woman, has rheumatoid arthritis and recently told her daughter that death would be a welcome escape from a life of chronic pain and limited mobility. She is admitted to hospital in a confused state and a chest X-ray shows a mass in her right lung and a lobar pneumonia.
>
> a. How do you decide whether to treat her with antibiotics?

Mental capacity is the ability to make decisions. This section describes how to assess capacity and how to protect the rights of people who lack it and is based on The Mental Capacity Act 2005, which applies to England and Wales only. The Act focuses on decisions about health, social welfare and finances, but its principles can be applied to any decision.

## Assessment of capacity

A person is considered to have capacity to make a decision if they are able to do all four of the following:

- to understand the information relevant to the decision
- to retain that information
- to use or weigh that information as part of the process of making the decision
- to communicate any decision (whether by talking, using sign language, writing, or any other means).

Figure 1 shows an imagined conversation between a doctor and a person who is considering whether to go ahead with treatment as advised and illustrates the factors that demonstrate capacity.

It is important to remember when carrying out assessments of capacity that someone may have the capacity to make some decisions, but not others. For example, a woman with dementia might be able to remember details of two nursing homes for long enough to choose which she would prefer, but might not be able to weigh up the risks and benefits of chemotherapy for breast cancer. A man with delusional disorder who believed that his teeth were being used by the government to transmit signals to aliens would probably not have capacity to make decisions about his dental care but might be fit to make choices about other aspects of his health.

## The five principles of capacity

The Mental Capacity Act describes five principles that should guide all work in this area – these are summarised in Figure 2. If you don't apply these principles to the assessment of capacity and to decisions concerning people who lack capacity in England and Wales, then you will be breaching people's statutory rights.

## Best interests

When a person doesn't have capacity to make a decision, other people must act in their best interests. It is the responsibility of the person who will be carrying out the intervention under consideration to decide whether to go ahead. In the case of healthcare, this will usually be the doctor or nurse in charge of the person's treatment. Their decision should be made on the basis of what is known as a 'best interests assessment', the aim of which is to determine, as best as possible, what the person would have decided for themselves if they had the capacity to do so. The Mental Capacity Act specifies several ways of seeking the information required to make this deci-

RETAIN
"Last time I saw you, you said it might help my blood pressure if I lost weight. I didn't like the sound of the side effects the blood pressure tablets might have"
USE OR WEIGH
"I don't want to take the tablets if I can avoid it. I think I could try harder to lose weight. Even if I do nothing I've got a good chance of being OK"
UNDERSTAND
"If I take the tablets, my risk of having a heart attack or stroke in the next 10 years will go down from 15% to 10%"
COMMUNICATE
"I've decided not to take the tablets. I'm going to make more effort to lose weight and come to see you again in a few months"

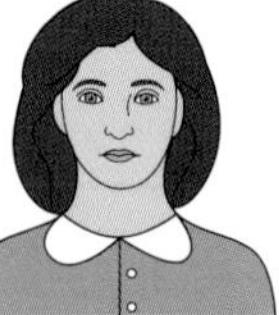

Fig. 1 **A person with capacity to decide about treatment for high blood pressure.**

| DO | PRINCIPLE | DON'T |
|---|---|---|
| Formally assess capacity | ASSUME PEOPLE HAVE CAPACITY UNLESS PROVED OTHERWISE | Assume someone lacks capacity on the basis of factors such as their age or diagnosis |
| Take the time to help people understand and make decisions. If they may regain capacity and it is possible to wait, then do so | HELP PEOPLE MAKE THEIR OWN DECISIONS | View capacity as a static phenomenon – it will change over time and will be affected by the way in which you communicate information |
| Base your assessment of capacity on how the person arrives at their decision, not on what they decide | PEOPLE HAVE THE RIGHT TO MAKE WHAT YOU THINK ARE UNWISE DECISIONS | Conclude that someone doesn't have capacity because you disagree with their decision |
| Use whatever means available to decide what the person would have wanted for themselves if they had capacity | WHEN SOMEONE LACKS CAPACITY, ACT IN THEIR BEST INTERESTS | Assume you know what is best for other people |
| Think about the least intrusive and restrictive means of achieving what is in the person's best interests | WHEN SOMEONE LACKS CAPACITY, DO NOT RESTRICT THEIR LIBERTY MORE THAN IS NECESSARY | Do more than is necessary |

Fig. 2 **The Five Principles of Capacity.**

sion, as illustrated in Figure 3. The decision maker, for example the doctor treating the person concerned, must follow this process and take into account all the views expressed, as well as their own, before making a decision about what to do.

## Advance Decisions

The Mental Capacity Act allows people to specify in advance treatments they would not want in certain circumstances, in case they lose the capacity to make the decision for themselves. These are known as Advance Decisions. For example, a man with Motor Neurone Disease might make an Advance Decision refusing life-prolonging treatment of any sort. If he later developed pneumonia, for example, and as a result lost consciousness and so couldn't make decisions for himself, the implication of the Advance Decision would be that palliative treatment should be given, but antibiotics should not.

## Who should speak on a person's behalf?

Most decisions that need to be made in a person's best interests will not be covered by a valid Advance Decision and so the decision maker will need to find people who can speak on the person's behalf. It may be that the person has given someone the power to make decisions on their behalf, in the form of Lasting Power of Attorney (LPA). These powers can cover Personal Welfare, Property and Affairs or both, so in the case of decisions about medical treatment, it is important to establish whether a LPA for Personal Welfare has been conferred.

If there is no valid Advance Decision or person with LPA, then the decision maker will seek the views of relatives and close friends. If there is nobody to speak on behalf of the person without capacity, then an Independent Mental Capacity Advocate (IMCA) should be asked to do so. IMCAs are people who have been trained to speak on behalf of people without capacity. It is also helpful to involve them when there is disagreement over what is in the best interests of the person concerned.

The decision maker should do their best to seek other people's views, in the ways described above and in Figure 3, but when people are acutely unwell there will not always be time to do so. Treatment that is required urgently should not be delayed if the person will be harmed as a result. In such circumstances, the doctor making the decision will have to do so on the basis of the information available to them at the time.

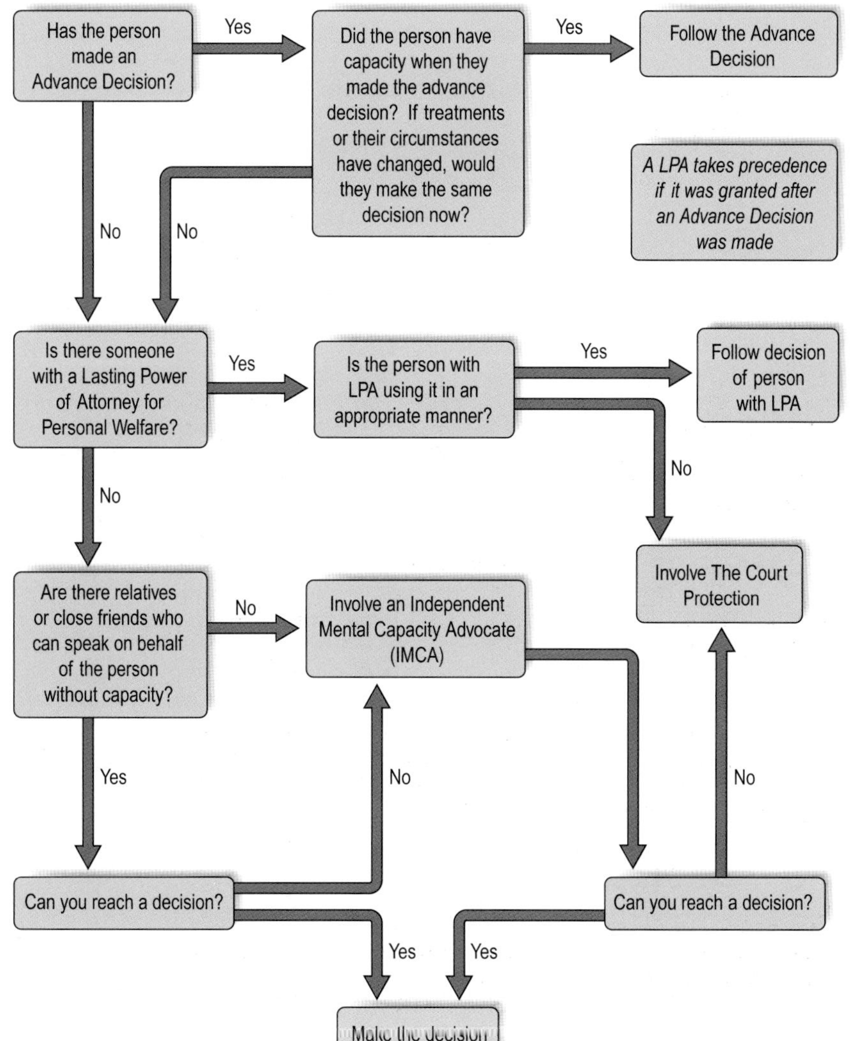


Fig. 3 **How to determine best interests when making decisions about medical treatment.**

## The Court of Protection

If decisions need to be made about a person's Property and Affairs and they do not have the capacity to do so, and if there is nobody with LPA for these matters, then the case must be referred to The Court of Protection. Decisions regarding medical treatment and other matters of Personal Welfare can usually be resolved in the ways described earlier but, if there is substantial disagreement, The Court of Protection can be asked to rule on the case.

## Deprivation of Liberty Safeguards (DOLS)

The Mental Capacity Act does not authorise the deprivation of a person's liberty, in contrast to legislation such as The Mental Health Act. Usually, the steps taken to act in the best interests of a person without capacity do not involve depriving them of their liberty. For example, making sure someone without capacity stays in a general hospital for a short period of time and receives treatment for an acute medical condition is considered to be a restriction of liberty, not a deprivation. If, though, a person without capacity is deprived of their liberty, for example during a prolonged hospital admission in which their movements and contact with the outside world are curtailed, then authorisation is required. This is obtained by the hospital making an application for a Deprivation of Liberty assessment, which will usually be carried out by a 'Best Interests Assessor', who typically will be a psychiatric nurse or social worker, and a psychiatrist. Those doing these assessments will have had special training and will assess the person's mental health, mental capacity and best interests before deciding whether the deprivation of liberty should be authorised.

### Mental capacity

- Always assess capacity when making decisions about medical treatment
- If someone lacks capacity, determine what is in their best interests by talking to the people who know them best

# The Mental Health Act

## *Case history 5*

A 35-year-old woman has become increasingly withdrawn and pre-occupied over the last month. She is beginning to neglect herself and it appears that she has not eaten for several days. She doesn't think she is unwell and refuses to come into hospital.

a. Are there grounds for compulsory admission?
b. If so, how would you arrange this?

The Mental Health Act (MHA) for England and Wales allows for the admission and treatment of people with mental disorder without their consent. The MHA 1983 established these powers and was modified by a further piece of legislation, the MHA 2007. Civil sections of the MHA are discussed in this chapter and the commonly used powers are summarised in Table 1. There is a description on pages 94–95 of the powers granted by the MHA to Courts and the Ministry of Justice, allowing for the detention in hospital of people facing trial and those serving prison sentences.

### Admission and treatment under the MHA

The decisions that need to be made when considering the use of the MHA are shown in Figure 1. It will be seen from this that people can only be admitted and treated against their will if they have a 'mental disorder', which is defined in the MHA 2007 as 'any disorder or disability of the mind'. Detention should only be authorised if it is in the interests of the person's health or safety, or for the protection of others, and if there is no less restrictive way available to deal safely and effectively with their problems. Detention under the MHA should not be prolonged longer than is absolutely necessary, so the detained person should be regraded to informal status by the responsible clinician (i.e. taken off section and treated on a voluntary basis) if they regain insight and agree to receive the treatment required, or if treatment is no longer needed.

Section 2 is used to assess the nature and severity of the detained person's condition. It cannot be renewed but can if necessary be converted to Section 3. Section 3 is used when the nature of a person's mental disorder has been established and compulsory treatment is needed. People can only be detained under Section 3 if the doctors recommending detention in hospital believe there will be appropriate treatment available for them there. For example, it might be in the interests of a person's health to detain them in a general adult psychiatric unit for treatment of residual schizophrenia with antipsychotic medication, but it might not be appropriate if past experience suggested they would be highly distressed by hospital admission and would only improve to a limited extent. It might though be appropriate to detain them in a specialised psychiatric rehabilitation unit. Section 3 can be renewed, initially for six months and subsequently for periods of one year.

Sections 2 and 3 both require written recommendations from two doctors. One doctor must be approved by the Secretary of State as having expertise in the assessment and treatment of mental disorder, as described in section 12 of the MHA. This will usually be a psychiatrist. The other doctor should, if possible, have previous knowledge of the patient and ideally will be their general practitioner. Once these medical recommendations have been made, an application is made to the managers of the hospital by an Approved Mental Health Practitioner (AMHP), who will be a qualified practitioner, such as a social worker, nurse or occupational therapist, who has experience in the mental health field and has gone on to complete special training for the role. The AMHP will form their own opinion about whether use of the MHA is appropriate and will also consult with the person's nearest relative. The application can also be made by the nearest relative, although this is unusual.

All this means that, before being placed on Section 2 or 3, the patient is assessed by a doctor who knows them and by a psychiatrist and another mental health practitioner with extensive experience, and in addition their nearest relative is consulted. This process is designed to safeguard the rights of people assessed under the MHA and ensure that these compulsory powers are not used inappropriately. In light of this, either Section 2 or Section 3 should be used whenever possible if compulsory admission is required. However, it can take time to assemble the AMHP and two doctors required for these sections and, if it is not

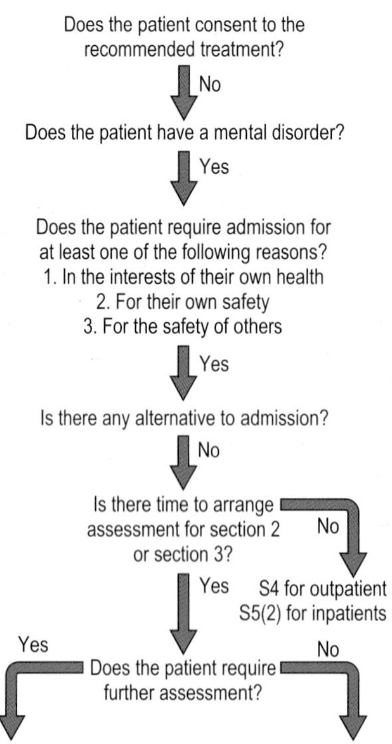


Fig. 1 **Deciding when to use the Mental Health Act.**

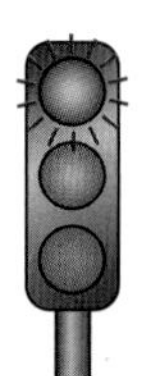

- Treatment outside hospital cannot be given by force
- Treatment for conditions not caused by mental disorder cannot be given without consent
- People cannot be detained in hospital under section 3 if appropriate treatment for them is not available there
- ECT cannot be given to a patient with capacity to refuse

- Some treatments require agreement from a Second Opinion Appointed Doctor:
  1. ECT for a patient without capacity to consent
  2. Medication after 3 months of detention, if the person still refuses
- Some treatments require agreement from the patient and a Second Opinion Appointed Doctor:
  1. Psychosurgery
  2. Hormone implants to reduce sex drive

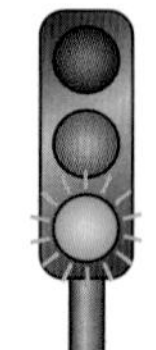

Covers admission and detention in any hospital, not just psychiatric hospitals

- Can be applied to people with any form of mental disorder
- Can be applied to people of any age (but alternative powers exist for children)

Fig. 2 **Extent and limits of the Mental Health Act.**

safe to wait, then there are other sections that can be used to detain the person in hospital until an assessment for Section 2 or Section 3 can take place. Section 4 and Section 136 can be used to admit people from the community and Sections 5(2) and 5(4) to detain informal inpatients who want to leave the ward; details of these powers are shown in Table 1.

Table 1 **Compulsory admission procedures under the Mental Health Act**

| Section | Powers | Recommendation | Applicant | Duration | Termination |
|---|---|---|---|---|---|
| 2 | Admission for assessment and treatment | Two doctors, one approved | AMHP or nearest relative | 28 days | 1. Regrade informal<br>2. Section 3 |
| 3 | Admission for treatment | Two doctors, one approved | AMHP or nearest relative | 6 months | 1. Regrade informal<br>2. Renew Section 3 |
| 4 | Emergency admission | Any doctor | AMHP or nearest relative | 72 hours | 1. Regrade informal<br>2. Section 2 or 3 |
| 136 | Removal to a place of safety | Any police officer | None | 72 hours | 1. Regrade informal<br>2. Section 2 or 3 |
| 5(2) | Detention of inpatient | Doctor in charge or nominated deputy | None | 72 hours | 1. Regrade informal<br>2. Section 2 or 3 |
| 5(4) | Detention of inpatient | Qualified nurse | None | 6 hours | 1. Regrade informal<br>2. Section 5(2) |

## Right of appeal and other safeguards

Patients can appeal against being detained under Section 2 or Section 3. Their appeal will be heard by a Mental Health Review Tribunal, which consists of a lawyer, a psychiatrist and a lay person. The Tribunal will hear evidence from the patient, their legal representative, the responsible medical officer, an AMHP or other professional able to comment on their social circumstances, and other relevant parties and has the power to discharge the patient from their section. A detained person's nearest relative can also request they are discharged from a Section – this can be blocked by the responsible clinician in the case of Section 2, but the only way in which a nearest relative can be prevented from having Section 3 revoked is for an application to be made to a Court to have them displaced from this role. A hospital's use of the MHA is monitored by regular visits from the Care Quality Commission, which also appoints second opinion appointed doctors (SOADs, see Fig. 2).

### *Powers available for supervision outside hospital*

- **Section 17.** Gives the Responsible Medical Officer power to place the patient on leave. Used to allow a gradual transition from hospital to community as the patient begins to recover. If periods of Section 17 leave of more than seven days are being considered, then a CTO may be more appropriate.
- **Community Treatment Order (CTO).** Sets conditions under which a patient detained under Section 3 can be allowed to leave hospital, such as compliance with medication and attendance of appointments. If the conditions are breached, the patient can be recalled to hospital, following which a decision about whether to continue the CTO must be made within 72 hours. If the CTO is revoked, the patient reverts to being detained under Section 3.
- **Guardianship (Section 7).** Gives power to specify where the patient lives and compels them to give professionals involved in their care access to the home.

## Limits of the MHA

The extent of powers contained in the MHA is shown in Figure 2. Two aspects of this merit further discussion. The first is that the MHA contains no power to forcibly give treatment outside hospital. There are however powers that can be used to supervise detained patients outside hospital and these are described in the Box on this page.

Another important limit of the MHA is that it only allows for compulsory treatment of mental disorder. Court rulings have determined that 'manifestations' of a mental disorder can be treated under the MHA, which allows for the treatment of self harm and the force feeding of people with anorexia nervosa. However, the MHA cannot be used to force people to have medical or surgical treatment for conditions other than mental disorder, even if they are refusing it because of their abnormal mental state. In such situations, the Mental Capacity Act 2005 (MCA) will often apply (see pages 16–17).

## Common law

Occasionally, there will be situations not covered by the MHA, the MCA or other powers created by Acts of Parliament, where it may be necessary to force someone to do something against their will. A simple example would be staff in a Casualty Department preventing a person leaving, because they believed the person was at immediate risk as a result of mental disorder and were waiting for an AMHP and psychiatrist to arrive. Such circumstances, in which statutory (or parliamentary) law doesn't apply, are governed by common law. In practice, this means that if the person held against their will in Casualty in the example above brought a prosecution for assault against the staff involved, the Court hearing the case would consider previous rulings in similar cases and, if there was no legal precedent, would base their decision on the likely opinion of an average person. Courts are much more likely to find health professionals negligent for allowing serious harm to come to their patients than they are to rule against those who have documented in their notes why the MHA and MCA did not apply to the situation they faced and why they felt it necessary to act against the patient's will on a common law basis.

### The Mental Health Act

- The Mental Health Act is used to admit people with mental disorders to hospital against their will
- These powers can be used in the interests of the person's health or safety, or for the protection of others

# Introduction to drug treatments

The drugs used to treat mental illnesses are known as 'psychotropics'. Psychotropic drugs exert their effects on neurotransmitter systems within the central nervous system (CNS). This section will begin with an overview of the functioning of the main neurotransmitter systems and chemical theories for the major psychiatric illnesses. In the following pages principles of prescribing psychotropics, antipsychotic drugs, antidepressants, mood stabilisers, anxiolytics and drugs for dementia will be described. How these and other drugs are used in the treatment of specific disorders will be described in the relevant chapters later in the book.

## Neurotransmitter systems

### *Neurotransmitters*

Neurotransmitters are chemicals in the central nervous system that relay signals between neurons by crossing the small gap (synapse) between neurons. The neurotransmitters are stored in vesicles close to the synaptic membrane, and when they are released into the synapse they bind to receptors in the synaptic membrane of the opposite neuron. The effect of this depends upon the properties of the receptor. In most cases receptor binding causes depolarisation of the receptor site. In general this results in the cell firing an action potential, and therefore has an excitatory effect. Some neurotransmitters cause hyperpolarisation of the receptor site, and this results in inhibition of the target neuron.

For a chemical to be regarded as a neurotransmitter it must fulfil a number of criteria (Fig. 1). There must be evidence that it is synthesised in the presynaptic neuron. The precursors and enzymes associated with synthesis must be found in the presynaptic neuron. It must be released when the presynaptic receptor is stimulated, and bind to the postsynaptic receptor, causing a biological effect. There must also be evidence of a mechanism for deactivating the chemical in the synapse, or for its reuptake.

The first neurotransmitter to be described was acetylcholine, in 1914. Since then a wide variety of neurotransmitters have been identified. The most common neurotransmitter in the CNS is glutamate, present in more than 80% of synapses in the brain. Gamma-aminobutyric acid (GABA) is present in the majority of other synapses. Other neurotransmitters are present in fewer synapses, but are of greater significance in the aetiology and treatment of mental illness – in particular dopamine, serotonin, noradrenaline and acetylcholine.

## Dopamine systems

Dopamine is found exclusively in the neural networks coming from the frontal areas of the brain to the amygdala and hippocampus in the limbic system. Synthesis of dopamine is shown in Figure 2A. There are four major dopaminergic systems in the brain (Fig. 3):

1. Dopaminergic neurons in the substantia nigra are responsible for controlling the initiation of and maintenance of movement, resting muscle tone and targeted movement. It is these cells that degenerate in Parkinson's disease.
2. The tuberoinfundibular tracts are neurons in the arcuate nucleus of the hypothalamus that project to the median eminence. They have an inhibitory role in regulating prolactin release from the anterior pituitary.
3. The mesocortical system connects the ventral tegmentum to the frontal cortex. It plays a role in cognitive processes, including motivation and emotional responses.
4. The mesolimbic system projects from the ventral tegmentum to the limbic system, including the amygdala, hippocampus and nucleus accumbens. It is thought that dopamine has a role in modulating feelings of reward and desire, and therefore affects behavioural responses to stimuli.

### *Dopamine hypothesis of schizophrenia*

The dopamine hypothesis was developed as a consequence of the observation that typical (i.e. older) antipsychotic drugs are dopamine antagonists. The hypothesis is that schizophrenia is due to overactivity of dopamine in the mesocortical and mesolimbic systems. This also explains some of the common side effects associated with typical antipsychotic drugs (Fig. 3). Inhibition of dopamine receptors in the substantia nigra results in so called 'extrapyramidal side effects', including Parkinsonian symptoms of tremor and increased muscle tone. Inhibition of dopamine receptors in the tuberoinfundibular tract results in raised prolactin levels which may cause galactorrhoea in women, or gynaecomastia in men.

It is likely that this is an oversimplification of the neurochemical basis of schizophrenia, and newer antipsychotic drugs have more complex modes of action.

## Monoamine systems

In addition to dopamine there are two other monoamines that have particular significance in psychiatry. They are the catecholamine noradrenaline (norepinephrine) and serotonin (5-hydroxytryptamine, 5-HT). Synthesis of these monoamines is shown in Figure 2B. Some adrenergic and noradrenergic neurons radiate from the limbic system to the frontal cortex, and are responsible for alertness, mood and stress (fight or flight) responses. The catecholamines also have peripheral effects. They are released from the adrenal glands in the 'fight or flight' response, and result in a wide range of physiological changes, including increased heart rate, dilation of pupils and increasing the blood supply to muscles.

Serotonin neurons project from the raphe nucleus to the frontal cortex. They control memory, mood, sex drive and appetite. There are three basic types of

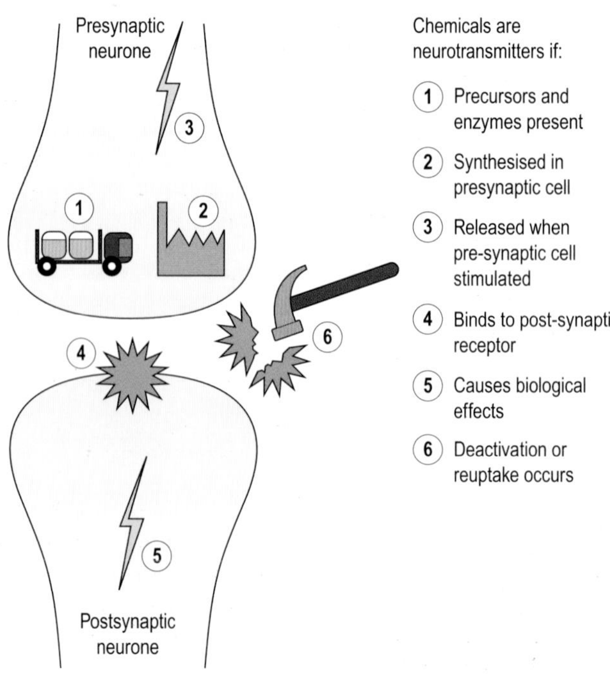


Fig. 1 **Properties of neurotransmitters.**

serotonin receptors: 5HT-1, 5HT-2, and 5HT-3. The first two are thought to be of most importance to psychiatry.

### *Monoamine theory of depression*

Like the dopamine hypothesis, the monoamine theory was developed from an understanding of the mode of action of antidepressant medication. Antidepressants increase monoamine activity in the brain. Some increase levels of serotonin alone (e.g. fluoxetine), some increase the levels of noradrenaline alone (e.g. reboxetine), and others increase both noradrenaline and serotonin (e.g. venlafaxine). This suggests that depression is associated with a depletion in the levels of serotonin and noradrenaline in the central nervous system.

## Acetylcholine system

Acetylcholine is an excitatory neurotransmitter found in both the peripheral and central nervous systems. Synthesis and deactivation of acetylcholine is shown in Figure 2C. It stimulates muscle movement in the peripheral sympathetic, parasympathetic systems and somatic nervous systems. It is found in several sites in the brain. Acetylcholine pathways form part of the reticular activating system, which control alertness, and also have projections to the hippocampus, which has a role in memory. There are acetylcholine neurons in the striatal complex. This is the site of action of anticholinergic medications used for Parkinsonian side effects of antipsychotic drugs.

### *Acetylcholine in Alzheimer's disease*

The dopamine and monoamine theories described above were developed from observation of drug effects, resulting in development of theoretical mechanisms and leading to a search for supporting evidence. The opposite is true of Alzheimer's, where anatomical discoveries led to a search for effective drug treatments. A loss of cholinergic neurons is a consistent finding on post-mortem examination of the brains of individuals who had died from Alzheimer's disease. This observation leads to the use of cholinesterase inhibitors in treatment. They work by reducing the breakdown of acetylcholine in the synaptic cleft, maximising the effects of the remaining cholinergic neurons. This has been shown to have benefits in reducing the symptoms and slowing the progress of Alzheimer's disease for a period.

## Gamma-aminobutyric acid (GABA) and glutamate

GABA is found throughout the brain, and is the principal inhibitory neurotransmitter in the CNS. It is synthesised from glutamate, which is itself an excitatory neurotransmitter. The balance between the effects of glutamate and GABA plays a key role in modulating much of the work of the brain, including the overall state of arousal.

GABA binds to two receptors, GABA-A and GABA-B, and causes hyperpolarisation of the receptor site, making it less likely that the neuron will fire an action potential. Benzodiazepines bind to GABA-A receptors, and increase the effects of GABA at these sites, resulting in an inhibitory effect. This explains the tranquillising and sedating effects of benzodiazepines.

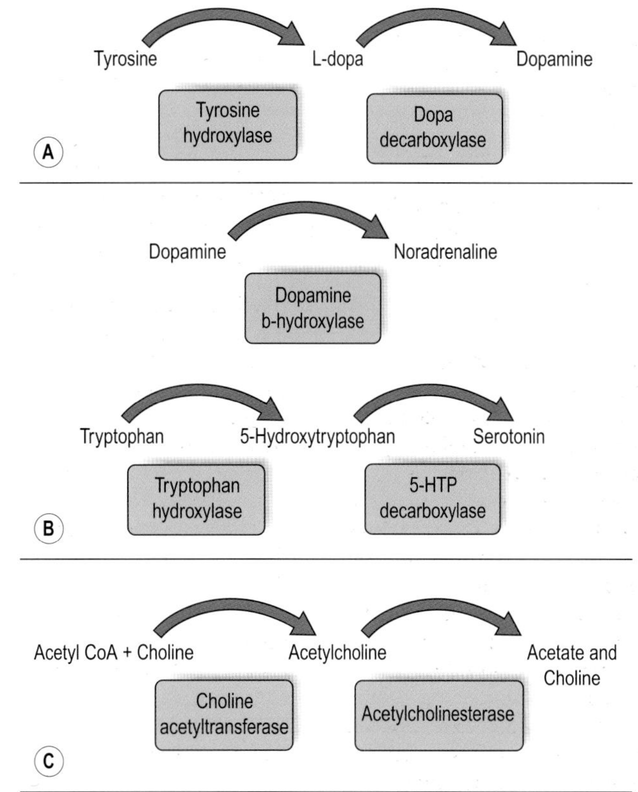


Fig. 2 **(A) Synthesis of dopamine. (B) Synthesis of noradrenaline and serotonin. (C) Synthesis and deactivation of acetylcholine.**

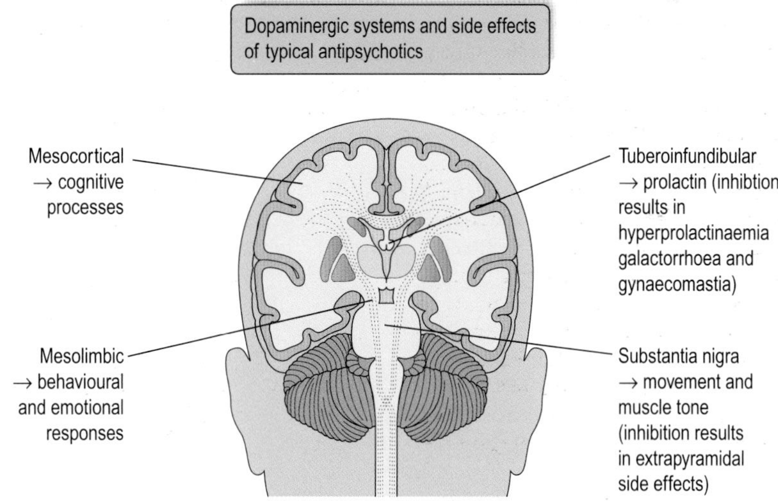


Fig. 3 **Dopaminergic systems and side effects of typical antipsychotic drugs.**

### Drug treatments

- Psychotropic drugs work on neurotransmitter systems in the central nervous system
- The neurotransmitters dopamine, serotonin (5HT), noradrenaline (norepinephrine) and acetylcholine have particular significance in the aetiology and treatment of mental illness
- The effects of antipsychotic and antidepressant drugs led to the development of the dopamine hypothesis of schizophrenia and the monoamine theory of depression

# Prescribing psychotropic drugs

## When to prescribe

A thorough assessment of the patient is required before a psychotropic drug can be prescribed. For the more severe mental illnesses, drugs are the most appropriate and effective treatment; for example, schizophrenia should be treated with an antipsychotic drug and severe depressive illness with an antidepressant. However, for the majority of disorders, effective non-drug treatments are also available. For example, depressive illness of moderate severity responds equally well to some forms of psychotherapy as to drugs. In these circumstances the appropriate treatment should be negotiated with the patient, taking into account their wishes and the available resources.

## Adherence to medication

Adherence is a measure of the extent to which patients follow the recommendations of the prescriber. The outdated paternalistic view of the relationship between doctor and patient – the former giving instructions, and the latter expected to follow them, is unhelpful. In prescribing any medication we should be aiming for 'concordance'. This implies a two-way process in which the doctor gives all of the information required to support the patient in reaching a decision that is mutually satisfactory. It is rare in psychiatry to be in a situation in which only one drug option is available. Where there are several options there are likely to be variations in side effects, dosing regimes and mode of delivery for which the patient may have a preference. For example, given the choice of taking an oral antipsychotic drug daily or having a depot antipsychotic injection once a fortnight, some patients with schizophrenia will choose the depot. This may be counter-intuitive from the doctor's perspective, and so the best decision can only be made by reaching concordance.

Adherence with psychotropic drugs is known to be poor (Fig. 1). Up to half of all patients on prescribed medication for chronic conditions do not take the medication as prescribed. Many patients fail to take the drug at all; others take it at a lower dose or for a shorter period than recommended.

### *Reasons for non-adherence to medication*

Some patients will make a decision to not take their prescribed medication. In many instances this will be because side effects are considered to be unacceptable. Attitudes to psychotropic drugs amongst the general population are generally negative. They are often thought of as causing dependency, and patients may need specific reassurance about this. Patients may also express concerns about stigma and attitudes of family, friends and employers. The degree of insight a patient has into his illness will clearly have an impact on a decision to accept medication. Often patients will accept treatment while they are experiencing active symptoms, but be very reluctant to continue treatment as prophylaxis against relapse. Sometimes it takes several cycles of relapse, successful reinstatement of treatment, and relapse on stopping treatment before an individual will decide to take medication longer term. Others may reasonably decide that infrequent relapses are preferable to constantly taking medication and having to cope with side effects all of the time.

Non-adherence may also occur for reasons beyond the patients' control. They may have difficulties with memory, or have not understood the instructions given. Some are unable to afford prescription fees.

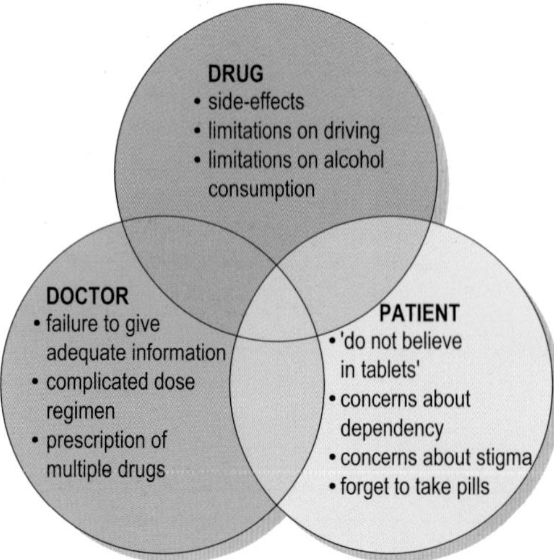


Fig. 1 **Reasons for poor compliance.**

### *Improving adherence*

The first step is to identify that there is a problem, and to understand fully the reasons for it. A 'no blame' attitude is essential; after all, non-adherence to medication is common enough to be virtually the norm! All decisions about treatment should be made in collaboration with the patient. Drug treatment of psychiatric disorders will usually continue for 6 months and in some cases over many years. Some patients will need lifelong treatment to prevent serious relapses of mental illness. Embarking on drug treatment is therefore a serious undertaking, and if it is going to be successful the patient needs to be fully engaged. They need to have a good understanding of the reason for prescription, the consequences of not using drug treatment. They also need to know whether there are non-drug alternatives, and if so their availability and effectiveness. If possible they should be given a choice of drugs, and need guidance about how the choices available to them compare in terms of efficacy and side effects (Fig. 2). Doctors have a responsibility to educate patients about their diagnosis and treatment options, and to listen and respond to their concerns, allowing them to take an active and informed role in decision making. Information leaflets and videotapes are available for the common illnesses and are often helpful.

Maintaining concordance over long periods is a challenge. Reviewing the effectiveness and side effects of the drug, and patient's views about it at regular intervals is helpful. It is also important to keep medication regimes simple, and minimise the number of times in the day when they need to be taken. It is also usually possible to allow flexibility of timing of medication – if it suits an individual to take their night-time medication at 7pm every day, except for the one evening they go out, and then take it at 11pm, then agreeing to this regime is more likely to achieve concordance than a rigid insistence that, for example, night time medications must be taken at 10pm. When mental health professionals visit patients at home there may be opportunities to check that they have the drug packets open and available, and that an appropriate number of tablets have been taken from the packets. Boxes with separate compartments for doses of

- Milder illness
- Serious illness, but no insight
- Low risk of relapse
- Significant side-effects
- Concern about stigma
- Treatment ineffective
- Poor relationship with services

- Serious illness
- High risk of relapse
- Risk to self or others when ill
- Treatment effective
- Good relationship with services

Fig. 2 **Weighing up a decision to accept treatment.**

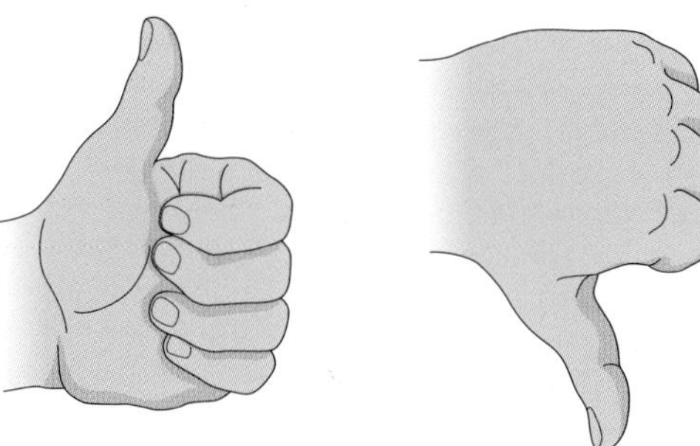

- Convenient, don't have to remember tablets
- Prescriber knows exactly what patient is receiving
- Mental state can be monitored each time depot is given

- Patients don't feel in control of their medication
- Slow dose titration
- Drug present for up to six months following cessation
- Local reactions at injection site

Fig. 3 **Advantages and disadvantages of depot medication.**

medication, or pharmacists packaging medication in blister packs can help patients on complex regimes, or those who are likely to forget. Simple reminders, such as setting a daily mobile phone alarm or putting a note on the fridge door can be very effective. For some drugs (e.g. lithium, clozapine) it is possible to monitor plasma levels, and this provides reassurance both that an appropriate dose is prescribed and that the patient is taking the medication. Depot antipsychotic medications are slow release drugs, given intramuscularly, usually every 2 weeks. They can be a very effective aid to concordance over long periods, in part because the responsibility for delivering the medication lies with the health professional. The pros and cons of depot antipsychotics are summarised in Figure 3. Depots can also be useful in the treatment of acute episodes if compliance is poor, especially if the dose required is known from previous episodes.

There will be circumstances in which the doctor feels that drug treatment is an essential part of the treatment plan, but the patient refuses to accept it. In addition to the reasons for non-concordance already mentioned the refusal may also be because they have no insight into the illness when acutely unwell, or because the symptoms of illness prevent them from taking medication (e.g. persecutory delusions that the drug prescribed is poison). Some of these patients will meet the criteria for treatment under the Mental Health Act because they pose a risk to themselves or others. They may then be treated, if necessary, against their will. Even in these circumstances it is important to engage with the patient as far as is possible, giving them explanations and reassurance about what they are being treated with and why. It may be possible to negotiate to some extent with them about the medication given. In general treatment in these acute circumstances will be with intramuscular injections of antipsychotic drugs or benzodiazepines (see page 44, Rapid Tranquillisation).

Some patients who refuse treatment will not meet criteria for treatment under the Mental Health Act, and their wishes with regards to treatment must be respected. Refusal of drug treatment should not exclude the patient from receiving a service. It is important to engage them, and offer support throughout their period of illness. It may be that the development of a more trusting relationship will result in them feeling able to accept medication. It will also allow a more rapid intervention should their mental state deteriorate to the point that admission under the Mental Health Act becomes necessary. Even when this is not the case it may be possible to offer psychosocial interventions that can be of some benefit.

## Monitoring drug treatment

Response to treatment should be carefully monitored. In many cases, drugs are prescribed at a low dose initially and increased according to the response, aiming to achieve maximum effectiveness with minimal side effects. Patients must therefore be seen regularly during this period in order to monitor their mental state, ensure that they are taking the medication as prescribed, and discuss any problems with treatment. The need for physical health monitoring is now better understood, and the specific requirements will be described in the appropriate drug treatment sections.

### Drug treatments

- Drug treatments cannot be provided in isolation – psychosocial options must always be considered
- Treatment should be negotiated with the patient
- Compliance is often poor and may be improved by providing the patient with adequate information

# Antipsychotic drugs

Antipsychotic drugs are also known as 'major tranquillisers' or 'neuroleptics'. There are now two distinct groups of antipsychotics: the older 'typical' drugs such as chlorpromazine and haloperidol, and the newer 'atypical' drugs, such as risperidone and olanzapine. They are used to treat psychotic disorders, such as schizophrenia, psychotic depression and mania, and to calm severe agitation. The atypical antipsychotic drugs also have mood stabilising effects, and are increasingly used in the treatment of bipolar disorder, both in the acute phase and prophylactically.

Antipsychotic drugs were first discovered in the 1950s. The tranquillising properties of chlorpromazine were noticed when it was used as a sedative prior to surgery, and this led to trials of its effects in patients with mental illness. The results were startling, with patients who had been chronically ill and untreatable in some cases able to recover normal functioning. The use of chlorpromazine, and other drugs that were rapidly developed, became widespread. The impact of this, the first effective treatment for schizophrenia, was profound. It made possible the closure of psychiatric inpatient beds, and the move to treatment of patients with serious mental illness in their own homes, that continues today. In the 1990s the atypical drugs were developed, and in general were better tolerated, and therefore more acceptable to patients. They are now more commonly prescribed than typical antipsychotics. Typicals are still used in depot medications, as there are limited atypical alternatives, and for patients who have been well on typical medications over many years. It is now considered to be good practice to offer atypicals to patients starting on antipsychotic drugs for the first time. The most effective antipsychotic, clozapine, is an atypical that was first discovered in the 1950s, but was thought to be too dangerous to use because it can cause agranulocytosis. The development of effective systems for monitoring patients on clozapine has allowed this drug to be reintroduced for the treatment of patients who do not respond to other antipsychotic drugs.

All antipsychotics have a calming effect which begins quickly, and they can provide rapid relief for an extremely distressed patient. The action on psychotic symptoms is slower, over a period of one or two weeks. In treatment of acute symptoms low doses are used initially, either orally or by intramuscular injection, and increased according to the patient's response, and side effects. In the long-term treatment of chronic schizophrenia, antipsychotics control continuing symptoms and prevent acute relapse.

## How do antipsychotics work?

The older antipsychotics act by blocking dopamine receptors in the brain. The mechanism of action of the atypical antipsychotics varies from drug to drug. They generally have a specific dopaminergic action, blocking a subtype of dopamine receptors known as D2. They also have serotonergic and alpha-adrenergic effects, and some work selectively in the mesolimbic cortex. This gives them a significant advantage over the older drugs in that they produce few or no extrapyramidal effects (see below). However they do have other side effects that can limit their use in some patients, and are significantly more expensive than typical antipsychotics. In general the atypicals are no more effective than the older drugs in treating psychotic symptoms. The important exception to this is clozapine, which is reserved for treatment-resistant schizophrenia (see below).

## Side effects

Typical antipsychotics have a characteristic side-effect profile, as follows:

- Extrapyramidal effects. There are four types:
  - Acute dystonia: severe muscle spasms occur, often affecting the neck or eyes (oculogyric crisis). This can be painful and distressing and occurs in up to 10% or patients, usually in the first few days of treatment.
  - Parkinsonian symptoms: lack of facial expression, increased muscle tone and tremor, occurring in about a third of patients.
  - Akathisia: a distressing side effect characterised by physical and psychological restlessness. It is present in up to a third of patients.
  - Tardive dyskinesia: a late onset side effect in which involuntary movements of the tongue and mouth occur. It emerges in about a fifth of patients on continuous treatment for five years or more. In some cases it is irreversible. The best management for tardive dyskinesia is to reduce or stop the antipsychotic drug, but this may not be possible in all patients.
- Autonomic effects. These are shown in Figure 1 and may be particularly problematic in the elderly. Chlorpromazine and thioridazine have prominent autonomic side effects; haloperidol and the newer drugs are relatively free of them.
- Endocrine effects. Raised prolactin levels may cause galactorrhoea in women, or gynaecomastia in men.
- Raised seizure threshold may result in fits.

The side effect profiles for atypicals varies enormously (Fig. 2). They tend to be well tolerated, but most can cause sedation and weight gain (aripiprazole is the exception to this, and can cause insomnia, restlessness and weight loss). They can also cause postural hypotension, particularly when they are first prescribed, and the dose is increasing. Extra-pyramidal side effects are rare, but can occur. Amisulpride, risperidone and zotepine can all raise prolactin levels. Olanzapine and risperidone are associated with increased risk of stroke in the elderly with dementia, and should not be used in these patients. Side effects of clozapine are described further below.

Both typical and atypical antipsychotics can, rarely, cause prolongation of the QT interval. The QT interval is the time from the start of the Q wave to the end of the T wave on the ECG. There is a rare link between prolonged QT interval and ventricular arrhythmia that may cause sudden death.

Neuroleptic malignant syndrome is a rare side effect of treatment with antipsychotic drugs. It is more likely to occur if high doses are used, or the doses are escalated rapidly. It presents with a raised temperature, fluctuating level of consciousness, muscle rigidity, and autonomic dysfunction. It is associated with elevated creatinine phosphokinase (CPK). This syndrome is associated with a mortality rate of up to 20%, and needs to be treated as a matter of urgency. The antipsychotic drug must be stopped, and general medical admission is usually required.

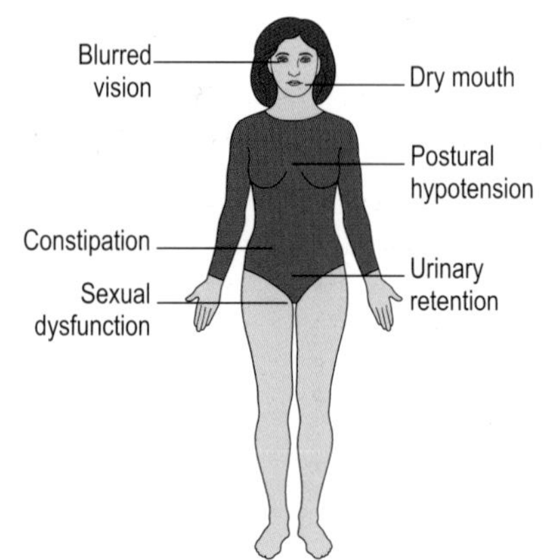


Fig. 1 **Autonomic side effects.**

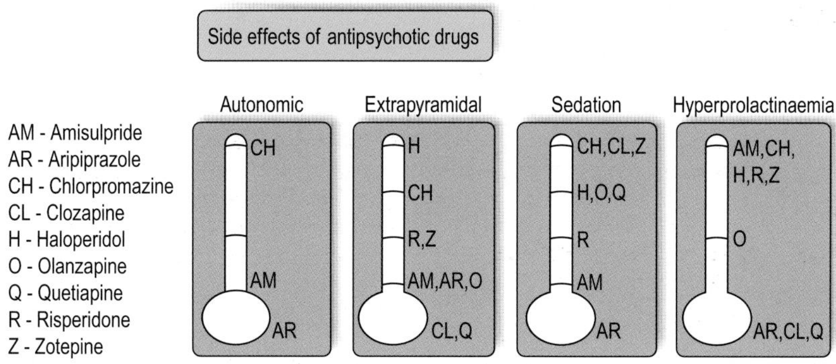

Fig. 2 **Side effects of antipsychotic drugs.**

## Clozapine

Clozapine is the most effective antipsychotic drug, is free of extrapyramidal side effects and does not cause tardive dyskinesia. It is used to treat patients who do not respond to treatment with two or more other antipsychotics, or those who are particularly sensitive to extrapyramidal side effects. It cannot be prescribed as a first-line treatment because of the risks of serious side effects. It is associated with a 3% incidence of neutropenia and 0.8% incidence of agranulocytosis. A very strict monitoring regime has been established by the Clozapine Patient Monitoring Service (CPMS). Full blood counts are done weekly for the first 18 weeks of treatment and fortnightly until a full year of treatment has been completed. Thereafter blood tests are done monthly, and by this time the risk of agranulocytosis has reduced to a level comparable with that of other antipsychotic drugs. CPMS ensures that clozapine is not dispensed unless a normal blood test result has been recorded, and the quantities dispensed are limited to fit in with the frequency of blood tests to ensure treatment can be stopped promptly in the event of an abnormal result.

There are other less serious, but more frequent side effects associated with clozapine, including seizures, particularly at higher doses. Prophylaxis with sodium valproate is sometimes required. Excessive salivation can be a problem, and tends to be worse at night. It can be managed with anticholinergic medication. There is also an association with cardiac problems, including hypersensitivity myocarditis and cardiomyopathy.

## Depot antipsychotic drugs

Depot antipsychotic drugs have been used since the 1960s, generally for the long-term treatment of schizophrenia. They are long-acting medications, given intramuscularly every 1–4 weeks. There are several typical antipsychotic depots, but currently only one atypical, risperidone. The typical depots are in an oily solution, and are gradually released from the solution from the time of the injection, resulting in a steady plasma level. Risperidone depot works in a different way. The active drug is contained within 'microspheres' made of a biodegradable polymer. The polymer breaks down in the muscle over several weeks. There is, as a consequence, a delay of several weeks between the first injection of this drug, and the plasma level rising. Over time a steady plasma level is achieved, although the same delay in effect occurs if the dose is changed. Depot injections are used to aid adherence with medication for patients who may find it difficult to take oral medication regularly.

## Monitoring

Patients who are prescribed antipsychotic drugs should be monitored physically. The medication in itself can cause physical health problems, but it is also known that patients with serious mental illness are more liable than the general population to have physical health problems, and may be less likely to seek help for these difficulties. The body mass index (see p. 76), blood pressure, pulse rate, fasting blood glucose, liver function tests, full blood count and lipids should be checked before starting antipsychotics, when the dose is changed, and in long-term treatment at least annually. Regular review of the medication is important. This should include a discussion to check continued adherence, and that the medication is still indicated. Side effects should be identified, and the dose adjusted as necessary.

In some circumstances consultant psychiatrists will prescribe antipsychotic drugs in high doses, that is, in doses above the maximum recommended licensed dose. This requires special monitoring. In addition to the monitoring described above, an ECG should be done before the high dose is given, and repeated periodically. Pulse, blood pressure and temperature should be checked at baseline and regularly during treatment.

## Antipsychotics drugs and diabetes

There is evidence of an association between antipsychotic drugs and diabetes, although it is not a straightforward relationship. It is known that patients with schizophrenia have an increased risk of diabetes, and this was evident before the advent of antipsychotic drugs. The risk increases with antipsychotic drug treatment, and there appears to be higher risk with olanzapine, clozapine and the typical antipsychotics. There is clearly an association between the development of diabetes and weight gain which may occur with some antipsychotics. However, there appears to also be a mechanism that is independent of the weight gain, and is probably mediated by a direct effect on insulin action in muscle by these drugs. It is good practice to monitor fasting blood glucose in patients on antipsychotic medication. Patients who have diabetes before the medication is started may find their diabetic control is worse, and will need careful monitoring.

### Antipsychotics

- There are two groups of antipsychotics: the older 'typical' drugs such as chlorpromazine and haloperidol, and the newer 'atypical' drugs, such as risperidone and olanzapine
- Antipsychotic drugs take 2 weeks to have an effect on psychotic symptoms
- Clozapine is the most effective antipsychotic drug, but can cause neutropenia and agranulocytosis, so requires careful monitoring
- Depot antipsychotic drugs can be used to improve adherence to medication
- There is an association between antipsychotic drugs and diabetes

# Antidepressant drugs

## *Case history 6*

Nilanjan is a 52-year-old year old man who presents with a moderate to severe depressive episode. He is despondent and hopeless, with fatigue, poor motivation and impaired sleep. He smokes cigarettes and is overweight. He found amitriptyline helpful during a previous depressive episode and wants to take antidepressants again. He was prescribed citalopram a few weeks ago but stopped it because of nausea and agitation.

a. What options would you discuss with him?

Antidepressant drugs, as their name suggests, were developed for the treatment of depressive disorders. They are most effective in the treatment of moderate and severe depressive episodes. It is uncertain whether they are helpful in mild depressive episodes and any efficacy they have in this condition is probably outweighed by the risk of adverse effects, as these milder illnesses often improve spontaneously or with simple non-pharmacological interventions (see p. 54). Antidepressants are also effective in the treatment of anxiety disorders and obsessive–compulsive disorder. Tricyclic antidepressants are used in low doses for the treatment of some chronic pain syndromes.

There are three main classes of antidepressants: tricyclics, selective serotonin reuptake inhibitors (SSRIs) and monoamine oxidase inhibitors (MAOIs). There are other drugs that have similar modes of action to tricyclics but are said to have a better side effect profile, such as serotonin and noradrenaline reuptake inhibitors (SNRIs), venlafaxine and duloxetine, and the noradrenaline reuptake inhibitor (NARI) reboxetine.

### How do antidepressants work?

In 1954, trials of iproniazid for tuberculosis showed that the mood of some subjects improved during treatment. Iproniazid was found to inhibit monoamine oxidase activity and other drugs that replicated this effect turned out to have an antidepressant action. Monoamine oxidase was known to be involved in the breakdown of monoamine neurotransmitters in the brain and the theory that increases in serotonin activity were important in the treatment of depression was suggested by the finding that the antidepressant effect of MAOIs was enhanced by oral supplements of the serotonin precursor, tryptophan.

In 1958, trials of a tricyclic drug, imipramine, in schizophrenia, showed it to be of no help in the treatment of psychotic symptoms but to have an antidepressant effects in subjects with depressive symptoms. Imipramine was found to inhibit the reuptake of noradrenaline into presynaptic neurons, which suggested that noradrenaline was also involved in depression.

All the antidepressants developed since have an effect on either noradrenaline or serotonin, as illustrated in Figure 1. The relative effects of the monoamine reuptake inhibitors are shown in Figure 2. Some antidepressant drugs affect monoamines in novel ways, such as mirtazapine, which antagonises the presynaptic adrenergic autoreceptors that inhibit serotonin and noradrenaline release.

There is a problem with the theory that antidepressants work as a result of their effect on serotonin and noradrenaline. The levels of these monoamines in the synaptic cleft increase within a few hours of the first dose of reuptake inhibitors, whereas it usually takes one or two weeks of treatment before any antidepressant effect is apparent clinically. One explanation for this is that the therapeutic effect of antidepressants depends on a decrease in the sensitivity of some receptors, such as presynaptic serotonergic autoreceptors, that occurs gradually during the first few weeks of treatment. Alternatively, it may be that increases in monoamine transmission have secondary effects that help relieve depression, such as regulation of the hypothalamic pituitary axis, or production of neurotrophic factors that promote healing of damaged neurones.

### SSRIs

The introduction of these drugs during the 1980s was an important development in the treatment of depression. The four most widely prescribed SSRIs are sertraline, citalopram, fluoxetine and paroxetine. They are generally better tolerated than tricyclics and are less dangerous in overdose. Their main disadvantage at first was cost, but patent expiry means that they have become relatively cheap. The SSRIs are not without problems. Gastrointestinal effects such as nausea and diarrhoea are common, particularly early in treatment, although less so if the drug is taken after food and the dose is increased gradually. Sweating, headaches and sexual dysfunction can all occur. Anxiety and agitation may occur in the early stages of treatment and occasionally are severe.

### Tricyclics

For many years, tricyclics were the most commonly prescribed antidepressant drugs, but their use was limited by a number of adverse effects, which are summarised in Figure 3. They include amitriptyline, clomipramine, dosulepin, imipramine, and lofepramine. Most tricyclics are sedating, with the exception of lofepramine and, to a lesser extent, imipramine. This can be helpful when sleep disturbance or anxiety is a particular problem, but daytime sedation is a common reason for people stopping these drugs. They have antimuscarinic effects and so can exacerbate glaucoma, prostatism and problems associated with reduced gastrointestinal motility, such as constipation. Weight gain and erectile dysfunction also occur. Tricyclics cause hypotension, tachycardia and arrhythmias, so can be problematic for people with cardiovascular disease or cardiovascular risk factors. The tricyclics are dangerous in overdose, because of their cardiotoxic effects – the overdose risk is greatest for dosulepin and amitriptyline and so these drugs should be prescribed only under specialist supervision. Lofepramine

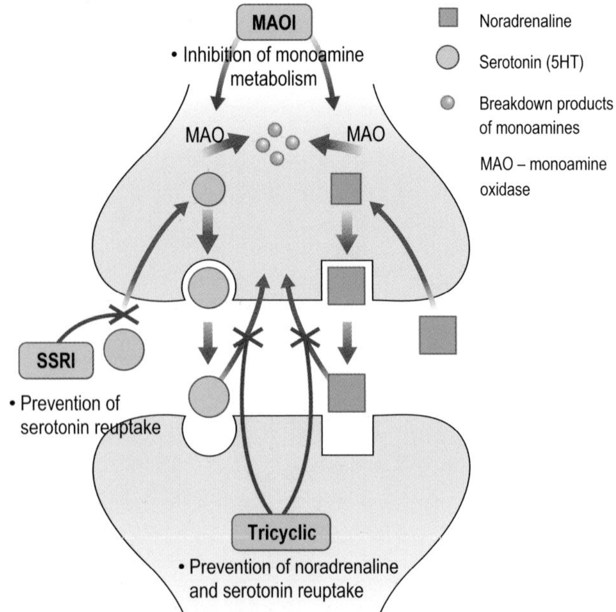


Fig. 1 **Antidepressant drug action.**

| SEROTONIN | DUAL ACTION | | NORADRENALINE |
|---|---|---|---|
| | (mostly 5HT) | (mostly NA) | |
| | Duloxetine | Lofepramine | |
| Sertraline | Venlafaxine | Imipramine | |
| Citalopram | Paroxetine | Dosulepin | Reboxetine |
| Fluoxetine | Clomipramine | Amitriptyline | Desipramine |

- Specific serotonin reuptake inhibitors (SSRIs)
- Tricyclic antidepressants (TCAs)
- Serotonin and noradrenaline reuptake inhibitors (SNRIs)
- Noradrenaline reuptake inhibitors (NARIs)

Fig. 2 **Relative effects of monoamine reuptake inhibitors on serotonin (5HT) and noradrenaline (NA).**

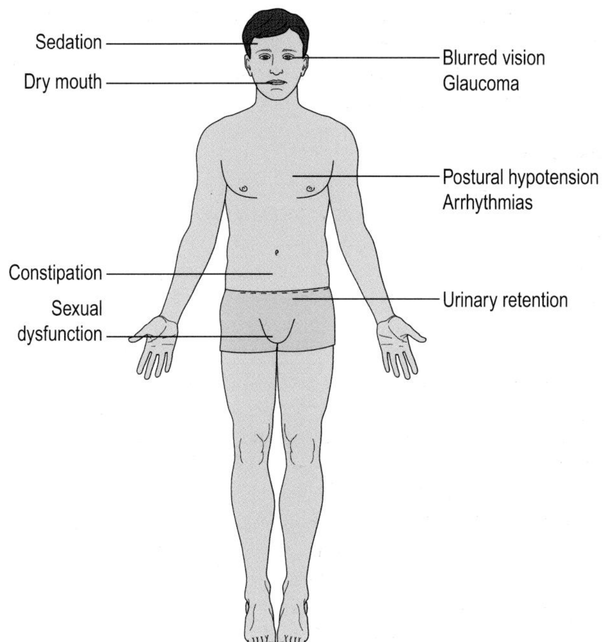


Fig. 3 **Adverse effects of tricyclic antidepressants.**

is a modified tricyclic that causes fewer of these adverse effects and is safer in overdose.

## SNRIs

Venlafaxine and duloxetine are drugs that have been developed to have the dual action of tricyclics, with fewer of the adverse effects. In low doses, venlafaxine acts mainly on serotonin. At higher doses, it has more of a dual action and starts to exhibit the antimuscarinic and cardiotoxic effects associated with tricyclics, but is still better tolerated by most people. Duloxetine has a dual action at all doses and antimuscarinic side effects are fairly common.

## MAOIs

The antidepressant effect of MAOIs occurs through the inhibition of monoamine oxidase A within neurones. This enzyme is involved in the breakdown of serotonin, noradrenaline and adrenaline. It can also break down dopamine, but in vivo this is achieved mostly by monoamine oxidase B. The MAOIs first developed for use in depression include phenelzine and tranylcypromine. These drugs are non-selective and bind irreversibly to both types of monoamine oxidase. They can cause a potentially life-threatening hypertensive crisis if taken with foods containing tyramine, such as cheese, yeast extracts, hung meats and red wine, or certain drugs, including dopaminergic drugs, sympathomimetics and amphetamines. MAOIs can also interact with serotonergic drugs, such as other antidepressants and pethidine, to cause the serotonin syndrome, which can present with agitation, shivering, sweating, nausea, diarrhoea, raised temperature, myoclonus, hyper-reflexia, tachycardia and hypertension, and can progress to confusion, seizures, hyperpyrexia, cardiovascular shock and death. As a result, before starting and after stopping MAOIs, no other antidepressant should be taken for two weeks. These interactions are much less of a concern with moclobemide, a MAOI that is selective for monoamine oxidase A and is displaced from the enzyme by high levels of monoamines. Tyramine containing foods can be eaten in moderation with moclobemide.

## Other drugs

Mirtazapine has sedative effects which can be helpful for people with depression who identify poor sleep as a particular problem. It is often associated with weight gain. Trazodone is a tetracyclic drug which has similar side effects to tricyclics, with antimuscarinic and cardiotoxic effects occurring to a lesser degree. It is sedating, so is often considered when sleep disturbance and anxiety are present. The NARI reboxetine is not widely used but can be a useful option for people who are particularly sensitive to the serotonergic side effects of other antidepressants. Antimuscarinic side effects commonly occur.

## Antidepressant discontinuation syndrome

About one in six people develop discontinuation symptoms after stopping or reducing the dose of antidepressants. Common symptoms are anorexia, nausea, vomiting, headache, feeling hot and cold, insomnia, anxiety and restlessness. In the case of SSRI discontinuation, additional symptoms of fatigue, influenza-like symptoms and paraesthesiae often described as feeling like electric shocks, have been reported. The syndrome is usually mild and it is unusual for it to last more than a few days. However, severe cases do sometimes occur and the syndrome tends to be worse following cessation of drugs with a short half-life, such as paroxetine and venlafaxine.

## Suicidality and antidepressants

There is evidence that antidepressants, particularly SSRIs, increase the incidence of suicidal thoughts and acts in young people. This phenomenon usually occurs early in treatment and in many cases is linked to the anxiety and agitation that can develop following initiation of these drugs. Whether antidepressants increase suicidality in other ways is a matter of debate. It is also not certain whether this phenomenon occurs in older people – it may be that people of all ages can be affected and that young people included in drug trials are less likely to experience the benefits of antidepressants that would counterbalance any increase in suicidality. In light of all this, anyone prescribed an antidepressant should be warned that the drug may cause an increase in suicidal thoughts, so they should seek advice immediately if this occurs. People below the age of 30 years should be reviewed within a week of starting an SSRI.

### Antidepressant drugs

- SSRIs are usually well tolerated and safe in overdose
- Antidepressants, particularly SSRIs, can cause agitation and increased suicidality
- Tricyclics and SNRIs are commonly used second line drugs

# Mood stabilisers and ECT

## Mood stabilisers

The discovery that lithium reduces the risk of both manic and depressive relapse in bipolar affective disorder has resulted in it being viewed as a mood stabilising drug. Some anticonvulsants, such as valproate salts and carbamazepine, have similar effects and have also come to be thought of as 'mood stabilisers'. In some ways, this is an unhelpful term. It wrongly implies that drugs such as lithium will help in other conditions in which there is instability of mood, such as emotionally unstable personality disorder. It does not take account of the fact that lithium is widely used to augment antidepressants in cases of treatment resistant unipolar depression. There is the additional issue of what to call the atypical antipsychotic drugs, such as quetiapine, that are effective in both the depressive and manic phases of bipolar disorder. It is probably more helpful to remember the indications for individual drugs (e.g. Table 1 on p. 51), rather than categorise them in a potentially misleading way, and we have only used the term 'mood stabilisers' as a heading for this chapter because it is conventional to do so.

### *Lithium*

Lithium is a naturally occurring ion and a member of group one of the periodic table, the alkali metals. Compared with other drugs, the ratio of toxic to therapeutic levels is low, so lithium can only be used safely if blood levels are monitored. At therapeutic levels, lithium has a number of benign side effects, as shown in Figure 1. It can cause nephrogenic diabetes insipidus early in treatment, which is reversible at first but can become permanent if lithium is not stopped soon enough. Chronic kidney disease is an uncommon but important long-term effect of treatment with lithium – the cases that do occur are usually in people who have taken the drug for 20–30 years. Hypothyroidism affects about 10% of people who take lithium, usually after several years of treatment and more frequently in people with other risk factors for hypothyroidism, such as female gender and family history. Hyperparathyroidism and hypercalcaemia can also occur. Lithium toxicity is usually associated with levels of 1.5 mmol/L or more. People taking lithium should be advised to stop the drug if they develop a coarse tremor, vomiting or diarrhoea, and to drink plenty of fluid and seek medical advice. Toxicity can be precipitated by dehydration, for example during hot weather, and prescription of drugs that increase lithium levels, such as NSAIDs and thiazide diuretics. Some people will develop abnormalities of cardiac conduction after starting lithium. The monitoring required during lithium treatment is summarised in Table 1.

Lithium reduces the risk of manic recurrence in bipolar affective disorder, and to a lesser extent depressive episodes. Lithium levels of 0.4–0.6 mmol/L are sufficient for a prophylactic effect, with levels closer to 1 mmol/L being almost three times as likely to prevent recurrence, but also being associated with three times the risk of discontinuation due to side effects.

Lithium has antimanic effects during acute episodes, but it is not the treatment of choice in severe episodes or when a quick response is needed, and levels close to 1 mmol/L are required. Long-term lithium treatment for bipolar disorder is associated with a reduced suicide rate. The drug is best avoided in people with bipolar disorder who are likely to stop it abruptly, as one-third of those who do will develop a manic episode within a few months. Lithium has antidepressant effects in unipolar depression, particularly when combined with an antidepressant.

### *Anticonvulsant drugs*

**Sodium valproate** and **valproic acid** are effective antimanic drugs with a relatively fast onset of action, particularly if the highest tolerated dose is used. They reduce the risk of manic recurrence and to a lesser extent depressive episodes. Blood levels give an indication of whether the person is taking treatment as advised but are not a good predictor of response. Gastrointestinal side effects are common and weight gain, sedation and ataxia can occur. There is a risk of blood dyscrasias and hepatic dysfunction, so full blood count and liver function should be checked annually.

**Carbamazepine** reduces the risk of recurrence in bipolar disorder and has antimanic effects. It is not a first-line treatment, because it can cause blood dyscrasias, hepatic dysfunction and skin reactions. It is a hepatic enzyme inducer and reduces the levels of a variety of other drugs.

**Lamotrigine** can be useful in the treatment of bipolar depression. It needs to be introduced slowly, because of a risk of skin reactions that include Stevens–Johnson syndrome and it can take six weeks to achieve a therapeutic dose.

## Electroconvulsive therapy (ECT)

ECT is a safe and effective treatment, most often used for patients with severe depressive illness, but also in catatonic schizophrenia and severe manic episodes. In most cases, these conditions can be effectively managed with medication, but ECT has the advantage of a rapid onset of action, often within two or three treatments, so is useful when a quick response is needed. ECT can also be helpful when medication has been ineffective. ECT enhances monoamine function in the brain, and its mode of action therefore fits with the monoamine theory of depression (see p. 26). Figure 2 shows the circumstances in which ECT should be considered.

When a person is treated with ECT, a current is applied across the brain by placing two electrodes on the person's head, with one placed on each temple (bilateral), or both over the non-dominant hemisphere of the brain (unilateral). Unilateral application has fewer side effects, but probably requires more treatments to produce the same degree of improvement. The effectiveness of ECT relies upon the induction of a convulsion and the effectiveness of each treatment is judged by the length of the seizure that follows, measured by observation of tonic–clonic movements and electroencephalography (EEG). In the past, the electrical stimulus required to produce a seizure of adequate duration was calculated on the basis of the person's age and gender, but it was a crude method that did not allow for the substantial variations in seizure threshold between individuals. This resulted in some people being treated with unnecessarily high doses of electricity and experiencing cognitive impairment as a result. Now, the method of

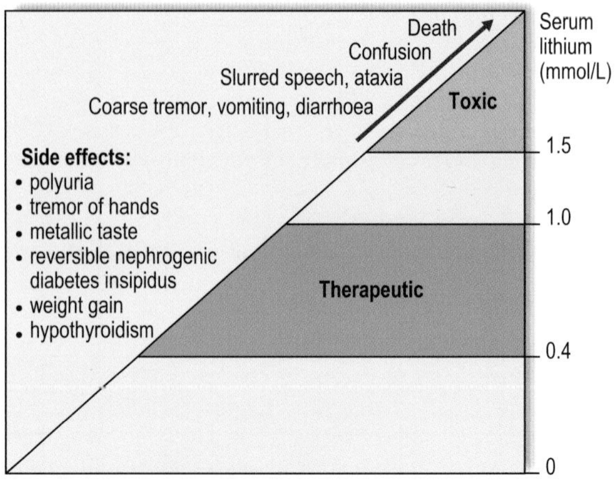


Fig. 1 **Side effects and toxic effects of lithium.**

Table 1 **Monitoring of people taking lithium**

| Test | When? | Why? |
|---|---|---|
| Lithium level | 5–7 days after initiation<br>Following change of dose<br>If drug interactions possible<br>Routinely every six months | Narrow therapeutic range<br>Risk of toxicity |
| Serum creatinine | Before initiation<br>Routinely every six months | Risk of chronic kidney disease<br>Renal function affects lithium levels |
| Thyroid function | Before initiation<br>Routinely every six months | Risk of hypothyroidism |
| ECG | Before and after initiation | Risk of conduction defects |
| Serum calcium | Routinely every year | Risk of hyperparathyroidism/hypercalcaemia |
| Urine volume | If polyuria occurs | Risk of diabetes insipidus |

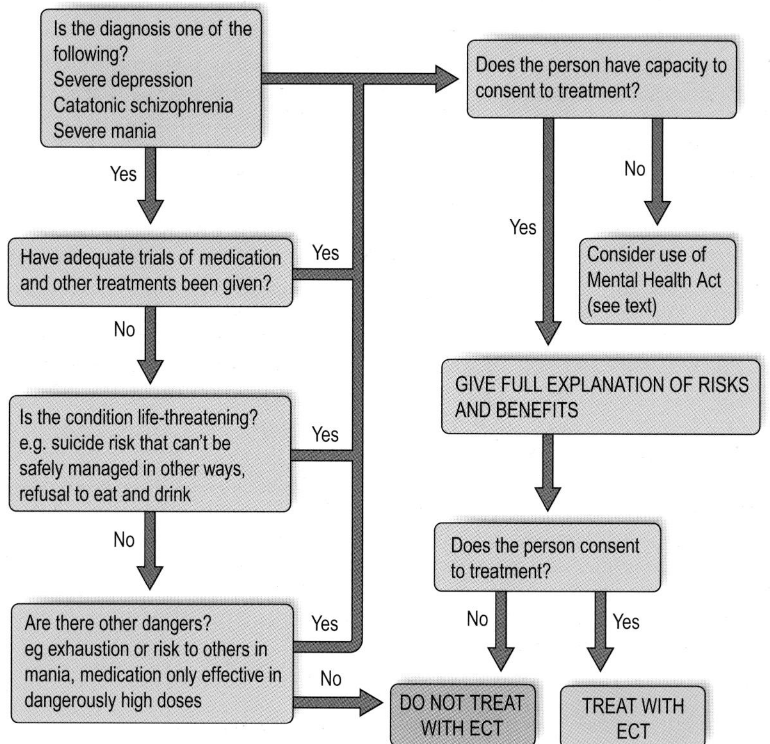


Fig. 2 **Circumstances in which ECT should be considered.**

stimulus dosing is widely used, in which the seizure threshold is determined at the first treatment session, by giving increasing doses of electricity until a seizure occurs.

All ECT is now 'modified' by the use of muscle relaxants given with a general anaesthetic, which limit the vigour of the convulsion and prevent injury. Treatment is given two or three times per week, with improvement usually beginning after two or three treatments. On average, a course of six to eight treatments is needed to achieve a full response. ECT is only effective in the acute phase of the conditions for which it is used, so when the course of treatment has finished, medication is usually continued to improve the person's chances of staying well. Very occasionally, maintenance ECT is used when medication does not prevent relapse.

The main side effect of treatment is loss of memory for recent events occurring over a short period before and after treatment. This usually resolves within two weeks of treatment ending, but can persist, usually to a mild degree, for several months. The only permanent cognitive impairment that can be caused by ECT is deficits in autobiographical memory. This is not usually problematic but causes some people to regret having ECT. Other side effects encountered are headaches, muscle pains and those due to the general anaesthetic.

Normally, a person must give written consent before undergoing a course of ECT. If the person does not have the mental capacity to give such consent, treatment can be given under Section 3 of the Mental Health Act, but only if authorised by an independent consultant psychiatrist.

## Mood stabilisers and ECT

- Lithium is often used in bipolar disorder and is associated with a reduced suicide rate
- Some anticonvulsants are also used in bipolar disorder
- ECT is used in life-threatening situations and when other treatments have been ineffective

# Benzodiazepines and drugs for dementia

## Benzodiazepines

The benzodiazepines are known as 'minor tranquillisers'. During the 1960s and 1970s they were enormously popular, but as the risk of dependence has been better understood they have been much less frequently prescribed. They are generally subdivided into two groups – the short acting hypnotics (e.g. temazepam), and the longer acting anxiolytics (e.g. diazepam).

### *How do benzodiazepines work?*

Benzodiazepines are gamma-amino butyric acid (GABA) receptor agonists. GABA receptors occur throughout the cortex and limbic system in the brain, and act to inhibit neuronal activity.

### *Indications*

Currently there are five main psychiatric indications for prescription of benzodiazepines:

1. Severe acute emotional distress, for example following a bereavement or assault, where short-term sedation can provide relief. The prescription should be for as short a period and as low a dose as possible.
2. Medical management of withdrawal from alcohol. Chlordiazepoxide is most commonly used, starting with a dose that is high enough to control all withdrawal symptoms, and reducing over 7–10 days.
3. As an adjunct to antipsychotic medication in patients with marked agitation due to severe mental illness, such as mania. Again the prescription should be short-term, although when used in these circumstances is unlikely to lead to dependency. Benzodiazepines are used in combination with antipsychotic drugs in rapid tranquillisation.
4. For patients who are dependent upon benzodiazepines prescribed to them over many years. These patients should be given opportunities to stop the drugs completely, by prescribing a slowly reducing course. Some, however, are unable to manage complete withdrawal.
5. For people with generalised anxiety disorder who continue to experience high levels of distress and disability despite having tried all other treatments and who understand and accept the risks of tolerance and dependence.

### *Side effects*

The main side effects of benzodiazepines are sedation and psychomotor impairment which may affect driving ability. They can also cause headaches, confusion, ataxia, and dysarthria. Some patients have a paradoxical reaction to benzodiazepines, and become disinhibited, excited or aggressive. This appears to be a particular risk in patients who have poor impulse control associated with brain injury, learning disability or personality disorder, and in younger and older patients. Respiratory depression is rare with oral formulations but can occur if benzodiazepines are used intravenously. In this event, the benzodiazepine antagonist, flumazenil, may be used.

Tolerance and dependency can develop rapidly, although are more likely after long-term treatment.

### *Management of benzodiazepine withdrawal*

It is thought that about half of all benzodiazepine users experience withdrawal symptoms. This is more likely if benzodiazepines with short half-lives are used (particularly lorazepam); they are used for a long time, at high dose; the patient has alcohol or other drug dependency, or a personality disorder; or they are used without medical supervision. Withdrawal symptoms vary widely. Some patients are able to withdraw without difficulty, even after many years of treatment, others suffer severe symptoms with insomnia, anxiety, agitation, depressed mood and perceptual changes. Withdrawal should be managed by first of all switching to an equivalent dose of diazepam, as withdrawal symptoms tend to be less severe with this longer-acting drug. The dose is then slowly reduced, titrating the speed of reduction against the patient's symptoms. The aim is to allow withdrawal symptoms to settle fully before attempting the next reduction in dose. The reductions in dose become smaller as the withdrawal proceeds.

### *Hypnotic drugs*

Hypnotic drugs induce sleep and are used to treat insomnia. Insomnia is a change to the normal sleep pattern, due to difficulty in either getting to sleep or maintaining sleep. What is regarded as a 'normal' sleep pattern varies enormously from one individual to another, although most healthy adults sleep between 7 and 9 hours each night. The causes of insomnia are shown in Table 1.

| Table 1 **Causes of insomnia** |
|---|
| Life events |
| Physical illness (e.g. pain, discomfort) |
| Mental illness (e.g. depression, mania) |
| Substance abuse (e.g. alcohol, nicotine, illicit drugs) |
| Prescribed drugs (e.g. SSRIs) |

The most appropriate way to manage insomnia is to treat any comorbid problems (for example, depression or pain), and encourage a routine that is more likely to result in good sleep. Key elements of this include keeping regular sleeping hours (including a focus on a regular time to wake up), avoiding alcohol and stimulants such as caffeine, sleeping in a dark and quiet room, and getting some regular physical exercise during the day.

Hypnotic drugs should only be used to treat severe insomnia that is resistant to non-drug treatments and is causing acute emotional distress. It should be treated with the lowest possible dose, and for no more than 4 weeks. Hypnotics provide symptomatic relief only, that is they induce sleep, but do not treat any underlying cause for the insomnia. Benzodiazepines and the so-called 'Z drugs' (zaleplon, zolpidem and zopiclone) are most commonly used as hypnotics.

The benzodiazepines with shorter half-lives, such as temazepam, tend to be used for insomnia, as they are less likely to cause side effects the following day. However, as with all benzodiazepine use there is a risk of developing tolerance and dependence. Insomnia is often a symptom of withdrawal, and can be worse than the original insomnia the benzodiazepine was prescribed for (known as 'rebound insomnia').

The Z drugs are non-benzodiazepine hypnotic drugs. Their structure is very different from the benzodiazepines, but their mode of action is similar – they act as GABA receptor agonists, and therefore increase GABA neuronal inhibition. All three have short half-lives, although have the potential to cause daytime sedation. There is a risk that they may be associated with tolerance and dependence, and their prescription should be restricted in the same way as benzodiazepines, with the additional caveat that they may be more costly.

## Drugs for dementia

### *How do drugs for dementia work?*

Acetylcholinesterase (AChE) inhibitors work by preventing the breakdown of acetylcholine in the synaptic cleft, resulting in more acetylcholine availability for neurotransmission.

Donepezil was the first acetylcholinesterase inhibitor to be licensed in the UK, in 1997. It is a reversible inhibitor of acetylcholinesterase. Galantamine is a competitive and reversible inhibitor of acetylcholinesterase. It was originally derived from extracts of snowdrop and daffodil bulbs, but is now produced synthetically. Rivastigmine is an acetylcholinesterase and butyrylcholinesterase inhibitor.

### Prescribing drugs for dementia

The acetylcholinesterase inhibitors donepezil, galantamine and rivastigmine are used in the management of Alzheimer's disease. In general they are prescribed in clearly defined circumstances by specialist services in secondary care (including psychiatric, learning disability, neurology and medical services). Their use is limited to patients with an illness of moderate severity. Severity of illness is assessed in various ways (Fig. 1), and usually includes the use of a standardised tool to measure cognitive function. This provides an objective measure that can be used to track progress. These assessments must be repeated at least every 6 months. When the assessments indicate that the illness is severe, or the drug no longer appears to be having a worthwhile effect on the functioning or behaviour of the patient, the acetylcholinesterase inhibitor should be stopped.

There is some evidence for the benefits of acetylcholinesterase inhibitor drugs in other forms of dementia, particularly Lewy body dementia, and research is continuing into this area to establish whether they should be used, and if so how. Until this research is completed these drugs are, in the main, restricted to treatment of Alzheimer's disease.

There is good evidence to show that acetylcholinesterase inhibitors can cause improvements in cognitive functioning, and other aspects of general functioning and behaviour. However the effects are often relatively small, and can be short-term. There is evidence from placebo controlled trials that improvement in cognitive function can be maintained over a period of 2 years. These medications do not appear to alter the underlying disease process, and this is apparent when they are withdrawn in drug trials, as the patients' condition deteriorates to that of those in the placebo group within 6 weeks of stopping treatment. It is also clear that some patients respond better to treatment than others. Currently it is not possible to predict which patients are likely to be in this group.

The high costs of these treatments have led to controversy about how they should best be used. It is thought that life expectancy is not changed with treatment, but as functioning is improved for a period it is likely that treated patients will maintain a degree of independence for a greater proportion of their illness. The overall cost of caring for treated patients may therefore be reduced. However, the prospect of treatment for what was in the past an untreatable condition may result in many more patients being diagnosed and referred to secondary care than before, pushing up costs for the health service.

### Side effects

The most common side effects are nausea and vomiting. Although these effects are usually short-term they may lead to non-adherence.

### Memory clinics

Memory clinics have been established to manage the increasing demand for treatment for dementia following the advent of these new drug treatments. They are community based services, run by multidisciplinary teams including psychiatrists, community mental health nurses, support workers and psychologists. Their role is to assess patients referred by GPs, establishing a diagnosis of dementia, and excluding other potential causes for memory impairment. They work closely with patients and their carers, providing information, advice and support. Treatment is planned and delivered by the memory clinics, and includes but is not limited to treatment with acetylcholinesterase inhibitors. Those who are prescribed these drugs are carefully monitored at regular intervals.

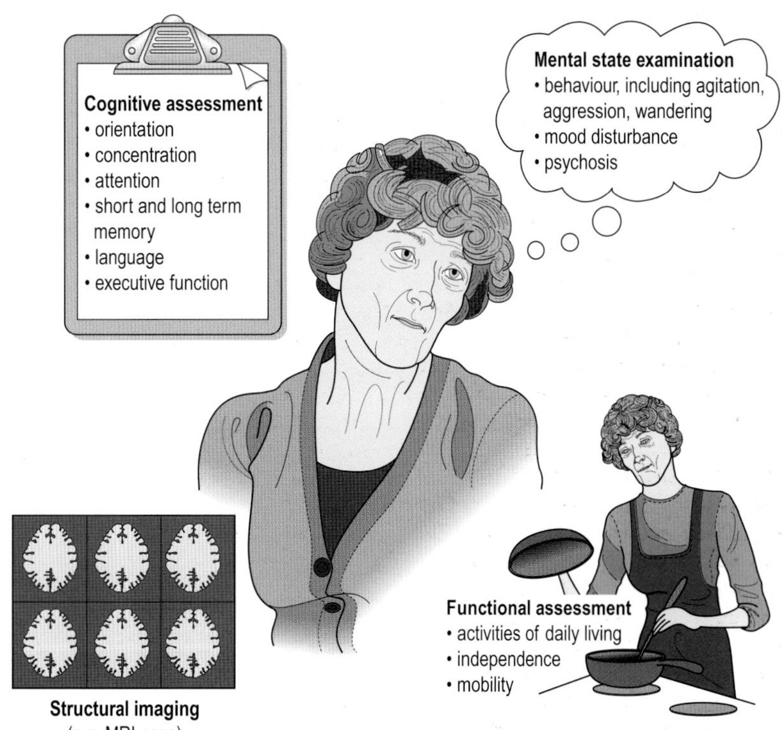


Fig. 1 **Assessing severity of dementia.**

## Benzodiazepines and drugs for dementia

**Benzodiazepines**

- should only be used to manage acute emotional distress, withdrawal from alcohol, treatment of the acute phase of severe mental illness, and for patients with chronic dependence
- withdrawal should be managed by switching to an equivalent dose of diazepam and reducing the dose slowly

**Drugs for dementia**

- increase the availability of acetylcholine in the central nervous system by inhibiting the enzyme acetylcholinesterase
- can improve the cognitive and behavioural functioning of patients with Alzheimer's disease over a period of 2 years, but do not alter the underlying disease process

# Psychological treatments

## *Case history 7*

Mary is a 32-year-old woman who presents with despondency, low self-esteem, lethargy and other depressive symptoms following a period of prolonged marital and financial difficulties. She has fallen behind at work and has panic attacks when colleagues appear to be observing her. She was brought up by her father and stepmother after her mother's death and always felt her half-sister's needs were put ahead of her own.

a. What psychological treatments would be useful in this case?

Psychological treatments may be used alone or in combination with physical treatments. They provide some of the most powerful means of treating many types of mental illness. The three main types of psychological treatment are dynamic psychotherapy, behavioural psychotherapy and cognitive psychotherapy. There is much debate about the relative merits of these and, as will be seen in this section, all appear to have a role. In deciding which psychotherapy, if any, to recommend to patients, it is important to consider the nature of their problems, as well as how receptive they are likely to be to the different approaches.

### Behavioural psychotherapy

The term behavioural psychotherapy covers a range of treatments, all of which make unwanted behaviours the focus of treatment. They include relatively simple techniques such as relaxation training, in which participants learn to reduce the somatic symptoms of anxiety through controlled breathing and muscle relaxation. Most other behavioural techniques are based on the psychological theory of operant conditioning which states that a behaviour is reinforced (i.e. is more likely to be repeated) if it has positive consequences. Positive reinforcement is when a behaviour increases because something good happens as a result, whereas with negative reinforcement a behaviour increases because it causes something unpleasant to go away. It will be seen from this description that negative reinforcement is not the same as punishment. When operant conditioning is involved in the development of mental illness, it is usually through negative conditioning. For instance, avoidance of going outside in agoraphobia or carrying out compulsions in obsessive–compulsive disorder are associated with a reduction in levels of anxiety and so these behaviours increase in frequency. Similarly, during depressive episodes, routine activities can lead to increased fatigue and feelings of failure if the patient finds them difficult to complete. In such cases, activity levels decrease because of negative reinforcement.

Operant conditioning is also important during treatment. For instance, in *exposure therapy* for agoraphobia, the therapist will explain to the patient that, if they force themselves to endure the anxiety associated with going out, it will eventually subside. When the patient discovers this to be true, negative reinforcement occurs, and they become less likely to give in to the anxiety next time it occurs. Common ways in which operant conditioning is applied to clinical situations are shown in Table 1.

### Cognitive therapy

Cognitive therapy is based on the principle that the way people perceive events has more effect on how they feel than the event itself. For instance, if you are woken by a banging noise during the night, you may believe that a burglar is breaking into your house and so feel frightened. Alternatively, you may believe that a housemate has returned home drunk and so feel angry, or you may believe that a draught has caused a door to slam, in which case you probably won't feel any particular emotion. This shows how the same **A**ntecedent has been responded to with different **B**eliefs, each resulting in different **C**onsequences, and is an example of the ABC model used in cognitive therapy. This process can often become self-perpetuating. In the example above, if you had become frightened, you would be more likely to attribute any further noises to a burglar.

The first stage of cognitive therapy is to teach patients to recognise their symptoms and then to apply the ABC model. This will reveal a number of *thinking errors* that cause them to appraise events in a way that leads to unpleasant consequences. For instance, a patient with an anxiety disorder will tend to view situations as threatening. As a result, they will become anxious, which will increase the chances of them viewing subsequent events in a similar way. Patients with depressive disorder will favour negative rather than positive explanations of events. This causes low mood which makes them view events in an even more negative way. Learning to spot and challenge these thinking errors is the key process in cognitive therapy. Patients keep diaries, to enable them and their therapist to monitor their progress and to discuss the issues that arise between treatment sessions when they put cognitive techniques into practice.

Thinking errors are a reflection of people's assumptions about themselves and their world, which are also known as *cognitive schema*. Understanding such schema and how they originated helps people avoid thinking errors. Diagrams like the one in Figure 1 are used to help patients gain this understanding.

**Cognitive behaviour therapy** combines cognitive and behavioural techniques. For instance, a patient with agoraphobia would be helped by exposure therapy and cognitive techniques that address the thinking errors that lead

Table 1 **Use of operant conditioning in behaviour therapy**

| Technique | Indications | Process |
|---|---|---|
| Exposure therapy | Simple phobia, agoraphobia | Identify things or places which lead to anxiety |
| | | List these in order, i.e. a *hierarchy* with most anxiety-provoking situations at the top |
| | | Expose patient to situation at bottom of hierarchy until no longer causes anxiety |
| | | Move on to next situation in hierarchy |
| Response prevention | Obsessive–compulsive disorder | Gradually reduce the number of times the person carries out the unwanted act, e.g. for compulsive handwashing, make the patient repeatedly 'contaminate' their hands and gradually reduce the time they spend washing them afterwards |
| Behavioural activation | Depressive disorder | Patient avoids doing things as they think they will not enjoy them or will feel a failure if they do not complete them |
| | | Make realistic and achievable plans to carry out activity each day |
| | | Gradually increase the amount of activity |

to anxiety when they go out. A patient with depression would be helped by both behavioural activation and cognitive techniques that deal with their negative thinking style. In **cognitive analytic therapy**, a psychodynamic approach is used to help the patient understand why they developed interpersonal difficulties and problematic cognitive schemata, with cognitive techniques being used to change these ways of thinking.

## Dynamic psychotherapy

Dynamic (or analytic) psychotherapy is derived from Sigmund Freud's descriptions of psychoanalysis. Freud's theories and the practice of dynamic psychotherapy have been adapted considerably and there are now many different forms of treatment available. It is only possible to describe here the key components of these therapies.

Psychodynamic theory states that the mind is divided into conscious and subconscious parts. When faced with overwhelming anxiety or distress, the conscious mind uses psychological defence mechanisms, such as repression, to push these feelings into the subconscious. These feelings may remain in the subconscious for many years and yet still influence the way the person views themselves and others. Situations similar to those which caused the original distress may cause the repressed feelings to re-enter the conscious mind. Alternatively, the conscious mind may respond by using other defence mechanisms, such as projection in which the distressing feelings are attributed to other people, thereby reducing the distress that would be caused if the person acknowledged that these feelings actually related to him or herself.

A psychodynamic therapist helps the patient to understand and alter these processes. At the centre of this therapeutic process is the assumption that the way the patient interacts with the therapist reflects the way they interact with others outside therapy, a process known as transference. Therapists are affected by the powerful emotions felt by the patient during therapy, which means that feelings the therapist has about the patient actually reflect what the patient is feeling. This is known as counter-transference. As the therapeutic relationship becomes more trusting and secure, the therapist is able to use transference and counter-transference to help the patient discover the repressed reasons for their current distress. An example of this process is given in Figure 2.

The shortest form of dynamic psychotherapy is brief focal therapy, which consists of 12–30 weekly sessions, each lasting 50 minutes. In some cases, treatment can continue for years. There is evidence that shorter forms of treatment are effective but longer-term therapy has not been properly evaluated.

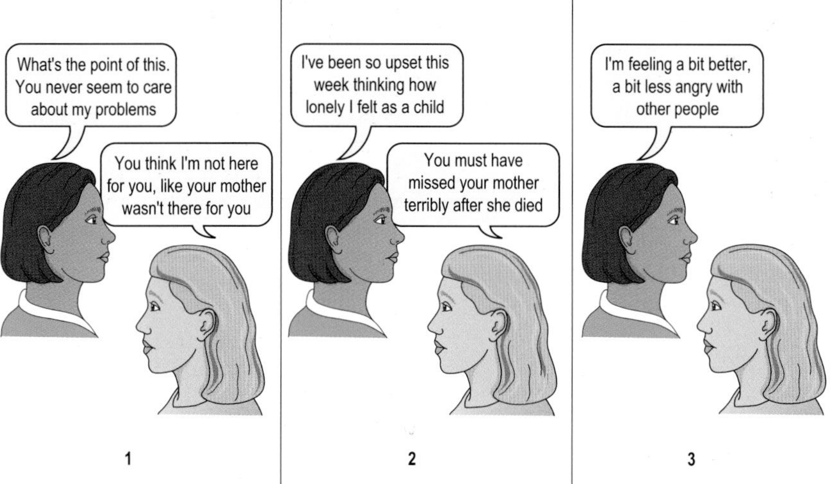


Fig. 1 **How childhood experience leads to cognitive schemata which increase the chance of thinking errors.** The alternative belief could be used to challenge the thinking errors.

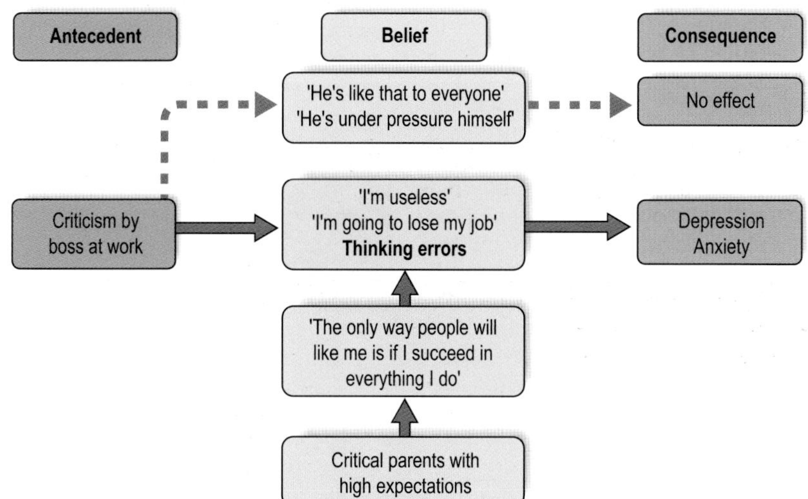


Fig. 2 **Helping the patient come to terms with repressed emotions by interpreting transference towards the therapist in dynamic psychotherapy.**

### Psychological treatments

- Dynamic psychotherapy helps patients understand how relationships and events from the past affect them in the present
- Behavioural psychotherapy focuses on dysfunctional patterns of behaviour
- Cognitive therapy helps patients identify and challenge thinking errors

# Family and social treatments

## *Case history 8*

Rose has chronic schizophrenia and has lived in a hostel with 24-hour nursing staff for 7 years, since she was 26 years old. She copes well in this environment and requires little support from staff. She still experiences auditory hallucinations most days, but these are not distressing to her. She has no friends outside the hostel, and little contact with her family. She is keen to gain more independence.

a. What type of accommodation may be suitable for her?
b. How would you decide between these options?

Episodes of mental illness are often precipitated or prolonged by family and social problems. To make matters worse, family life and social function is often adversely affected by mental illness. Dealing with these issues can be as effective as drug and psychological treatments and should be considered in the management of anyone with a mental disorder.

## Family treatments

### *Family therapy*

All forms of family therapy are based on the principle that it is helpful to involve families when treating mental illness, regardless of whether the problem is considered to lie within an individual family member or be a consequence of disturbed family dynamics. In family therapy for schizophrenia, education is provided about the condition, with the aim of encouraging family members to be realistic in their expectations and to help them reduce the levels of expressed emotion within the family. Family therapy is commonly used in the treatment of childhood psychiatric disorders. Therapists will see families together and look for patterns of interaction that may be maintaining the presenting problems, rather than looking at the behaviour of individual family members.

### *Couples therapy*

Many patients describe a poor relationship with their partner. In some cases this is secondary to their mental illness, which may place a strain upon the relationship or alter their perception of it. In such cases, treatment of the mental illness may be enough, along with carers' support, as described below. In some cases though, relationship problems will be a cause of mental illness and couples therapy may be needed.

Couples therapy is often provided by organisations outside the health service, such as 'Relate'. Although a variety of therapeutic techniques are used, most treatment is based on the fact that relationships usually deteriorate because couples start to communicate poorly and problems build up as a result. Addressing their differences with the help of a third person helps couples improve their communication and regain a sense of togetherness. Making the time to do enjoyable things together reinforces this process.

### *Families with young children*

Caring for young children can be very demanding, especially for parents with a mental illness. Additional support from health visitors may be required, and parenting resource centres, which give support and guidance for parents, are a useful source of help where available. Support with child care costs can provide respite for parents. Parental mental disorder can be a cause or effect of emotional and conduct problems in children, and it will sometimes be necessary for adult and child psychiatry services to work jointly.

### *Working with carers*

The term 'carer' is used to describe those who provide care for relatives or friends who are unwell. Usually they are the patient's spouse, parent or child. They are often the primary caregiver, especially if they live with the patient. They face the distress of seeing someone close to them becoming mentally ill and the burden of looking after them. As a result, they may stop providing care and may become mentally ill themselves. Most carers want to provide care however and are able to do so effectively if given adequate levels of support, as summarised in Figure 1.

## Social treatments

### *Problem solving*

It is always best if patients can sort out their own financial and social problems as much as possible. Doing so will give them a sense of autonomy and achievement and improve their chances of dealing effectively with similar problems in the future. In some cases, encouragement and advice will be all that is needed. However, some patients may not approach their problems in a realistic way or may have become completely overwhelmed by them. In such cases, the technique of problem solving is often helpful. This involves helping the patient to make a list of all their problems and then prioritise them. Problems that can be sorted out quickly or will become worse if left too long should be dealt with first. Problems should be dealt with in turn, with the patient planning what they need to do to sort out each problem and whether they need to obtain help from other people. The role of the professional in this process is to help the person approach their problems in this structured way and give encouragement. An example of problem solving is shown in Figure 2.

### *Accommodation and finances*

The range of accommodation available to people with mental health problems is shown in Figure 3 and mental health services usually work closely with local providers of both independent and supported housing. Most patients live in independent accommodation and some may need help to maintain their tenancy, for example setting up direct debits for bills, providing support in keeping the property in reasonable condition and intervening at an early stage if changes in their mental state threaten their relationships with neighbours. Supported accommodation is usually necessary only for those with severe illness, especially those who require frequent or lengthy admission to hospital. Very occasionally, The Mental Health Act is used to compel people to live in a par-

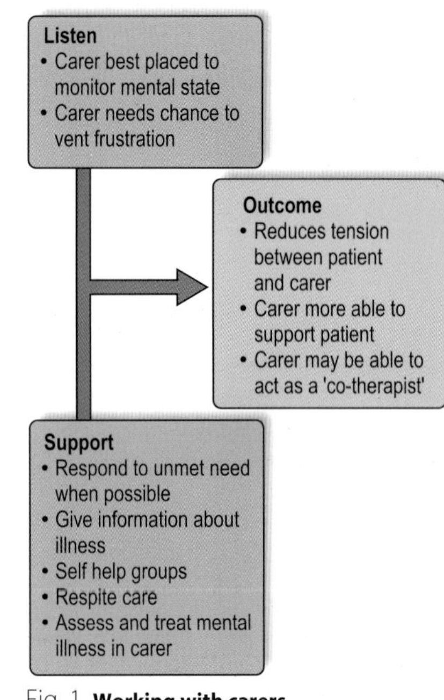


Fig. 1 **Working with carers.**

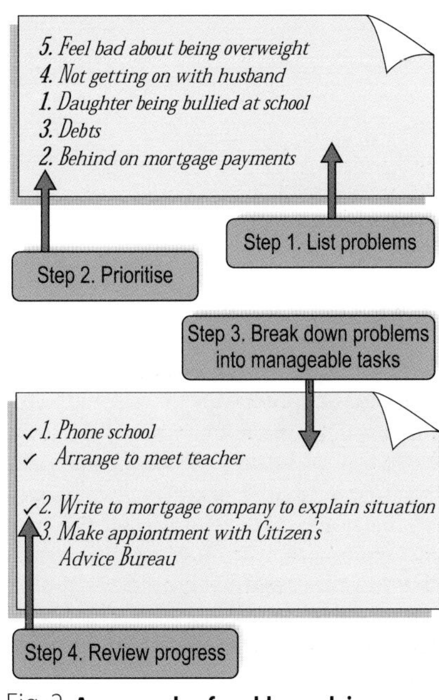


Fig. 2 **An example of problem solving.**

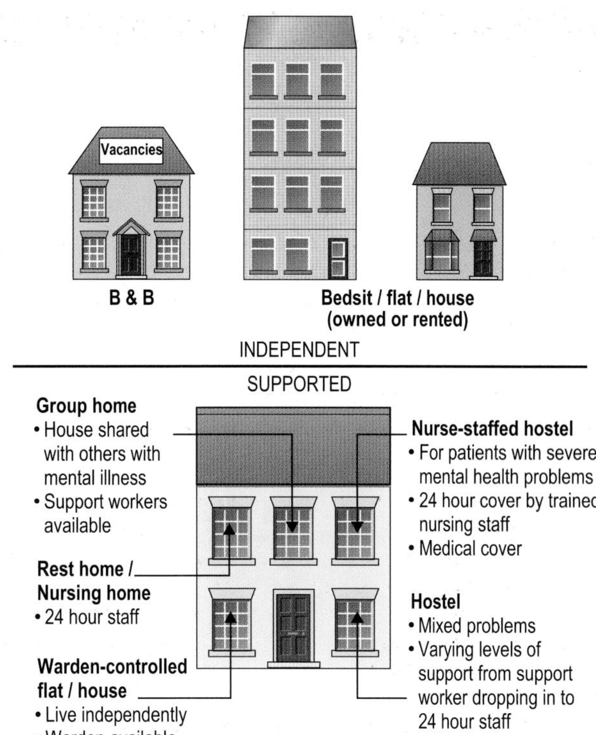


Fig. 3 **Examples of accommodation for patients with mental illness.**

ticular place, either through a Guardianship Order or as a condition of a Community Treatment Order.

Many psychiatric patients live in poverty and many more have financial problems of some sort. Financial worries can be a precipitating and maintaining factor in most mental illnesses. They are also associated with other causes of mental illness, such as conflict within the family and poor physical health. Mental illness can be the cause of financial problems, as it reduces people's ability to earn money and manage their financial affairs. Supporting people in maintaining employment or providing routes into education, training and work will boost their finances as well as self-esteem. For those not in work, help should be given to ensure that they receive all the statutory benefits to which they are entitled. Mental health staff can work with patients to improve their budgeting skills. Organisations such as the Citizen's Advice Bureau can give guidance on financial matters and debt.

## Occupational therapy

Occupational therapists improve the mental health of their patients by helping them identify, establish and maintain activities that provide their life with structure, enjoyment and meaning. They work on inpatient units, day hospitals and in community teams, carrying out group and individual sessions. They use structured assessment processes to help patients identify their priorities and goals. They carry out functional assessments to identify aspects of daily living with which the patient needs help and they address problems such as lack of confidence and motivation and impairment of daily living skills. They sometimes provide activities but their aim is usually to help patients re-establish themselves in their local community, through work, leisure and social activities. They will often establish close links with providers of education and training, and organisations that help people find and maintain employment.

## Rehabilitation

Psychiatric rehabilitation services began to develop in the 1960s, around the time the large psychiatric asylums started to be closed down. Until then, patients with chronic mental illnesses often spent most of their life in hospital. They became isolated from the outside world, learning to adhere to hospital rules and routines and relying on staff to do things for them. This process, known as institutionalisation, meant that even if patients were well enough to be discharged from hospital, it was difficult for them to adjust to life in the community. The secondary handicap caused by institutionalisation added to the primary handicap caused by mental illness. Psychiatric rehabilitation services were introduced to help overcome these problems.

Even though patients now spend much shorter periods of time in hospital, institutionalisation still occurs and the primary handicap caused by mental illness is as great as it was 40 years ago. Therefore, rehabilitation is often needed before discharge from hospital. The aim is to teach patients the skills they need to cope outside hospital and then gradually reintroduce them to life in the community. During this process, the strengths and weaknesses of each patient can be assessed, with a view to providing appropriate accommodation, support and treatment once they are discharged. The principles of rehabilitation are also applied to the care of patients outside hospital who are coping poorly in the community and those who are functioning well in supported accommodation and want to move on.

### Family and social treatments

- Social problems can precipitate and maintain mental illness, or may be created or made worse by the illness
- Caring for carers of individuals with mental illness is an important role of mental health services
- All patients should have an assessment of their housing, financial and occupational needs

# Recovery and social inclusion

## The recovery model

Mental illness can affect all aspects of the individual's life, and that of those close to them. The personal journey of these individuals in coping with the effects of mental illness is termed 'recovery'. Many patients feel that as a consequence of struggling with mental illness they learn more about themselves and others, and ultimately benefit from this experience. In this context recovery does not necessarily mean 'cure'; in fact for the majority of people with severe mental illness cure is unlikely. In the recovery model of mental health care patients (or 'service users') are not passive recipients of treatment. Instead there is recognition that many aspects of recovery occur without the input of professionals, and that where professional treatment is needed it is most effectively delivered in collaboration with the patient. Mental health professionals are most effective in promoting recovery if they have a positive and optimistic attitude towards treatment.

The key elements of recovery are shown in Figure 1. An important component of recovery is that patients feel they gain control over the symptoms of mental illness. However, gaining control over wider aspects of life, such as relationships, home life, employment and money is often even more important to a sense of wellbeing and quality of life. It is essential, therefore, that in treating mental illness these broader issues are taken into account, and given the same consideration as the medical treatments.

## Social inclusion

People with mental illness continue to experience negative attitudes and discrimination in many aspects of their lives. The consequence of this is that they become excluded from aspects of life that others take for granted. An essential component of the recovery model is supporting patients to improve their social inclusion. The barriers to social inclusion are diverse; some of the key ones are described below:

1. **Stigma and discrimination**. There is ample evidence of stigma and discrimination against people with mental illness. The consequences of this are that people with mental illness are more likely to have a low income, insecure housing, be unemployed and denied access to education, and have limited social networks. Negative attitudes and fear of mental illness are reinforced by media portrayals of people with schizophrenia being violent or having a split personality. Sadly, discrimination also occurs within health services. Diagnoses of mental illness are commonly cited on sick certificates, but in many cases no active treatment is delivered. The physical healthcare of people with serious mental illness is often inadequate. People with schizophrenia have a life expectancy that is 10 years shorter than average, mainly as a consequence of physical health problems. Patients report that their physical health concerns are not taken seriously by doctors, or are assumed to be manifestations of their mental illness, and this leads to reluctance to disclose symptoms. One way of addressing these issues is to involve patients (in this context the term 'service user' is usually used) in the running and development of services. Examples of service user involvements are shown in Figure 2.

2. **Unemployment**. Lack of meaningful activity is generally detrimental to mental health. Unfortunately only a quarter of people with long-term mental health problems are in employment. While it is true that some are too unwell to work, for many others work would be an option if the opportunities were there. The barriers to employment include negative attitudes amongst employers, the benefits system creating disincentives to work, low expectations of professionals and carers, and the individual's lack of confidence. There is evidence that

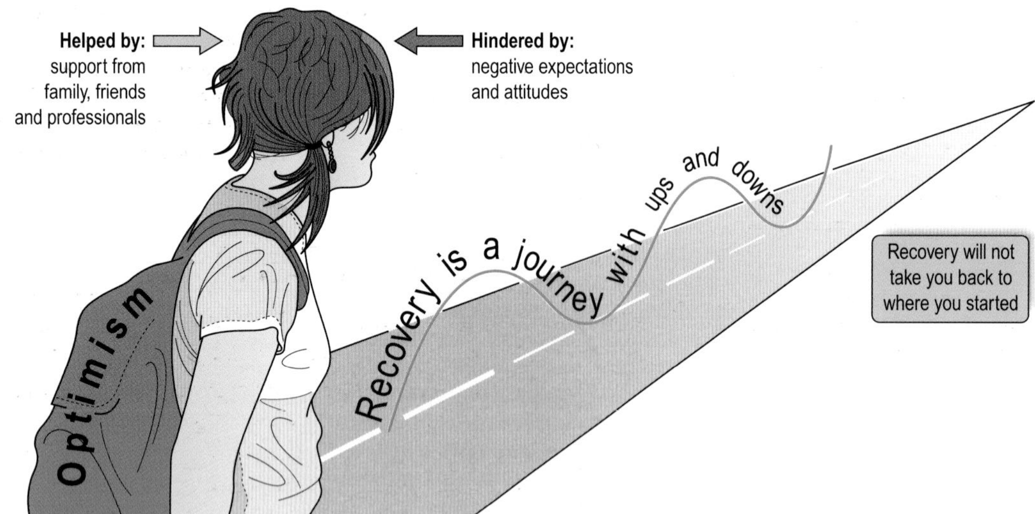


Fig. 1 **The recovery model.**



Fig. 2 **Service user involvement in mental health services.**

employers are less likely to employ someone with a history of mental health problems than someone with a physical disability. Many mental health services have tackled some of these issues by employing vocational advisors who work both with individuals to identify and support appropriate employment, and with employers to tackle negative attitudes.

3. **Lack of secure housing**. The majority of people with severe mental illness live in independent housing, with fewer than 20% living in accommodation that includes some form of residential support. Of those living independently about half live alone. They are more likely than the general population to live in rented accommodation and to feel their housing is not secure. About one in five of all homeless people has a mental illness often complicated by substance misuse, and of those who sleep rough about half are mentally ill. Mental health services work with housing departments and housing associations to support patients to stay in their accommodation, and some have specialist homeless teams that provide flexible outreach services.

4. **Low educational achievement**. About a third of people with mental health problems have no academic qualifications. The barriers to accessing education or training are similar to those for employment. Low expectations, lack of confidence and false assumptions about the potential benefits of education all play a part. With encouragement and support from within educational institutions, and provided externally by mental health and other agencies, many people with mental illness are able to participate in mainstream education.

5. **Ethnic minorities**. The prevalence of most severe mental illnesses is similar across different ethnic groups. However there is evidence that people from black and minority ethnic groups access help from services late, and are more likely to be detained under the Mental Health Act than white people. In general terms people from ethnic minority groups are more likely to experience social deprivation, social isolation and racism, which may act as precipitating and maintaining factors in mental illness. Refugees may have particularly complex or severe mental health issues. They may have come from war zones, and been subject to torture or other traumatic experiences. Language barriers can make assessment and treatment difficult, and access to interpreters is essential. Family members and friends are rarely able to interpret for someone with mental illness in a reliable way. Ideally interpreters should have some training in mental illness so that they are able to communicate abnormalities in the mental state. An holistic, person-centred approach that is sensitive to the cultural and spiritual needs of all patients is needed to overcome some of these difficulties.

This is my Advance Statement in case I have a manic episode and cannot make decisions about my care:

- I prefer to be treated at home if at all possible.
- Previously treatment with quetiapine and diazepam has worked well.
- Treatment with valproate has not worked well in the past, and I prefer to avoid it.

If I do need to be admitted to hospital:

- I would like my friend, David Smith, and my neighbour June Taylor to be informed immediately.
- David Smith will contact my work. I do not want any health professionals to contact my work.
- I have a dog, and prefer that he go to my neighbour, June Taylor, during my time in hospital.
- I do not want my parents to be informed of any admissions.
- I am a vegetarian, and it is important to me to maintain a strict vegetarian diet throughout any stay in hospital, even if I say this is not important when I am ill.
- My neighbour, June Taylor, has a key to my house, and will make sure my home is secure.

Signed: Mark Evans

Fig. 3 **An advance statement.**

## Advance decisions and statements

One of the key principles of the recovery model of mental health care is that patients regain control over their lives. However, for people with severe mental illness there may be an ongoing risk of relapsing into acute mental illness, and as a consequence losing the capacity to make appropriate decisions. They risk losing control at these times, as services may step in and impose treatment under the Mental Health Act or Mental Capacity Act (see pp. 16–19). Advance decisions and statements (sometimes called 'living wills') have been developed as tools to allow patients to state what type of treatment they wish to receive in these circumstances. Advance decisions are defined in the Mental Capacity Act, and allow the patient to make a decision in advance to refuse a specified type of medical treatment. Advance statements do not carry the same statutory power, but can contain positive decisions about treatments or broader aspects of care they wish to receive. Ideally they should be developed with support from the care co-ordinator or other mental health professional, and a copy should be kept in the clinical notes, so that it can be taken into account when decisions about treatment are being made. The issues that may be included in an advance statement are shown in Figure 3.

### Recovery and social inclusion

- 'Recovery' is the term used to describe the personal journey of individuals in coping with the effects of mental illness
- A positive and optimistic attitude on the part of mental health professionals is essential to promoting recovery
- Stigma and discrimination against people with mental illness results in social exclusion, and prevents recovery

# Diagnosis and classification of schizophrenia

Schizophrenia is the illness most readily associated with psychiatry. It has a variable course and in some cases may involve only a few short episodes of illness. However, in about one-third of cases the illness is severe, chronic and disabling. Because of this, care for people with schizophrenia accounts for a large proportion of the workload of mental health services.

Schizophrenia is characterised by two types of symptoms: positive (type 1) and negative (type 2). Positive symptoms are those which are added on to pre-existing functions, whereas negative symptoms are those which involve a loss of function. There are four main groups of positive symptoms:

- delusions (false beliefs)
- hallucinations (false perceptions)
- thought disorder (disorganised thinking)
- catatonic symptoms (abnormalities of movement and muscle tone).

The main negative symptoms are apathy, avolition, alogia and affective blunting or incongruity (best remembered as the four As). Apathy is lack of interest in personal and other events. Avolition describes an inability to initiate tasks or see them through, which causes the patient to avoid activities and spend long periods of time doing nothing. Alogia is another term for poverty of speech in which the patient says little spontaneously and gives brief replies to questions. Blunting of affect is a reduction in emotional expression which is manifested by a reduction in facial expression, eye contact and body language. Incongruity of affect is the exhibition of emotions which are clearly inappropriate to the situation, often leading the person to appear silly or strange.

## Diagnosis

### *Duration*

In ICD10, symptoms must have been present for at least one month before a diagnosis of schizophrenia can be made. If symptoms have been present for less than this time, a diagnosis of acute schizophrenia-like psychotic disorder should be made with the diagnosis being revised to schizophrenia if symptoms persist beyond one month.

There is often evidence of changes in behaviour and mood for months or even years before the onset of clear cut symptoms but this should not be taken into account when deciding whether the illness has lasted long enough to make the diagnosis of schizophrenia. This is because symptoms occurring during the prodromal period are non-specific and so basing a diagnosis on these will often lead to mistakes.

## Symptoms

Symptoms required to make the diagnosis of schizophrenia are shown in Figure 1. It will be seen from this that some symptoms are virtually pathognomonic of schizophrenia. Most of these were described by Schneider and are known as *Schneider's first rank symptoms*. If any of these symptoms are clearly present for at least one month and there is no organic cause, then the likely diagnosis is schizophrenia, although 15% will turn out to have an illness other than schizophrenia, most commonly a mood disorder. Two symptoms also considered to be diagnostic of schizophrenia were not described by Schneider: hallucinatory voices which appear to emanate from a body part and bizarre delusions.

Schizophrenia can also be diagnosed if at least two of the other symptoms shown in Figure 1 are present. There are also symptoms which are very common in schizophrenia but are not diagnostic because they occur relatively often in other conditions. The most common of these are persecutory delusions and delusions of reference, and examples of these are given in Table 1, along with examples of some of the symptoms described above.

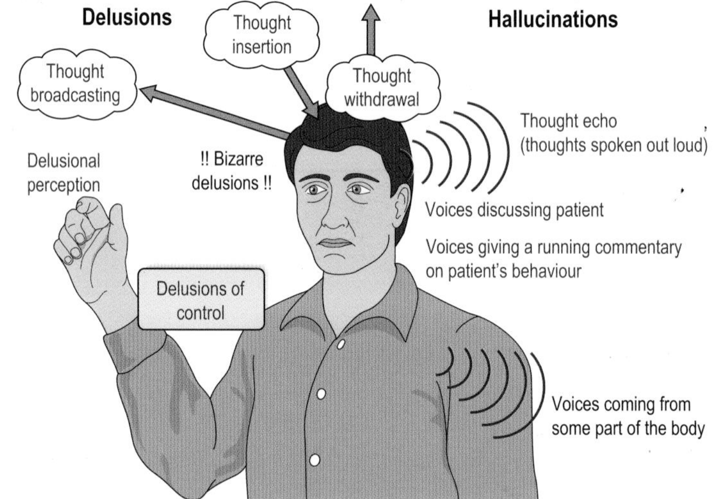


Fig. 1 **Symptoms of schizophrenia.** Schneider's first rank symptoms are in red; other symptoms are in black.

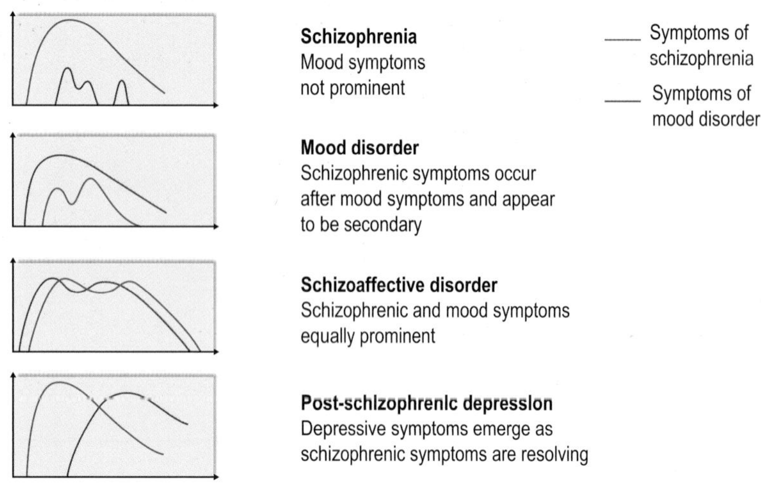


Fig. 2 **Differential diagnosis between schizophrenia and mood disorders.**

Table 1 **Examples of some common symptoms of schizophrenia**

| Symptom | Example |
|---|---|
| Third person auditory hallucination | *'I hear a voice saying "He's an idiot, I hate him" and another saying "I don't, he's not that bad"'* |
| Running commentary | *'I hear a voice talking about what I'm doing, saying things like "Look at him, walking across the room. Now he's making a cup of tea".'* |
| Thought echo | *'I hear my thoughts spoken out loud; it's like a tape recorder playing them back to me out loud.'* |
| Thought insertion/withdrawal | *'They put thoughts into my head and take them out.'* |
| Thought broadcasting | *'The thoughts go out of my head. Other people can pick them up and tell what I'm thinking.'* |
| Delusions of control (passivity) | *'They control my thoughts and make me feel sad. They must have some sort of machine to do it.' 'They create a force field that pushes me against the wall.'* |
| Delusional perception (delusional interpretation of a true perception) | *'I knew the police were after me when I saw that the lamp-post outside wasn't working.' 'When the postman opened the gate with his right hand, I knew the world would end tomorrow.'* |
| Bizarre delusions (delusions that could not possibly be true) | *'I'm observed from an alien space-ship, they use a scanner in my radio and beam the signal up using microwaves.' 'My neighbour sends poisonous gas through the walls and down the telephone line.'* |
| Persecutory delusions | *'My neighbour is spying on me for the government' (also an example of a non-bizarre delusion, i.e. a false belief that could conceivably happen).* |
| Delusions of reference (false belief that things refer to the patient) | *'There are messages for me hidden in what they say on TV and the radio' 'When I see people talking, I know they are talking about me.'* |
| Thought disorder and neologisms | *Patient says: 'I walk down through back to square one something like the mooncar judging up to the nimjet".'* |

Table 2 **Sub-types of schizophrenia**

| Sub-type | Clinical presentation | Comment |
|---|---|---|
| Paranoid schizophrenia | Delusions<br>Hallucinations | Commonest subtype in most parts of the world |
| Hebephrenic | Thought disorder<br>Blunting or incongruity of affect<br>Behaviour appears childlike or meaningless | Usually presents in early adulthood<br>Negative symptoms appear early |
| Catatonic | Stupor or mutism<br>Excitement<br>Stereotypies<br>Abnormalities of muscle tone and posture | Rare in developed countries |
| Residual | Negative symptoms dominate clinical picture<br>Previous positive symptoms less prominent | Occurs later in course of illness<br>Other subtypes may evolve into residual schizophrenia |
| Simple | Negative symptoms with no history of positive symptoms | Difficult to differentiate from abnormal personality |
| Undifferentiated | Mixed features of above | |

### *Mood changes in schizophrenia*

Changes in mood are a common feature of schizophrenia, and symptoms of schizophrenia can occur during episodes of mania or severe depression. As a result, there is often a difficult differential diagnosis between schizophrenia and mood disorders. Knowing when symptoms occurred and their relative severity is essential in making the correct diagnosis, as shown in Figure 2. **Schizoaffective disorder**, which is discussed in more detail on page 47, is diagnosed when first rank or other pathognomonic symptoms of schizophrenia occur at the same time as severe mood disturbance. **Post-schizophrenic depression** occurs as the acute psychotic phase is beginning to resolve. The depressive symptoms may seem to be an integral part of the illness or they may appear to be an understandable psychological reaction to having developed schizophrenia, but the diagnosis is the same in either case. It is an important condition to recognise, as it is associated with an increased risk of suicide.

## Subtypes of schizophrenia

Schizophrenia is a broad diagnosis which covers a wide range of clinical presentations. Because of this, ICD10 includes several subtypes of the disorder which are summarised in Table 2. **Schizotypal disorder** is a subsyndromal condition that presents with an odd eccentric affect, suspiciousness and unusual speech, ideas and perceptual experiences. It is more common among relatives of people with schizophrenia and runs a fluctuating course, sometimes with brief psychotic episodes.

## Delusional disorders

Some patients present with a single delusion or set of related delusions (delusional system) without having any of the symptoms required to make a diagnosis of schizophrenia. In such cases, a diagnosis of delusional disorder should be made. The content of the delusions is often of a persecutory, grandiose or hypochondriacal nature or may concern litigation or jealousy.

There are some differences with schizophrenia. Onset is usually in middle age or later. The onset and content of the delusions is more often understandable in terms of the patient's life circumstances. Symptoms respond to antipsychotic medication, but less often than positive symptoms of schizophrenia. However, these features occur in some cases of schizophrenia and not in all cases of delusional disorder, so there is debate about whether delusional disorder should be viewed as a separate condition or as a form of paranoid schizophrenia.

### *Case history 9*

Peter is a 22-year-old man who complains that the police are controlling his thoughts and giving him orders wherever he goes. Since these experiences began, his mood has become increasingly depressed. His family report that his speech has become difficult to follow and that he rarely leaves the house.

a. What is the most likely diagnosis?

### Diagnosis and classification of schizophrenia

- Schizophrenia is characterised by positive and negative symptoms
- The common types of positive symptoms are delusions, hallucinations and thought disorder
- The diagnosis should not be made if there is an organic cause or if mood symptoms are a central feature of the illness

# Epidemiology and aetiology of schizophrenia

Much is known about the aetiology of schizophrenia but the exact nature of the condition is still unclear. One problem in researching this area is that schizophrenia is defined on the basis of symptoms for which there are no biological markers and there may be more than one underlying disease process. This possibility should be kept in mind when reading this section, in which the epidemiology of schizophrenia will be described, followed by a discussion of factors thought to be of aetiological importance.

## Epidemiology

A striking finding of epidemiological surveys of schizophrenia is the similarity of prevalence in different countries. Most studies have found the lifetime prevalence of schizophrenia to be 7–9 per 1000 members of the population and, at any one time, 2–5 per 1000 population will have schizophrenia. There is not a great difference between these lifetime and point prevalence figures, which reflects the fact that schizophrenia is often a chronic illness. Men and women are affected equally. However, the average age of onset in men is usually late teens and twenties, whereas for women it is usually about 10 years later.

Although the prevalence of schizophrenia is similar in different countries, some studies have found an altered risk in different parts of the world. Some of these variations are probably the result of studies using different diagnostic criteria. They may also reflect *selective migration* of people with schizophrenia. For instance, the high prevalence found in Northern Sweden may indicate that people with schizophrenia are more likely than others to tolerate life in an isolated community. Selective migration may also explain the high rates of schizophrenia found in some immigrant groups. An exception to this is the raised rate found in men of Afro-Caribbean origin in the UK, which is most apparent not in those who migrated but in their children. One explanation for this finding is that young black men are more likely to be misdiagnosed with schizophrenia because of cultural differences, and are more likely to be admitted to hospital, which may give a false impression of true prevalence rates.

People with schizophrenia are more likely to be of lower social class than other members of the population. This is largely accounted for by *social drift*, a term used to describe the way people with schizophrenia drift down the social scale because of the effects of the illness. This phenomenon was demonstrated in a famous study which found that although people with schizophrenia were, on average, of lower social class, the social class of their fathers was representative of the general population. However, the social drift hypothesis may not be the only explanation. Some studies have shown that people with schizophrenia are more likely to have been born into deprived inner city areas. One explanation of this finding is that such environments may increase exposure to some of the risk factors for schizophrenia described later in this section.

## Aetiology

The aetiology of schizophrenia is summarised in Figure 1.

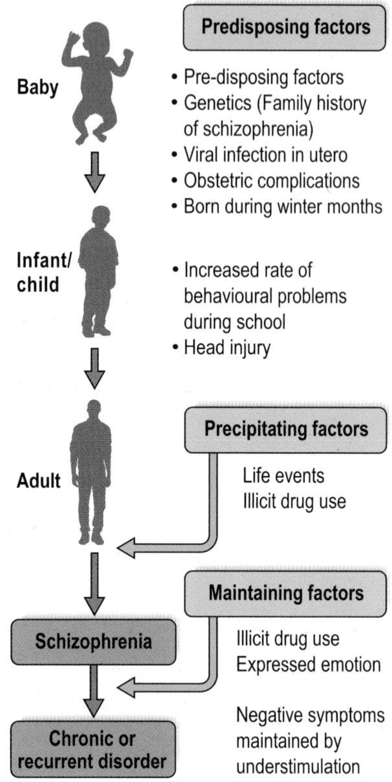

Fig. 1 **The aetiology of schizophrenia.**

### *Genetics*

The finding that schizophrenia has a similar prevalence in different countries suggests that there is a large genetic component to its aetiology. This is supported by family studies which show that 8% of siblings and 12% of children of people with schizophrenia will also develop the condition. Twin and adoption studies suggest that this familial pattern is the result of genetic factors rather than shared environment. Monozygotic twins show a concordance rate for schizophrenia of 50% whereas for dizygotic twins the rate is only 20%. Adoption studies show a raised risk in biological but not adoptive relatives.

A number of genetic variations have been found to be associated with schizophrenia. Most of these variations are common in the general population, and are responsible for only a small increase in risk. It is thought that when a number of these genetic variations occur together, and particularly in the presence of environmental risk factors, an individual's risk of developing schizophrenia rises significantly.

### *Environmental factors*

The incomplete concordance for schizophrenia between monozygotic twins suggests environmental factors are also important in its aetiology. There is much evidence that gestation may be the period of highest risk and this is summarised in Table 1. Raised rates of schizophrenia have been found among people born shortly after some viral epidemics and famines, and in cases of rhesus incompatibility. These findings have led to the *neurodevelopmental hypothesis of schizophrenia* which postulates that factors acting during gestation may increase the risk of schizophrenia through an effect on intra-uterine brain development.

There is an increased rate of obstetric complications in people who go on to develop schizophrenia, a finding for which there are at least two possible reasons. It may be that the risk of brain damage during difficult deliveries increases the risk of schizophrenia. However, another explanation for this finding is that the subtle abnormalities of prenatal brain development caused by the genetic or environmental factors discussed above may increase the risk of obstetric complications, rather than be caused by them.

There is little evidence that childhood environment is important in the aetiology of schizophrenia. Previous theories that schizophrenia was caused by particular styles of mothering or problems in the parents' relationship have since been discredited, although not before causing a great deal of distress to the families of people with schizophrenia. It is the case that people with schizophrenia are more likely to have had behavioural problems during childhood but this is thought to be another manifestation of the neurodevelopmental abnormalities described above, rather than the result of poor parenting.

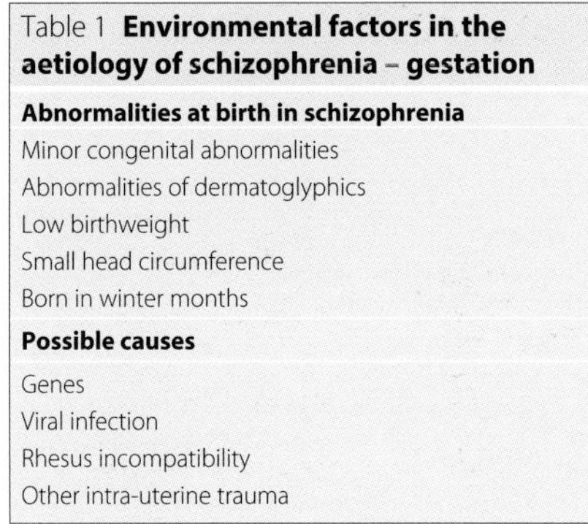

| Table 1 **Environmental factors in the aetiology of schizophrenia – gestation** |
|---|
| **Abnormalities at birth in schizophrenia** |
| Minor congenital abnormalities |
| Abnormalities of dermatoglyphics |
| Low birthweight |
| Small head circumference |
| Born in winter months |
| **Possible causes** |
| Genes |
| Viral infection |
| Rhesus incompatibility |
| Other intra-uterine trauma |

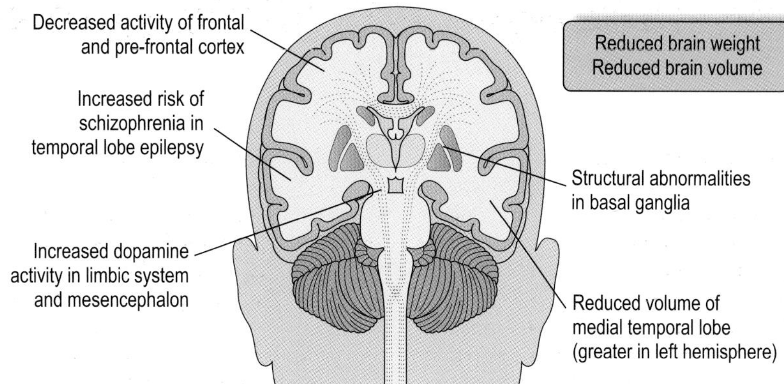


Fig. 2 **Brain abnormalities in schizophrenia.**

High expressed emotion
It really upsets me when you don't do your washing
Low expressed emotion
Come on. I'll give you a hand with your washing


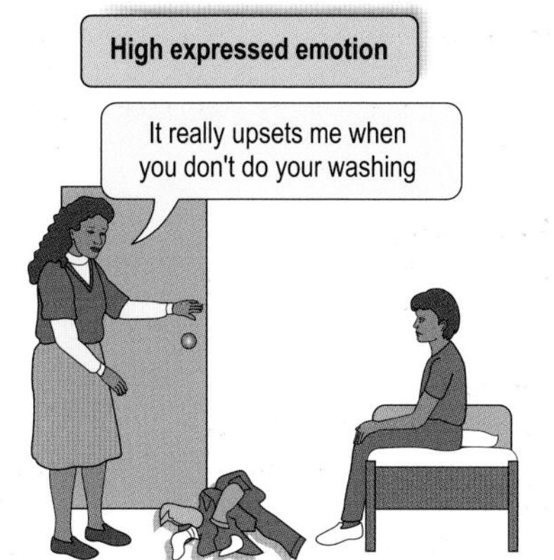

Fig. 3 **Different levels of expressed emotion.**

### *Neurological abnormalities*

There is a slightly raised risk of schizophrenia in people who have suffered head injuries and, in rare cases, clear-cut structural brain abnormalities are found in patients presenting with schizophrenia. In most cases though, such abnormalities are more subtle and only become apparent when groups of people with schizophrenia are compared with controls. Some of these abnormalities are summarised in Figure 2.

### *Neurochemical abnormalities*

Amphetamines, which cause increased dopamine release, can cause psychotic symptoms very similar to those seen in acute schizophrenia. Antipsychotic drugs, the most effective treatment for acute schizophrenia, are dopamine antagonists. These observations have given rise to the *dopamine hypothesis* of schizophrenia, which postulates that positive symptoms are caused by overactivity of dopamine in the mesolimbic area of the brain. Modern neuroimaging techniques such as positron emission tomography provide the opportunity to measure the activity of dopamine and its receptors in the brain and this approach has produced evidence to support the dopamine hypothesis. However, mesolimbic dopamine activity is regulated by other areas of the brain and, given that dopamine does not appear to have an important role in the development of negative symptoms, it is likely that abnormalities of dopamine in schizophrenia are secondary to other abnormalities, perhaps in the frontotemporal region (see Fig. 2).

### *Precipitating and maintaining factors*

Episodes of schizophrenia can be precipitated by illicit drug use. In most cases the drugs are triggering illness in vulnerable individuals. However there is evidence that heavy use of cannabis in adolescence can increase the risk of schizophrenia independently of other factors. Stress also can play a role in precipitating episodes. Once the illness has developed, it may be maintained by stress and illegal drug use. A particular type of stress known to maintain the illness is living in an emotionally charged environment in which people display high levels of what is known as *expressed emotion*. This is shown in Figure 3.

An interesting study of hospitals with very different treatment regimes showed that the amount of emotional and psychological stimulation to which patients with schizophrenia are exposed influences whether they have positive or negative symptoms. Patients in a hospital with an active rehabilitation programme in which they were encouraged to do as much as possible had more positive symptoms and fewer negative symptoms. In the hospital where patients received little encouragement and did very little as a result, there were more negative and fewer positive symptoms.

## *Case history 10*

The parents of Peter (see Case history 9) ask you what has caused his illness, as they are concerned that they are to blame.

a. What should you tell them?

## Epidemiology and aetiology of schizophrenia

- Schizophrenia is thought to be a neuropsychiatric disorder in which structural and neurochemical abnormalities of the brain cause psychiatric symptoms
- Genetic and early environmental factors are important in the aetiology of schizophrenia
- Social factors are important precipitating and maintaining factors

# Acute and chronic schizophrenia

## Acute schizophrenia

The first presentation of schizophrenia is usually with an acute episode, consisting of positive symptoms. In some cases, the patient has been well prior to the onset of these symptoms. In many, however, there will have been a prodromal phase lasting months or years, in which non-specific changes of behaviour such as social withdrawal and reduced level of function occur.

The acute episode often starts with delusional mood, in which the patient believes that something strange is going on but doesn't know what it is. The patient then begins to experience other positive symptoms. The most common are delusions, especially of reference and persecution, and auditory hallucinations, which may be in the 2nd or 3rd person. However, any combination of positive symptoms can occur.

Patients' behaviour can be affected by their positive symptoms in a number of different ways. If the patient is thought-disordered, their behaviour may become disorganised as a result. Unusual behaviour in acute schizophrenia may also be an understandable response to delusions and hallucinations. For instance, a patient may be suspicious or aggressive because of persecutory delusions, or may refuse medication they think is poisoned. They may smash a television because of frightening delusions of reference. They may refuse to remove a cycle helmet, feeling a need to protect themselves because of delusions of control. They may talk or laugh to themselves or appear preoccupied as a result of auditory hallucinations.

An example of a mental state examination of a patient with acute schizophrenia is shown in Figure 1. While most patients present with some of these abnormalities, it would be unusual for them to have quite so many. In fact, some patients may appear completely normal until they begin to discuss their delusions or hallucinations.

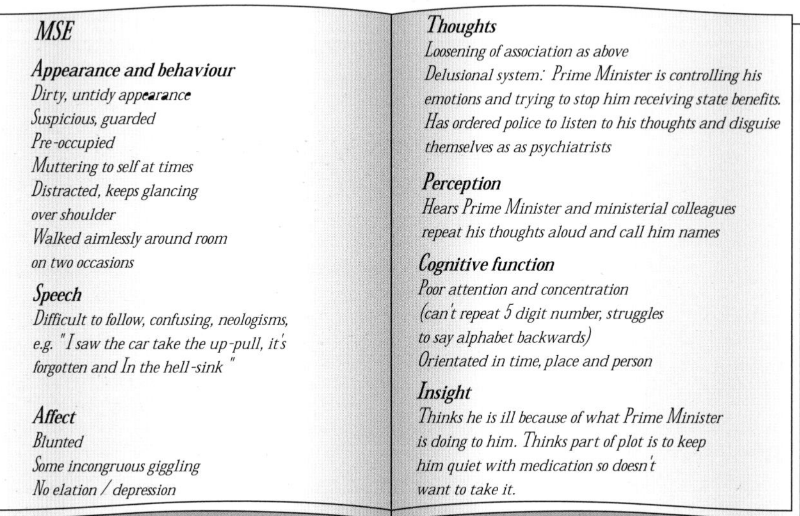


Fig. 1 **Mental state examination of patient with acute onset schizophrenia.**

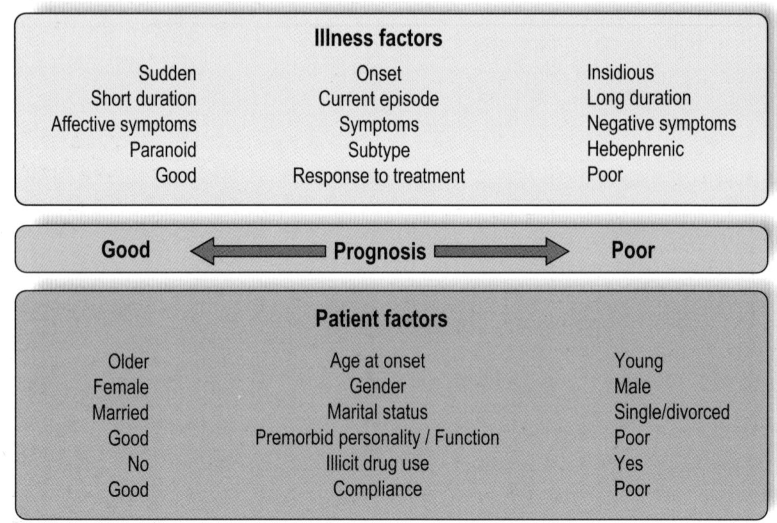


Fig. 2 **Prognostic factors in schizophrenia.**

## Chronic (residual) schizophrenia

Some patients make a good recovery from episodes of acute schizophrenia. Others are less fortunate, going on to develop a chronic unremitting illness in which function is markedly reduced. As discussed below, positive symptoms often continue in such patients but the clinical picture is usually dominated by the gradual emergence of negative symptoms and it is these which are usually the greatest cause of disability. Illnesses which run this chronic course are known as chronic or residual schizophrenia.

### *Negative symptoms*

Different combinations of the negative symptoms described in the previous pages occur in chronic schizophrenia. They develop insidiously and their severity varies. In some cases, they are mild but in others they dominate the patient's life. The patient will spend increasing amounts of time on their own, often doing very little. They avoid social contact and lose the ability to respond to verbal and non-verbal social cues. Their social skills deteriorate and they lose the ability to plan and carry out even simple tasks. They rarely make conversation spontaneously and their replies to questions are often limited to short, perfunctory sentences. They may show incongruity of affect, smirking or giggling inappropriately, or looking very sad and upset for no apparent reason. Their affect may be blunted, with little variation in emotion.

### *Positive symptoms*

Thought disorder is common in chronic schizophrenia and will often be the most obvious abnormality in the mental state examination. Hallucinations may persist and in some cases may continue to distract or distress the patient. More often, they will become less prominent, either because their intensity reduces or because the patient adapts to their pres-

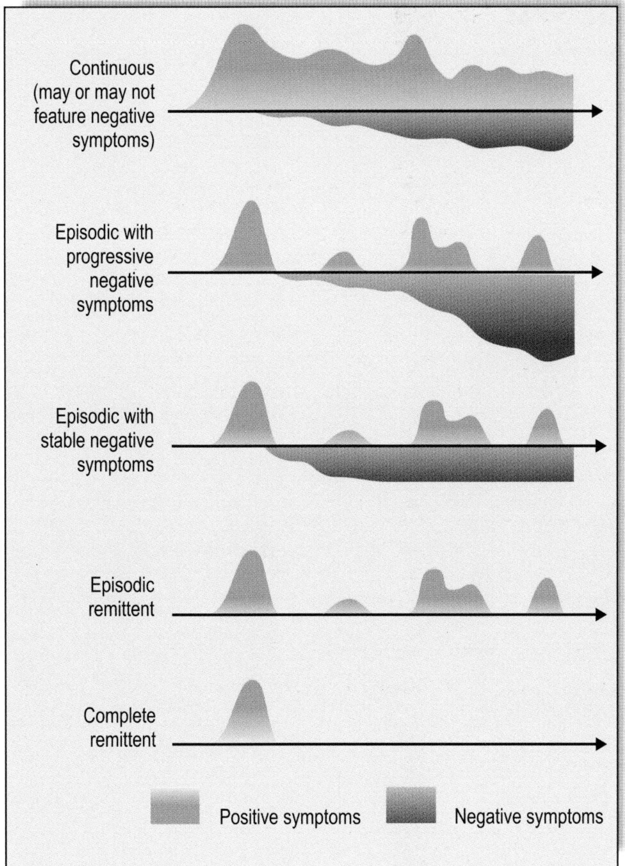


Fig. 3 **The varying course of positive and negative symptoms over time.**

ence. Delusions may also occur but tend not to be a prominent feature. In many patients, delusions and hallucinations will become prominent again during acute exacerbations of the illness. Such acute exacerbations occur most often early on in the course of illness, becoming less frequent with time.

There are two reasons why delusions and hallucinations become less prominent in chronic schizophrenia. The first is that they are the symptoms which respond best to antipsychotic medication. However, even before the development of antipsychotic drugs, chronic schizophrenia followed the course described here, which suggests that the change in the balance of symptoms is part of the natural course of the illness.

## Prognosis

Prognostic factors for schizophrenia are shown in Figure 2. An easy way of remembering most of these factors is that patients who present with acute episodes of positive symptoms but appear to have been functioning well previously have a good prognosis. Their positive symptoms are likely to respond well to treatment and they should return to their previous level of function. They will be at risk of acute episodes in the future, especially following life events or periods of stress and high expressed emotion. However, if they comply with treatment as recommended and avoid illicit drugs, their chances of remaining well are good. The longer they remain free of negative symptoms, the lower their chances of developing them.

Patients with a poor prognosis are likely to do badly because of negative symptoms, positive symptoms or a combination of the two. Patients who already show evidence of negative symptoms and poor function have a poor prognosis as negative symptoms are a cause of great disability and usually get worse with time. Positive symptoms also impair function and so compliance with treatment for these is an important prognostic factor. However, if positive symptoms have a gradual onset or have been present a long time, they will often not respond fully to treatment.

The varying course of positive and negative symptoms over time is shown in Figure 3. Assessment of prognosis aims to work out which of these is most likely to occur in a particular patient. This will give patients and their families an idea what to expect in the future so that they can plan accordingly. It also helps determine what social treatments and follow-up are likely to be required.

## Suicide risk

Up to 10% of patients with schizophrenia die by suicide. This is most likely to happen during the first few years of the illness, especially in the months following discharge from hospital. The suicide risk does not disappear later in the course of the illness but it does diminish with time. Possible reasons for this are the patient having time to come to terms with their illness and the relative increase of negative symptoms, compared with positive symptoms.

### *Case history 11*

Mr Dylan, a 20-year-old man who was previously well, presents acutely with persecutory delusions, delusions of thought insertion and third person auditory hallucinations.

a. Are these symptoms common in schizophrenia?
b. How is this illness likely to develop over the next 10 years?
c. What factors determine his prognosis?

### Acute and chronic schizophrenia

- Patients with schizophrenia have acute episodes consisting of positive symptoms from which they usually make a good recovery
- Some patients regain premorbid levels of function between episodes but others develop chronic schizophrenia in which their function is impaired by negative symptoms

# Management of schizophrenia

## Clinical assessment

The differential diagnoses shown in Figure 1 should be excluded by history and mental state examination, and by interviewing informants. If there is any suggestion of a drug-induced psychosis a urinary drug screen should be carried out. Apart from this, only those investigations suggested by the history and examination are likely to reveal abnormalities relevant to the diagnosis. There are two exceptions to this. In cases with an unusual presentation, such as onset in middle age, organic causes should be actively investigated. In cases which do not respond to treatment, the diagnosis should be reviewed and a wider range of investigations carried out.

It is important to assess whether inpatient treatment is required. This will depend on a number of factors including the severity of symptoms and their effect on carers, the level of support the patient has in the community, the patient's insight, the likelihood of them sticking to the advised treatment, and an assessment of risk to themselves or others. The majority of acute episodes can now be managed in the community with input from specialist teams such as CRHT, EIP and AOT (see p. 5). Chronic schizophrenia is usually managed in the community, sometimes after a period of rehabilitation as an inpatient. A small number of patients require long-term care in hospital or in 24-hour nurse-staffed community hostels.

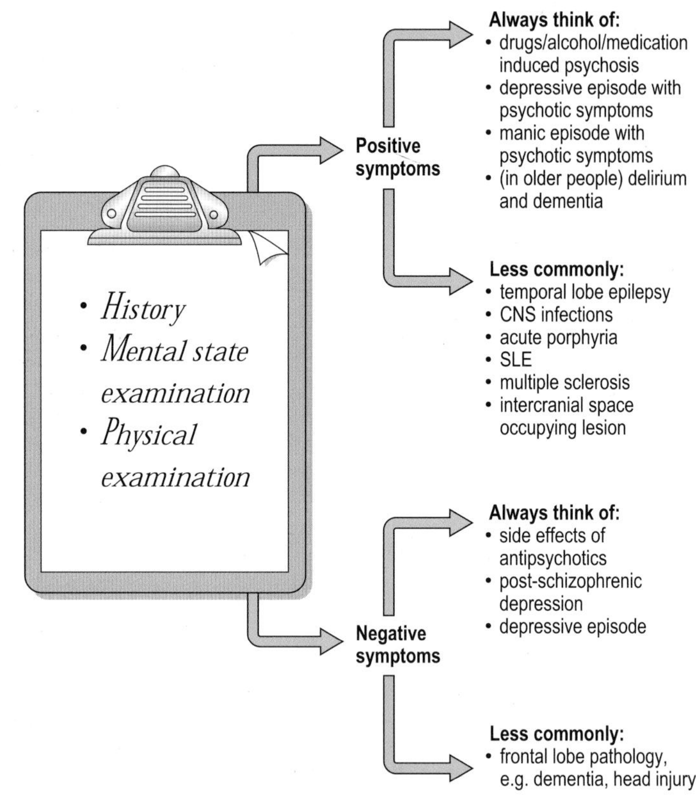


Fig. 1 **Differential diagnosis of positive and negative symptoms of schizophrenia.**

## Drug treatment

### Acute treatment

The standard treatment of schizophrenia is with antipsychotic drugs (see p. 24). In drug trials of antipsychotics in acute schizophrenia, up to three-quarters of patients receiving active treatment improve, with this improvement usually beginning after 2–3 weeks. Of patients receiving placebo medication, a small proportion will improve but most will either stay the same or get worse. Antipsychotic drugs are particularly effective in reducing positive symptoms.

Most of the commonly used antipsychotics are equally effective. The important exception is clozapine, which often reduces positive symptoms that have proved resistant to treatment with other antipsychotics. Negative symptoms are usually unaffected by antipsychotic drugs. If they appear to get worse, it is probably because the sedative and Parkinsonian effects of the antipsychotic are being mistaken for negative symptoms. If they appear to improve, it is probably because the patient is less distracted by positive symptoms. There is some evidence that the atypical antipsychotics have a direct effect on negative symptoms but this remains controversial.

Antipsychotics are usually given orally for the treatment of acute schizophrenia. Until recently, atypical antipsychotics were the usual treatment of choice, because of their lower propensity to cause movement side effects. However, the metabolic effects of these drugs, particularly weight gain and diabetes mellitus, have prompted a re-evaluation. The atypicals are still the most commonly prescribed drugs but conventional antipsychotics are coming back into favour. As the different drugs are equally likely to be effective, apart from clozapine, decisions about which drug to use should be based on their likely side effects. For instance, more sedative drugs may be preferred for a patient who is sleeping poorly or is very distressed or anxious, but not for one whose job involves driving motor vehicles.

### Rapid tranquillisation

During acute episodes of illness a few patients become so distressed that they pose a serious and immediate threat to themselves or others. There are many possible reasons for this. The risky behaviour may be a direct response to psychotic symptoms, such as a persecutory delusional belief that they are about to be attacked and need to defend themselves. Admission under section can be very distressing, particularly for a patient who has no insight into their illness, and some may respond violently to what they view as an unjustified restriction of their liberty. Intoxication with alcohol and drugs during an acute psychotic episode also makes risky behaviour more likely. Whatever the cause, the initial response should be to reduce the amount of stimulation around the patient, give them some space and a calm environment, listen to what they have to say and provide clear explanations and reassurance. An oral dose of antipsychotic or benzodiazepine should be offered. However, if the situation cannot be managed with these measures it is sometimes necessary to proceed to using rapid tranquillisation. This is medication, usually an antipsychotic or benzodiazepine and often a combination of the two, given intramuscularly. Most units have a local protocol of preferred drugs and doses and the advantages and disadvantages of the three most commonly used drugs in the UK are summarised in Table 1. In order to administer the injection the patient may need to be restrained. This is a potentially dangerous procedure for the patient, and

Table 1 **Drugs given intramuscularly for rapid tranquillisation**

| |
|---|
| **Lorazepam** (benzodiazepine) |
| Less accumulation than diazepam |
| Cardiorespiratory depression |
| Little effect on cardiac conduction |
| Can cause disinhibition |
| Other than sedation, effects usually acceptable |
| Can accentuate effects of alcohol |
| **Haloperidol** (conventional antipsychotic) |
| Little cardiorespiratory depression |
| Movement side effects |
| Less hypotensive effects than other antipsychotics |
| Small risk of arrhythmias |
| **Olanzapine** (atypical antipsychotic) |
| Few movement side effects |
| Cannot be given within 1 hour of benzodiazepine |
| ? smaller risk of arrhythmias than haloperidol |
| More sedating than haloperidol |

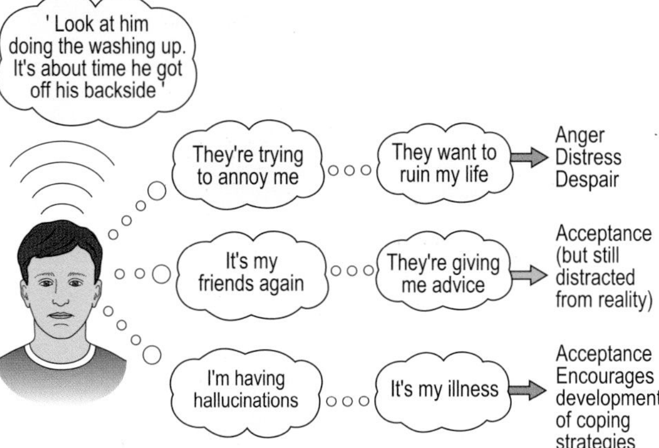


Fig. 2 **Examples of how cognitive response to auditory hallucinations influences their consequences.**

should only be done by appropriately trained staff. The aim is to reduce distress and arousal, not to send the patient to sleep. Following rapid tranquillisation, there is a risk of hypotension, arrhythmias and cardiorespiratory depression, so pulse, blood pressure and respiratory rate should be monitored regularly.

### *Continuation treatment and prophylaxis*

Once the acute episode has responded to treatment, it is important to continue with antipsychotic medication at normal therapeutic doses to prevent relapse. Even patients with a good prognosis should be advised to continue maintenance treatment for 1 to 2 years, before cautiously reducing and stopping it. In patients with a poorer prognosis, and those who relapse following cessation of treatment, long-term prophylaxis is required. In some cases it will be necessary for the patient to continue taking antipsychotic drugs for the rest of their lives.

Antipsychotic drugs given by long-acting (depot) injections are often used for maintenance and prophylactic treatment. The pros and cons of depot antipsychotics are summarised in Figure 3 on page 23. Depots can be useful in the treatment of acute episodes if compliance is poor, especially if the dose required is known from previous episodes.

## Psychological treatment

All patients with schizophrenia should be offered cognitive behavioural therapy. Figure 2 shows how a patient's response to auditory hallucinations can influence the consequences of these symptoms. As some patients continue to hear voices despite taking medication, helping them alter their cognitive response is a valuable treatment option. Cognitive therapists also use cognitive techniques to challenge delusions or alter the way in which patients respond to them. Positive symptoms can also be reduced by identifying activities and situations which exacerbate or relieve symptoms, and modifying these accordingly. There is evidence that this form of therapy can reduce distress and improve functioning.

## Family treatments

Carers of patients with schizophrenia tend to be family members, most commonly parents. Because schizophrenia is difficult to understand and can cause behaviour that is distressing, threatening or socially embarrassing, the burden on carers can be immense. Education and support is clearly important and carer groups, at which experiences and coping strategies can be shared, are particularly useful.

As discussed in the previous section, symptoms of schizophrenia can be exacerbated by households in which there are high levels of expressed emotion. This is usually reduced by helping carers understand and cope with the effects of the illness, using the measures outlined above. In addition, family therapy can be used to teach family members (or other members of the household) to recognise and reduce expressed emotion.

## Social treatments

Patients with schizophrenia often neglect themselves because of negative symptoms, or because they are distracted by positive symptoms. They may spend many years having their basic needs attended to by others, either in hospital or at home, and so may have forgotten or never have learned how to look after themselves. If they live in an understimulating environment, then any negative symptoms will worsen, but if the environment is overstimulating, then positive symptoms will become more of a problem. For all these reasons, it is essential that the full range of social treatments described on pages 34–37 is available to patients with schizophrenia.

### *Case history 12*

Dylan, the 20-year-old man described in the previous section, is admitted to hospital and treated with olanzapine. His positive symptoms respond partially to this treatment but he complains of weight gain and sedation. His family is supportive, but he does not want to live with them when he leaves hospital.

a. Devise a management plan for Dylan.

### Management of schizophrenia

- Antipsychotic drugs are an essential part of treatment and often need to be given long-term
- Cognitive therapy has an important role in reducing distress and improving functioning
- Family and social treatments are particularly important in schizophrenia, especially for patients with negative symptoms

# Classification of mood disorders

## *Case history 13*

Sarah is a 35-year-old woman who has been diagnosed with recurrent depressive disorder. She thinks this diagnosis is misleading, as each of her depressive episodes has occurred following adverse life events and she thinks it would be more accurate to view her problems as stress-related. In the course of your discussion, she describes episodes of elated mood and increased confidence, which she hasn't mentioned before, because she enjoys them.

a. What advice would you give her regarding diagnosis.

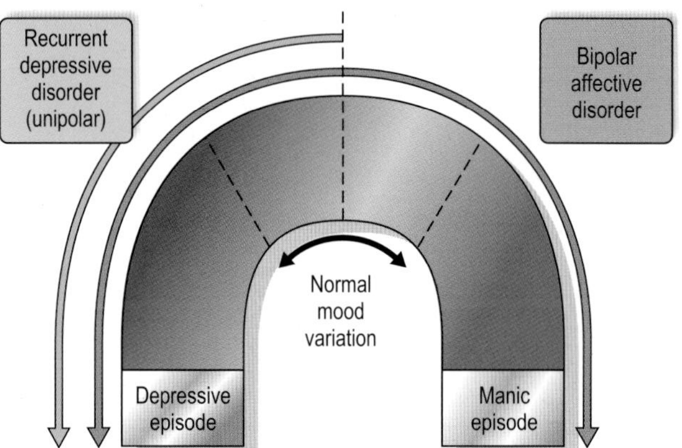


Fig. 1 **Classification of mood disorders.**

Many physical and mental disorders are accompanied by changes in mood. The term 'mood disorder', also known as affective disorder, is reserved for conditions in which an enduring change in mood is the predominant symptom. The mood state may be depression, occurring in depressive episodes, or elation, occurring in manic episodes. What follows is a general overview of the classification of mood disorders and more detail about the clinical presentation of depressive and manic episodes will be given in the following chapters.

## Bipolar affective disorder

In the most commonly used classification system of mood disorders, depression and mania are viewed as representing polar extremes, as illustrated in Figure 1. 'Bipolar' disorders are those in which both extremes of depression and elation occur, usually in separate depressive and manic episodes, but sometimes together in what are known as mixed affective episodes. Bipolar affective disorder, previously known as manic depression, is diagnosed when a person has had two or more episodes of mood disorder in total and at least one of these has been a manic or mixed affective episode. Any of the acute affective episodes shown in Table 1 can occur during the course of the condition and, at different times in their lives, some people with bipolar disorder will experience most, if not all, of these different mood states.

In some cases of bipolar disorder, only manic episodes occur. It might be expected that this presentation would be classified as 'unipolar' mania, but in fact a diagnosis of bipolar disorder is made even when there have been episodes of mania with no episodes of depression. The reason for this is the finding in cohort studies that most people with a history of manic episodes will eventually have a depressive episode. Also, people with bipolar disorder, including those who have had only manic episodes, have an increased rate of relatives with both bipolar and unipolar mood disorders. People with a history of depressive but not manic episodes tend to have a family history of unipolar depression only.

Manic episodes are divided into two types, hypomania and mania. Hypomania is milder and is only diagnosed if the person affected is able to maintain a reasonable level of social and occupational function. Mania involves a complete disruption of the person's usual activities and when diagnosed should be classified as occurring either with or without psychotic symptoms. People with bipolar disorder who have had at least one episode of mania are said to have bipolar I disorder. Those with a history of depressive and hypomanic episodes are classified as bipolar II. A final term used in the classification of bipolar disorder is 'rapid cycling', which denotes a phase of illness in which there is frequent switching of mood states, defined as four or more episodes of mania and depression occurring within a period of one year.

Table 1 **ICD10 classification of mood disorders**

| | |
|---|---|
| **Single episode** | |
| Manic episode | Hypomania |
| | Mania, without psychotic symptoms |
| | Mania, with psychotic symptoms |
| Depressive episode | Mild |
| | Moderate |
| | Severe, without psychotic symptoms |
| | Severe, with psychotic symptoms |
| Mixed affective episode | |
| **Recurrent episodes** | |
| Bipolar affective disorder | Current episode mania |
| | Current episode depressive |
| | Current episode mixed |
| Recurrent depressive disorder (Major Depressive Disorder in DSM4) | Current episode mild, moderate or severe |

## Unipolar disorders

As discussed above, people with a history of manic episodes are considered to have bipolar disorder and so the only unipolar mood disorders are those in which depression occurs. Recurrent depressive disorder is diagnosed when a person has had two or more depressive episodes. If a manic episode occurs subsequently, then the diagnosis should be changed to bipolar disorder.

Depressive episodes are classified on the basis of severity, as outlined in Table 1. Mild depressive episodes are distressing and cause some difficulty in continuing with ordinary work and social activities, but the person affected will probably not cease to function completely. Moderate depressive episodes cause considerable difficulty in continuing with social, work and domestic activities. During a severe depressive episode, the sufferer will be able to function to a very limited extent, if at all. Severe depressive episodes should be classified as occurring either with or without psychotic symptoms.

In the past, a distinction was made between 'endogenous' and 'reactive' depressive episodes. Endogenous depression was thought to be a more severe condition that tended to occur without precipitating factors, presented with somatic (or biological) symptoms such as weight loss, early morning waking and diurnal variation of mood, and responded well to physical treatments such as drugs or ECT. In contrast, reactive depression was seen as being a milder condition that occurred in response to a specific stress and responded better to psychosocial treatments. This categorisation of depression is not valid and the somatic syndrome can occur in depressive episodes of all severities, regardless of whether there were precipitating factors. You should always find out whether a depressive episode appears to have been a 'reactive' response to adverse life events and other social factors, because this can have a considerable bearing on treatment and prognosis, but diagnosis should be made solely on the basis of symptoms and their severity.

## Other persistent mood disorders

Cyclothymia is a condition in which there is a persistent instability of mood, involving numerous periods of mild depression and mild elation that fall short of meeting diagnostic criteria for depressive and manic episodes. It usually develops in early adult life and tends to run a chronic course. Cyclothymia is more common among relatives of people with bipolar affective disorder and some affected individuals will go on to develop bipolar disorder.

Some people experience chronic depressive symptoms of a severity that falls short of diagnostic criteria for depressive episodes. This condition is known as dysthymia and onset is typically during adolescence or early adulthood. When the onset is later in life, the disorder often occurs in the aftermath of a depressive episode, usually associated with bereavement or other obvious stress. Depressive episodes sometimes occur in the course of dysthymia and the combination of dysthymia and recurrent depressive disorder is sometimes referred to as 'double depression'.

## Seasonal affective disorder

Some people experience recurrent mood disorder at particular times of year and in the DSM4 classification the course specifier of 'seasonal type' can be added to a diagnosis of mood disorder. The only well established form of seasonal affective disorder is winter depression, which is described in Figure 2.

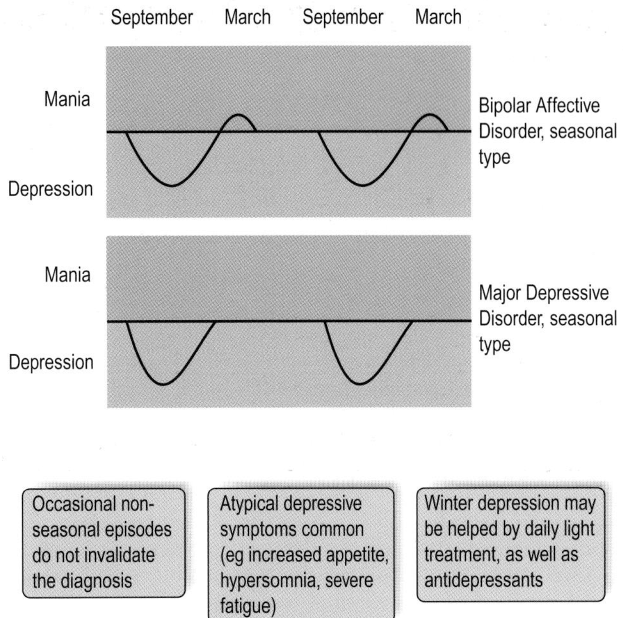


Fig. 2 **Seasonal affective disorder (DSM4 classification).**

## Schizoaffective disorder

When people present with a disturbance of mood that meets diagnostic criteria for a manic, mixed or depressive episode, and at the same time have one or more of the pathognomonic symptoms of schizophrenia (see Fig. 1 on p. 38), a diagnosis of schizoaffective disorder is made. The nature of the mood disturbance experienced by the patient determines the type of schizoaffective disorder diagnosed. For example, a woman might present with elated mood, increased energy, reduced sleep and the belief that ideas were being inserted into her mind that would enable her to earn a fortune and relieve famine throughout the world. This combination of symptoms meeting diagnostic criteria for a manic episode with psychotic symptoms and delusions of thought insertion should prompt a diagnosis of 'schizoaffective disorder, manic type'. A man who presents with loss of interest, severe fatigue, impaired sleep and appetite and auditory hallucinations consisting of several voices discussing his faults in the third person should be given a diagnosis of 'schizoaffective disorder, depressive type'. A woman who had the bizarre delusion that she had become pregnant by the long deceased King George III of England, as a result of reading an article in The Daily Mail newspaper, and who presented with agitation, tearfulness, marked emotional lability and a superior attitude towards others would be diagnosed as having 'schizoaffective disorder, mixed type'. Schizoaffective disorder is usually classified alongside schizophrenia, but represents part of a continuum between non-affective and affective psychoses, hence our mention of it here.

### Classification of mood disorders

- People with bipolar affective disorder have manic episodes and usually episodes of depression
- Recurrent depressive disorder is also known as unipolar mood disorder

# Epidemiology and aetiology of mood disorders

> **Case history 14**
>
> Kwame has bipolar affective disorder. He asks you whether his adult children are likely to develop the condition and if there is anything they can do to reduce the chances of this happening.
>
> a. What advice can you give him?

## Bipolar affective disorder

### *Aetiology*

Genetic factors play an important role in the aetiology of bipolar disorder. There are increased rates of both bipolar and unipolar affective disorders among the families of people with bipolar disorder, and their first degree relatives have a 12% risk of developing a bipolar illness. Most twin studies have found concordance rates of around 60% for monozygotes and 20% for dizygotes. Numerous candidate genes have been identified and the inheritance of bipolar disorder is likely to be polygenic, with a strong gene–environment interaction.

There is a raised rate of adverse life events prior to manic episodes, although social factors appear to play less of a part in precipitating mania once several episodes have occurred. Disruption of biological rhythms, for example as a result of travelling across time zones, can sometimes precipitate mania and many people with bipolar disorder find that the frequency of manic relapse can be reduced if they maintain a regular sleep pattern. There is a raised rate of manic episodes in spring and early summer. Childbirth is a common precipitant of affective episodes in women with bipolar disorder (see 'Puerperal psychosis' section on p. 78).

Little is known of the neurochemical basis of mania. There is some limited evidence of increased monoamine transmission during manic episodes, involving dopamine, serotonin and noradrenaline. The effectiveness of antipsychotic drugs in the treatment of manic episodes suggests that an increase in dopaminergic activity may be involved.

### *Epidemiology*

Bipolar disorder is much less common than unipolar depressive disorder, with a lifetime risk of around 1%. Women and men are at equal risk of developing bipolar disorder type I, but women are over-represented among type II cases. While some people are particularly creative and capable of high levels of achievement during periods of elevated mood, in general bipolar disorder is associated with high levels of functional impairment and is more common among people with low household incomes. Relatives of people with bipolar disorder are more likely to be high achievers than those of people with unipolar depression.

### *Course of illness*

The mean age of onset is the late teens, whereas mean age of diagnosis is late twenties. The delay in diagnosis often results from manic episodes not being recognised as a manifestation of mood disorder. In other cases, early episodes are depressive in nature and it is not until a manic episode occurs that the bipolar nature of the condition becomes apparent.

Manic episodes typically last between 4 and 6 months, although this can vary considerably. Once someone has experienced a manic episode, it is likely that they will go on to have further affective episodes. The frequency and nature of these episodes varies greatly between individuals and some examples of relapse patterns in bipolar disorder are shown in Figure 1. The duration of remission between episodes tends to decrease over time. Clustering of episodes also occurs, with several episodes of mania and depression occurring close together, followed by a relatively long period of full recovery. 'Rapid cycling' can be viewed as an extreme form of clustering.

Mania can be extremely disruptive, but most people with bipolar disorder will spend a greater proportion of their lives in a state of depression. This is the case in both forms of the disorder but is particularly so for bipolar II. There is also a high rate of anxiety disorders among people with bipolar disorder. The suicide rate is around 10%, with the greatest period of risk during depressive and mixed episodes. People with bipolar II disorder are at greater risk of suicide.

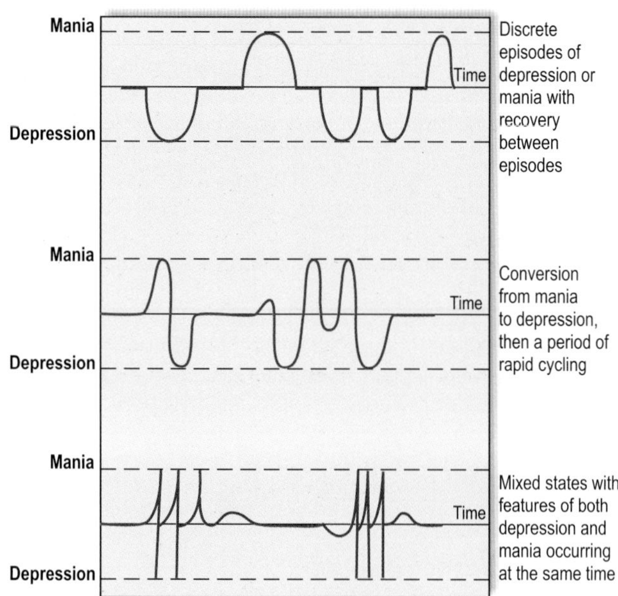


Fig. 1 **Patterns of illness found in bipolar disorder.**

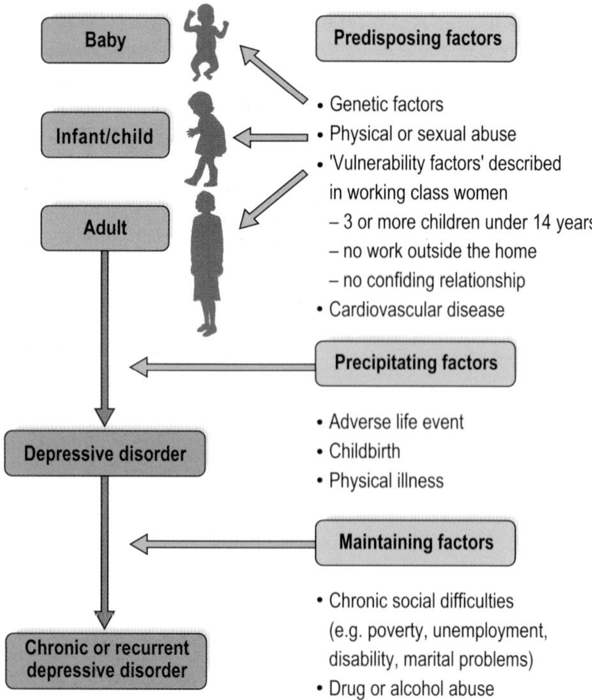


Fig. 2 **Aetiology of depressive disorder.**

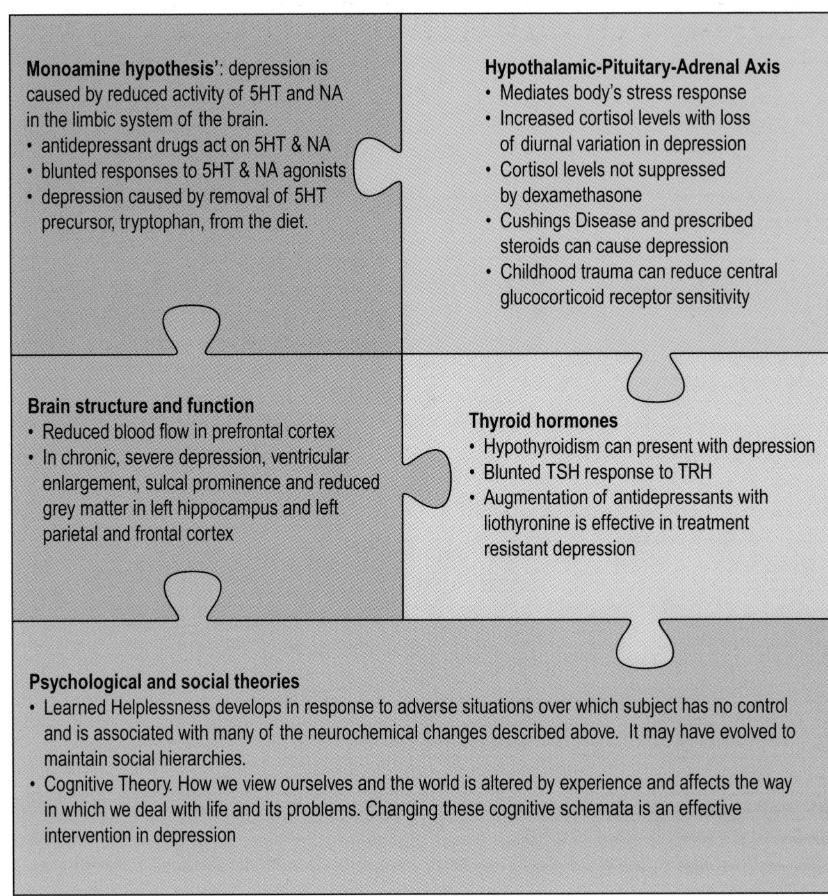


Fig. 3 **Proposed mechanisms in the aetiology of depression.**

# Depressive disorders

## Aetiology

Figure 2 shows some of the aetiological factors that have been identified for depressive disorders. Genetic factors and childhood adversity tend to play a greater role in the early-onset cases that begin in the first three to four decades of life. In later onset cases, there are raised rates of cardiovascular risk factors and an increased risk of later dementia, suggesting a neurodegenerative element to the pathogenesis.

Figure 3 summarises some of the aetiological theories proposed for depression and it is important to note that these hypotheses are not mutually exclusive. For example, administration of corticosteroids can cause many of the abnormalities of monoamine activity that occur in depression and antidepressants can reduce HPA overactivity via their effect on monoamines. Administration of a single dose of antidepressant can change the way in which people appraise facial expression and antidepressants can impede the development of learned helplessness.

### *Epidemiology*

Depressive disorder is extremely common, affecting about 3% of the population every year and having a lifetime prevalence of 10–30%. GPs treat the majority of those who seek medical help. They can expect to see an average of one moderate or severe case of depression in every surgery session. About 10% of the patients diagnosed with depression by GPs are referred on to psychiatrists, and 10% of these are admitted for inpatient psychiatric treatment.

Depressive disorder is more common among people with low household incomes and those who live in urban areas and are unemployed. The rate among women is twice that in men. The reasons for this are not fully understood, but may relate to differing social expectations of men and women and the effect of gender on the way distress is expressed and diagnosed. For example, there may be a greater tendency among men to seek recourse in alcohol at times of distress, as reflected in their higher rates of alcohol dependence. Also, it has been suggested that the syndrome of depressive disorders, in which feelings of sadness and unhappiness are a core symptom, is unduly restrictive. Some people, particularly men, may present with anger and irritability rather than low mood, but otherwise will have symptoms typical of the depressive syndrome.

### *Course of illness*

Among people admitted to hospital with depression, length of episodes tends to be around 5 months and 75% will recover within a year. Duration is shorter in community samples, with half recovering within 3 months. Chronic depressive episodes are defined as those lasting two years or more and the majority of people still depressed after one year will go on to experience a chronic course.

Unipolar disorders are usually recurrent and 85% of people who have had a depressive episode will have at least one more. Depressive episodes tend to become more frequent as time goes on and later episodes are less likely to be preceded by adverse life events. Various reasons have been suggested for this, such as the biological theory that the neurochemical changes associated with depressive episodes can lead to permanent neuronal damage, the psychological view that the experience of depression changes the way a person views themselves and responds to events, and the social perspective that depression has an enduring effect on a person's relationships and social circumstances.

**Aetiology and epidemiology of mood disorders**

- Mood disorders are usually recurrent conditions
- Genetic factors play a large role in bipolar disorder
- Depression is common and has a complex aetiology

# Bipolar disorder – clinical presentation and management

## Clinical presentation of mania

In manic episodes, there are characteristic changes in mood, biological functions and thinking, and in severe cases psychotic symptoms develop. The symptoms and signs commonly encountered are described below and a typical mental state examination of a person with mania is shown in Figure 1. A manic episode is not usually diagnosed until typical features of the illness have been present for at least a week.

*MSE*

***Appearance and behaviour***
*Has taken little care over appearance*
*Restless, active*
*Overfamiliar*
*Confident, superior manner*

***Speech***
*Pressured, difficult to interrupt*
*Flight of ideas*
*'So doctor, do you think I'm healthy? It's healthy to be wealthy. I don't like milk chocolate though, it's too rich'*

***Affect***
*Elated, jovial*
*Brief moments of irritability and tearfulness*

***Thoughts***
*Optimistic about everything*
*Believes he has discovered a solution to global warming and will become rich, despite having no relevant expertise*
*Wants to set up a hostel for homeless people*
***Perception***
*Colours seem vivid*
*No hallucinations*
***Cognitive function***
*Impaired attention and concentration*
*Fully orientated*
***Insight***
*Accepts he has been manic in the past but says he is currently well*
*Doesn't want to take medication because it slows him down*

Fig. 1 **Mental state examination of a person with mania.**

### *Changes in mood*

Manic episodes are characterised by an elated mood, described by some as 'feeling high'. Elation can, of course, be a normal mood state, and in mania is distinguished from normal cheerfulness because it is persistent, out of context and may be extreme.

People experiencing manic episodes are often infectiously happy. However, their mood can be labile, and brief periods of sadness, fearfulness, anger or irritability are common, typically lasting less than a minute and being followed by a rapid return to elation. In some cases, elation does not occur and irritability and anger are the predominant emotions.

### *Biological functions*

Energy is increased and can seem boundless. Sleep is reduced and typically the person affected doesn't feel tired or in need of rest. Appetite may be increased but the person's behaviour is often so frantic and disorganised that they end up eating less than usual. Increased energy and activity mean that weight loss may occur. Libido is usually increased.

### *Thinking*

Thinking becomes faster and more expansive. An early sign of this is prolixity of speech, in which the person talks more than usual and covers in their conversation an uncharacteristically broad range of topics. As the episode progresses and thinking speeds up more, the person may begin to exhibit pressure of speech, talking more forcefully and faster than usual and being difficult to interrupt. During episodes of mania, speech often reflects an underlying thought disorder called 'flight of ideas', in which thoughts progress from one topic to another in a logical way, but so quickly that it can be difficult to follow the train of thought. Puns and rhymes may be used to connect thoughts.

People experiencing hypomania become sociable, optimistic and confident. Their life may seem more vivid and interesting. During episodes of mania, they can become grandiose, thinking they are superior to other people and capable of great things. Impaired judgement and disinhibition occur. Attention and concentration are impaired.

These changes in thinking are manifest in the person's behaviour. They may be effusive, and wish to share their wonderful ideas with the world, but may also be self-important and pompous. A manic episode can be a time of great creativity, but often projects are started and not completed. Poor judgement can result in grandiose ideas being acted upon with disastrous consequences.

### *Psychotic symptoms*

Psychotic symptoms in mania are typically mood congruent. The most common are grandiose delusions and are an extension of the optimism and confidence that occur when manic episodes are less severe. The person may believe that they have superhuman powers, are very important or wealthy, or have a special mission to achieve. Persecutory delusions are also common, with the belief that others are against them usually being related to the person's sense of self-importance. Auditory hallucinations are unusual. If they do occur they are usually in the second person.

### *Depressive episodes*

Bipolar depression presents in the same way as unipolar depressive episodes, the clinical features of which are described on pages 52–53. The only way to establish whether a depressive episode is part of a unipolar or bipolar disorder is to check for a history of manic episodes. There are, however, features of depressive episodes that can suggest the possibility of bipolar disorder – psychotic symptoms, severe agitation suggestive of a mixed affective state, atypical symptoms such as increased sleep and appetite, and poor response to antidepressant drugs are all suggestive of bipolar depression and should prompt a review of the case, to check whether a history of manic episodes has been missed.

## Management of mania

The differential diagnoses to consider in a patient presenting with an elated mood are shown in Figure 2. Usually, the most important investigation when assessing someone suspected to have a manic episode is talking to informants. People with mania often co-operate poorly with clinical assessment, because they do not think they are ill and are overactive and distractible. In milder cases, people with mania may be able to exert enough control over their speech and behaviour to disguise any evidence of illness. The early signs of mania are often subtle and may only be apparent to someone with prior knowledge of the person concerned – for example, a mild-mannered quiet person who becomes more talkative and confident during manic episodes might not appear unwell to someone who has not met them before.

The risk assessment of someone with mania must consider overspending, sexual disinhibition, vulnerability to

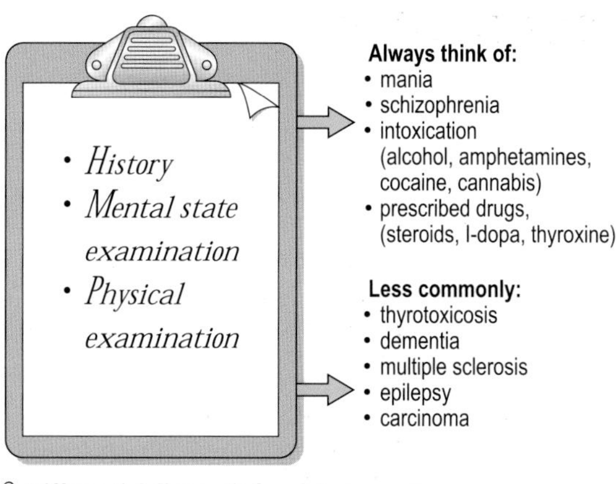

Fig. 2 **Differential diagnosis for elated mood.**

Table 1 **Physical treatments for the different phases of bipolar disorder**

| | Acute episodes | Prophylaxis |
|---|---|---|
| **Manic/mixed episodes** | Antipsychotic drugs | Lithium |
| | Valproate | Valproate |
| | Lithium (not for severe episodes) | Antipsychotic drugs |
| | Carbamazepine (not often used) | Carbamazepine |
| | ECT | |
| **Depressive episodes** | Antidepressant drugs (only with an antimanic drug) | Lithium |
| | Quetiapine | Valproate |
| | ?Other atypical antipsychotics | Antidepressant drugs (only with an antimanic drug) |
| | Lamotrigine | ?Carbamazepine |
| | ECT | ?Lamotrigine |
| | | ?Atypical antipsychotics |

sexual and financial exploitation, self-neglect and exhaustion, aggression and violence. People should not drive a car during manic episodes, because of impaired concentration and the risk of disinhibition and recklessness. Grandiose delusions concerning special powers, such as being indestructible or able to fly, carry obvious risks. When there is marked emotional lability, particularly during mixed episodes, the combination of depressive cognitions and manic disinhibition is associated with a high suicide risk.

## Treatment

Treatment in hospital is often required because of the risks described above and the disruptive effects of overactive chaotic behaviour. It may be necessary to arrange for compulsory admission under a section of the Mental Health Act (see pp. 18–19).

Table 1 shows the physical treatments thought to be effective in the different phases of bipolar disorder. Drug treatment is nearly always required during manic episodes, with antipsychotic drugs and valproate being the usual first choices. Antipsychotics are effective even in manic episodes without psychotic symptoms and they should be prescribed if psychosis is present. Combinations of drugs, for example an antipsychotic with either valproate or lithium, are often more effective and can bring about a quicker recovery, but there will be a greater likelihood of adverse effects (see pp. 18–19).

## Management of bipolar depression

The differential diagnosis, investigation and general treatment of depression in bipolar disorder are the same as described on pages 54–55 for unipolar disorders. The social and psychological interventions effective in unipolar episodes will often be helpful and it is physical treatments that require a different approach in bipolar depression. Antidepressant drugs have the potential to cause manic episodes and to trigger rapid cycling, so should always be prescribed with an antimanic drug. They are also less likely to be effective in bipolar depression than in unipolar episodes. Maintenance treatment following resolution of depressive symptoms is often not required, as the risk of relapse at this stage is not as great as in unipolar disorders. Stopping antidepressants soon after the person has recovered from depression reduces the risk of conversion to mania. The other main difference in bipolar depression is the effectiveness of quetiapine, possibly other atypical antipsychotics, and the anticonvulsant drug lamotrigine.

### *Prophylaxis in bipolar disorder*

Recovery from acute manic and depressive episodes in bipolar disorder is generally good, but the risk of relapse is high. The drug treatments that reduce the risk of manic and depressive recurrence are included in Table 1. Such treatment will not be appropriate for everyone with bipolar disorder and prophylaxis with medication is usually recommended in the following circumstances:

- after a manic episode that was associated with significant risk and adverse consequences
- when a person with bipolar I disorder has had two or more acute episodes
- when a person with bipolar II disorder has significant functional impairment, is at significant risk of suicide, or has frequent episodes.

### *Psychological and social interventions in bipolar disorder*

Psychological and social interventions help improve the quality of life of people with bipolar disorder and their families and may reduce the risk of recurrence. Social and family problems may precipitate episodes, and equally can be caused by the illness, so may need addressing. Psychological support and education about bipolar disorder are important and are often best provided by self-help and support groups such as the Manic-Depressive Fellowship. Interpersonal and Social Rhythm Therapy (IPSRT) emphasises the importance of sticking to social routines and avoiding the disrupted sleep that can lead to manic episodes, with diaries being used to spot early signs of recurrence, so that medication can be introduced at an early stage if needed.

### *Case history 15*

Anya has been taking antidepressants since becoming depressed 4 months ago. During a routine follow-up appointment the GP notices a change. She rushes into the room, speaks quickly and urges the doctor to hurry as she has a number of very important meetings to go to later in the day. She tells him that she only kept this appointment because she knows how much he looks forward to seeing her.

a. Which diagnoses should be considered?
b. How should the GP confirm the diagnosis?

### Assessment and management of bipolar disorder

- A manic episode is characterised by elevated mood for at least one week, poor sleep, overactivity, pressure of speech and grandiosity
- Different drug treatments are needed during different phases of the illness
- Antidepressants can trigger manic episodes

# Depressive disorder – clinical presentation

> ### Case history 16
>
> Sharon is a 26-year-old single woman who lives alone and works as a civil engineer. She is having problems at work as she has been forgetful, making errors and finding it difficult to talk to her colleagues. She dreads going to work and lies awake at night worrying about what the future holds for her. During the day she is tired and tearful.
>
> a. Sharon has symptoms of a depressive disorder: what are they?
> b. What questions would you ask her in order to confirm the diagnosis?

*Depressive symptoms* consist of persistent low mood that affects all aspects of a person's life, and other characteristic psychological and physical changes. *Depressive episodes* are psychiatric syndromes in which a specified number of symptoms are present for at least two weeks. Depressive symptoms occur in many other psychiatric conditions, such as dementia, schizophrenia, anxiety disorders, PTSD and adjustment disorders. Organic depressive disorders also occur, for example in hypothyroidism and Cushing's syndrome.

## Clinical presentation

People with depressive disorders may present with psychological symptoms, but for many the physical symptoms, such as fatigue, weight loss or insomnia, are the main concern. Patients with a coexisting physical illness may find this harder to bear when depressed and may complain about a flare up of physical symptoms. Hypochondriacal concerns are also common. As a result, people with depressive disorder may present to doctors in virtually every branch of medicine.

The symptoms that occur in depressive episodes are described below. Not all these symptoms are used to make a diagnosis and there are differences between ICD10 and DSM4 in the way the condition is classified, as shown in Figure 1. Depressive episodes are categorised as mild, moderate or severe, partly on the basis of the number of symptoms present. Mild episodes usually feature the minimum number of symptoms required to make a diagnosis of depressive episode, and in severe episodes most symptoms are present, with moderate episodes falling somewhere between. However, as was discussed on pages 4–6, the extent to which a person's life is disrupted by depression is also used to classify the severity of the episode.

## Core symptoms of depression

In ICD 10, three core symptoms of depression are described. As would be expected, one of these is **depressed mood**, which some patients describe as being the same as normal sadness, but more intense or prolonged, while others say it has a distinct quality, like a dark cloud. There is sometimes a 'diurnal variation of mood' in depressive episodes, with the person feeling worse in the morning and improving as the day progresses. The second of the core symptoms is **loss of interest and enjoyment**. Motivation is reduced. Hobbies cease to be of interest, and previously enjoyable encounters with friends and family may become chores to be avoided. Anhedonia, an inability to experience pleasure, often occurs. The final core symptom is reduced energy leading to **increased fatiguability**. People with depression can feel too tired to do things, or rapidly become fatigued and have to stop what they are doing.

### *Psychological symptoms*

Feelings of low self esteem, self blame and guilt occur, and patients tend to view everything in a negative light. The future often seems bleak to them and they can lose hope of their situation improving. It is not surprising that, in the face of such persistent unpleasant feelings, suicidal thoughts or actions may occur. Psychotic symptoms such as delusions and hallucinations can occur in severe episodes and typically are 'mood congruent'. Thus, delusions may be concerned with ideas of worthlessness, guilt, illness (hypochondriacal delusions), poverty or feelings that one has ceased to exist, or is rotting away (nihilistic delusions). Auditory hallucinations tend to be simple in nature. Typically, they consist of a single voice repeating a few words, speaking directly to the patient (second person hallucinations) and reinforcing their negative thoughts saying, for example 'it's all your fault, they would be better off without you'.

### *Biological symptoms*

Sleep disturbance is common in depressive episodes. Although increased sleep (hypersomnia) can occur, reduced sleep is more typical. Some people have difficulty falling asleep and others sleep rest-

| | ICD10 | DSM4 |
|---|---|---|
| Name | Depressive episode | Major Depressive Episode |
| Core Symptoms | Depressed mood | Depressed mood |
| | Loss of interest and enjoyment | Loss of interest and enjoyment |
| | Loss of energy/fatigue | Loss of energy/fatigue |
| Other Symptoms | Reduced concentration and attention | Reduced concentration and attention/indecisiveness |
| | Reduced self-esteem and self-confidence | Psychomotor agitation or retardation |
| | Ideas of guilt and unworthiness | Ideas of guilt and unworthiness |
| | Bleak/pessimistic views of the future | |
| | Ideas or acts of self-harm or suicide | Ideas or acts of self-harm or suicide/ thoughts of death |
| | Reduced concentration and attention | Reduced concentration and attention |
| | Disturbed sleep | Insomnia/hypersomnia |
| | Diminished appetite | Weight loss/weight gain |
| Minimum Number Of Symptoms | At least two core symptoms, at least two other symptoms | At least one core symptom, at least five symptoms in total |
| Minimum Duration | Symptoms must be present for most of the time for at least two weeks in both ICD10 and DSM4 | |

Fig. 1 **Comparison of diagnostic criteria for depressive episodes in ICD10 and DSM4.**

What's your confidence like at the moment? What are your good and bad points? How do you compare with other people?
Have you done anything you shouldn't have done? Do you feel guilty about anything?
Have you any concerns about your health at present? Is your body functioning properly?
What do you think the future holds for you? Do you ever think you would be better off dead?

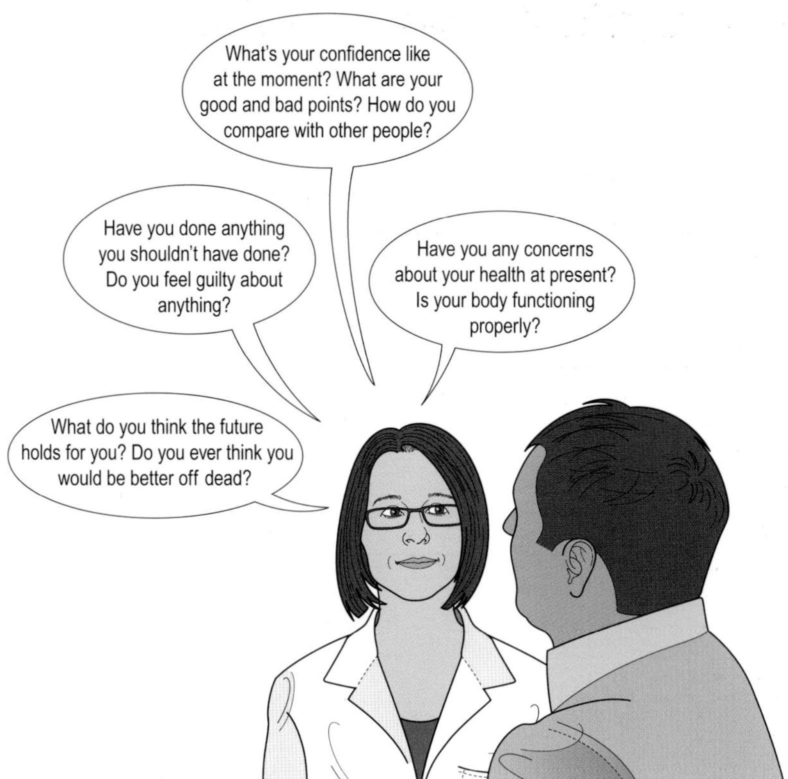

Fig. 2 **Asking about depressive thoughts.**

***MSE***

***Appearance and behaviour***
*Clothes creased, hair unbrushed, hasn't shaved for several days*
*Weary and lethargic*
*Head bowed, no eye contact, little facial expression*
*Sits very still, except for constant wringing of hands*

***Speech***
*No spontaneity*
*Slow to answer questions, long pauses*
*Monotonous tone*

***Affect***
*Very unhappy, seems close to tears*
*Mood does not pick up even when discussing happy events*

***Thoughts***
*Feels useless, says he must be weak to have allowed himself to get like this*
*Thinks his family would be better off without him and thinking of moving away.*
*'Suicide's too good for me, I deserve to suffer'*
***Perception***
*Occasionally hears his own voice inside his head saying 'Useless'*
*No hallucinations*
***Cognitive function***
*Impaired attention and concentration evident throughout interview*
*Doesn't feel capable of answering questions to test cognitive function*
***Insight***
*He views his condition as a consequence of his inadequacy, not as an illness, so doesn't see any point in receiving treatment*

Fig. 3 **Mental state examination of a man with a severe depressive episode.**

lessly and wake during the night. Another form of sleep disturbance is early morning waking, defined as waking at least two hours earlier than usual and then not being able to return to sleep. These different forms of sleep disturbance often coexist. Change of appetite is also a common feature of depressive disorders. Some patients lose their appetite and consequently lose weight; others have an increased appetite, and describe 'comfort eating', which may be accompanied by weight gain. Constipation can occur in depression, particularly in older people. Many patients lose their sex drive when depressed.

Loss of concentration is common and can be distressing. An inability to concentrate can lead to forgetfulness and older people sometimes present with **depressive pseudodementia**, in which an apparent memory loss leads to misfounded concerns that they are developing dementia. People with pseudodementia are usually worried about their cognitive function. They will tend to avoid testing of cognition because they believe they will not be able to give adequate answers but in casual conversation often demonstrate good recall. A diagnosis of depressive pseudodementia rather than dementia is also supported by an acute onset and the presence of other symptoms and signs of depression. It is important to remember that depressive episodes can occur in people with dementia, so you should bear in mind the possibility that some patients will have both conditions.

## Mental state examination

It can be seen from Figure 1 that depressive episodes are diagnosed primarily on the basis of symptoms. Mental state examination is important though, as it helps determine severity of depressive episodes and indeed whether depressive symptoms are extensive enough to make a diagnosis at all. Examination is also useful in identifying depression in a patient who is reluctant to discuss their symptoms.

Fatigue and poor motivation are likely to be manifest as poor self-care. Eye contact and social interaction are often limited and can be a sign of psychomotor retardation, which is a slowing of thought and movement. Psychomotor agitation can also occur, leading to restlessness and anxiety. The person often lacks spontaneity and their speech can be slow, with long pauses and reduced intonation. The depressed mood that occurs in depressive episodes is present most of the time, so sadness and despondency should be evident on examination and reactivity of mood will be reduced. Enquiry should be made about the negative thinking that is typical of depression, as suggested in Figure 2, and it is crucial to explore extensively any thoughts of hopelessness, self-harm or suicide. Check for psychotic symptoms and test cognitive function, as discussed earlier. Regarding insight, most people will recognise they are not their normal self, but some will view this is a reaction to their circumstances rather than an illness and others will find it hard to accept that their symptoms are not caused by a physical disorder. Insight in psychotic depression is usually poor.

### Depressive disorder

A depressive episode is characterised by:

- depressed mood, anhedonia and fatigue
- the patient thinking negatively about themselves and their future
- altered biological functions
- duration of at least two weeks

# Depressive disorder – management

The differential diagnosis of depressive episodes is shown in Figure 1. Physical causes of depression need to be excluded, through physical examination and, if indicated, physical investigations, such as blood tests and neuroimaging. Blood tests, particularly full blood count and liver function tests, are important if covert alcohol dependence is suspected. Except in severe cases, people with depression usually give a good description of their symptoms but it is still helpful to talk to informants, whose account will not be affected by the negative thinking that is typical of depressive episodes.

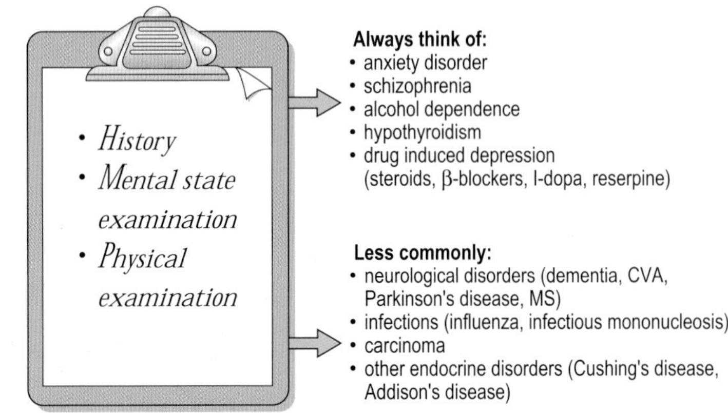


Fig. 1 **Differential diagnosis of depressed mood.**

| Step | Who | Treatment |
|---|---|---|
| 4 | Severe or psychotic depression<br>Risk to life<br>Severe self-neglect<br>Complex social circumstances<br>Treatment resistance<br>Dual diagnosis, eg with personality disorder, alcohol/substance misuse | Medication<br>High intensity psychological interventions<br>ECT<br>Combinations of treatment<br>Multidisciplinary care<br>Intensive Community Treatment /<br>Hospital treatment |
| 3 | Moderate to severe depression<br>Step 2 cases with inadequate response to treatment | Medication<br>High intensity psychological interventions<br>Combinations of treatment |
| 2 | Mild to moderate depression<br>Dysthymia | Low intensity psychosocial interventions<br>Sleep hygiene<br>Medication |
| 1 | All cases of depression | Assessment<br>Watchful waiting<br>Support<br>Monitoring<br>Education |

Fig. 2 **Stepped care of depression.**

## Treatment

Treatment for depression is currently delivered according to the stepped care model illustrated in Figure 2. In this model, all people with depression start at step 1 and most people with symptoms of mild to moderate severity will be managed at step 1 or 2, with the minority of cases that do not improve being referred on to step 3. People with moderate to severe depression should be referred immediately to step 3 or step 4, on the basis of the criteria shown in the figure.

Interventions at steps 1 and 2 are provided in primary care, and in many areas this is also the case for step 3. A typical arrangement is for a team of high intensity and low intensity mental health workers to be based at large GP surgeries, or across a cluster of smaller practices, with prescribing being carried out by GPs with advice from a psychiatrist when needed. Level 4 care is provided by mental health services, using the different methods of service delivery described on pages 2–5. Psychiatrists will take a lead in prescribing at level 4 and there will be access to more specialised or intensive psychological treatments.

The rest of this section outlines the treatments used at the different levels of the stepped care model.

### *Low intensity psychosocial interventions*

**Computerised cognitive behaviour therapy** consists of software packages that have been developed to deliver CBT through a computer, either on CD-Roms (e.g. Beating the Blues) or the internet (e.g. MoodGYM). The usual procedure is for the patient to be referred to a low intensity worker, who will introduce the programme and be available to give advice if need be.

**Guided self-help** involves the provision of self-help manuals and books about depression. A low intensity worker will help the person select the reading material most suitable for them and meet with them a few times, to advise and support them in their reading and to monitor their progress.

**Exercise** is an effective measure in the treatment of mild to moderate depression. The evidence base for this intervention is based on structured programmes, undertaken in groups or on an individual basis, and both aerobic and anaerobic exercise has been found to be effective. Whether it is sufficient for health professionals to give simple advice and encouragement regarding exercise is uncertain.

Poor sleep is often one of the greatest problems for people with depression and this can be helped by advice on **sleep hygiene.** Establishing a comfortable environment for sleep and sticking to regular sleep and wake times is essential. Habits such as waking late on days off work in order to 'catch up' on lost sleep will usually perpetuate the problem. Caffeine should not be consumed after 5pm. Advice should also include avoiding excess eating, cigarette smoking and alcohol before sleep. Physical exercise during the day improves the chances of sleeping well at night.

### *High intensity psychological treatments*

**Cognitive behaviour therapy** is often the first-line psychological intervention for moderate to severe depression and is usually the treatment in which high intensity mental health workers in primary care have received the most training. Cognitive therapy, the principles of which are described on page 32, aims to address the negative 'cognitions' or thoughts that are associated with depressive illness. People with depression develop negative thinking biases, such as minimisation of their achievements, a selective focus on things they could have done better, and overgeneralisation, so that a minor mistake, such as burning toast, leads them to jump to the conclu-

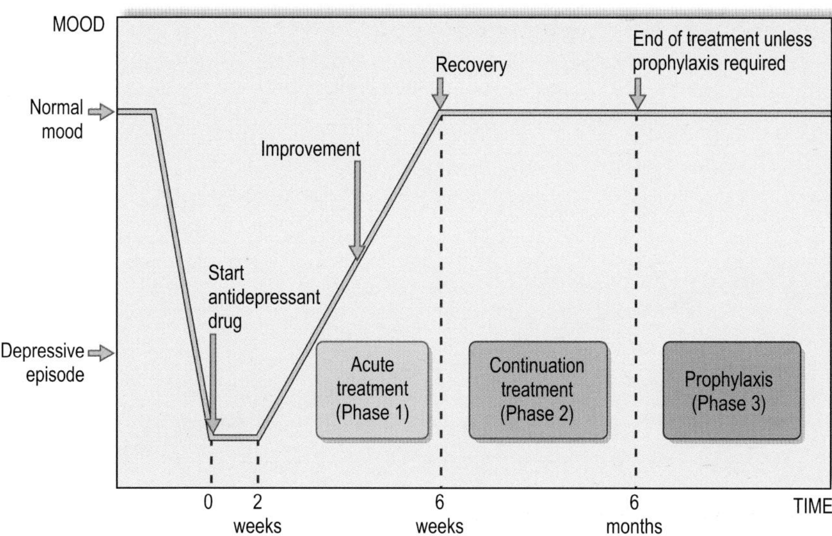


Fig. 3 **Phases of antidepressant drug treatment.**

sion that they are a terrible cook, wife and mother. In traditional cognitive therapy, people are taught to recognise and challenge such thoughts.

**Mindfulness Based Cognitive Therapy** is a variant of the treatment that draws on some of the principles and techniques of Eastern meditation practices. People are taught to recognise and acknowledge the bodily sensations, feelings and thoughts that occur during depression and, rather than reinforce this way of being by dwelling upon it, they learn to distance themselves and switch back to more healthy ways of thinking.

**Behavioural activation** is a component of cognitive therapy, but can be effective when delivered as a stand-alone treatment. It is a useful option for people who don't find the cognitive model of depression helpful and involves them collaborating with the therapist to identify how their behaviour affects their symptoms. It is based on the principle of operant conditioning that is described on page 32. Behavioural tasks are agreed (activity scheduling) that allow the person to gradually resume activities they have avoided (graded exposure). If these tasks result in a sense of achievement or improved wellbeing, they will be more likely to continue with these healthy behaviours (positive reinforcement).

**Problem solving** is described on page 34 and is helpful in depression in two ways. First, the structured approach of problem solving can help people resolve problems that may be maintaining their depression. Second, as a result of them dealing with these problems, any negative thoughts about being incapable and powerless are likely to change.

Other psychological interventions, such as **Couples therapy** (p. 34), and **Psychodynamic psychotherapy** (p. 33) are also used in the treatment of depression.

### *Physical treatments*

Antidepressant medication is effective in the treatment of moderate to severe depression. Trials of these drugs in mild depressive episodes have produced equivocal results, which may be a consequence of the high placebo response in these studies, and antidepressants are not a first-line treatment in such cases, unless there is a past history of progression to more severe forms of depression.

Drug treatment of depressive disorders can be divided into three distinct phases (Fig. 3):

1. **Acute treatment**. Drug trials usually find that 50–70% of subjects improve during the acute phase of treatment, although in real life settings, in which patients often have multiple problems, the response rate can be lower. All antidepressant drugs have a slow onset of action and patients should be warned that it may take up to two weeks before they start to notice any benefit and around six weeks for the full effects to occur. Adverse effects are usually at their worst in the first two weeks of treatment and so people will often stop medication at this stage if they are not given suitable support and advice. If there is no improvement after three to four weeks, then consideration should be given to increasing the dose of the antidepressant or switching to a different drug.

There are a variety of antidepressants to choose from, as described on pages 26–27. SSRIs are the usual first-line treatment. If depression does not improve after adequate trials of at least two antidepressant drugs at therapeutic doses, there are a variety of strategies that should be considered, such as augmentation of an antidepressant with lithium or an atypical antipsychotic, or treatment with high doses of the SNRI venlafaxine.

2. **Continuation treatment**. The continuation phase of treatment begins once the patient has recovered. It is important that they do not stop the drug suddenly once they feel better, as up to half will have an immediate relapse into depression. Instead the drug should be continued, at full dose, for 4–6 months before slow withdrawal. With continuation treatment, the relapse rate falls to about 20%. It is important that patients are monitored throughout this phase and following drug withdrawal, so that they can be re-established on the antidepressant quickly if symptoms of depression recur.

3. **Prophylaxis**. Many patients with depressive illness suffer recurrent episodes. Long-term prescription of antidepressant drugs can prevent or reduce the rate of recurrence in many cases. The full dose required to get the patient well initially should be maintained.

ECT is a highly effective and sometimes life saving treatment and its use in depressive disorders is described on pages 28–29.

### *Case history 17*

Janet has been diagnosed with depressive disorder by her GP. She has suicidal ideas, but no plans to act on them. The episode began 3 months after breaking up with her boyfriend of 2 years. No other aetiological factors are evident from the history. She has no previous psychiatric history.

a. What are the treatment options available in primary care?
b. What would influence your decision about which treatment to pursue?

### Management of depressive disorders

- Mild to moderate depressive episodes should be treated with low intensity psychosocial interventions
- Antidepressant drugs, high intensity psychological treatments and occasionally ECT are used to treat moderate to severe depressive episodes

# Anxiety disorders – clinical presentation and aetiology

The term 'neurotic' has slipped from popularity in psychiatry because of difficulties in agreeing upon a precise and useful definition, and because it tends to be used pejoratively to refer to people (usually women) who are perceived to be emotional and prone to unnecessary worry. In its broadest sense neurotic simply means 'not psychotic', and so could be applied to a very wide range of disorders. In the World Health Organization's tenth International Classification of Disease (ICD10) the term is reserved for disorders arising in response to stress, or in which symptoms of anxiety are prominent. This includes the anxiety disorders, obsessive–compulsive disorder, adjustment disorders, post-traumatic stress disorder and dissociative disorders.

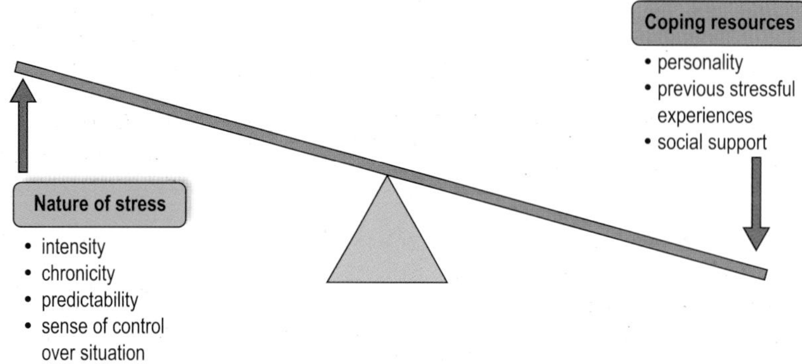


Fig. 1 **Factors which effect the response to stress.**

## Anxiety disorders

Anxiety occurs when an individual believes that the demands of a situation are greater than their abilities to cope with it. It is a subjective and variable phenomenon, as what is stressful for one person may be stimulating and enjoyable for another (Fig. 1). The symptoms of anxiety include feelings of fear, worrying thoughts, increased alertness or arousal, activation of the autonomic nervous system and increased muscle tension (Fig. 2). This is a normal reaction to stress that prepares us to defend ourselves or escape from a threatening situation ('fight or flight'). Of course, we are rarely confronted with stressful situations that literally require fight or flight, but anxiety can still be of value. It has been shown that we perform tasks better when more aroused, although as arousal levels increase, performance begins to decline (Fig. 3). You may be aware of this phenomenon at exam time when an overly laid-back approach is likely to be as ineffective as terror. Anxiety may be considered abnormal if it occurs in the absence of what most people would consider to be an adequate stress, or if it is so severe or long-standing that it interferes with day to day life.

Panic attacks can occur in any of the anxiety disorders. They are brief but very intense episodes of anxiety. An extreme sense of fear is usually present and may begin suddenly or build gradually to a crescendo. Hyperventilation is common, with shallow and rapid breathing that flushes carbon dioxide from the body resulting in a respiratory alkalosis. This causes symptoms of palpitations, chest pain, sweating, dizziness, feelings of pins and needles around the mouth and extremities, and muscle spasms. There is often a fear of losing control or, because similar symptoms occur in ischaemic heart disease, a fear of dying.

### Classification

Anxiety disorders can be divided into three broad categories, although in practice there is considerable overlap between them:

- phobic anxiety disorders, including agoraphobia, social phobia and specific phobia
- panic disorder
- generalised anxiety disorder.

#### *Phobic anxiety disorders*

In phobic anxiety disorders, symptoms of anxiety occur repeatedly and predictably in response to a particular object, situation or thought. The degree of anxiety is quite out of proportion to the circumstances. For example, while most people would be wary of approaching a large aggressive looking dog, an individual with a phobia about dogs might develop severe anxiety if they saw a small well-behaved dog across the street and might stop walking in public places in order to avoid dogs. *Avoidance* is a characteristic feature of phobias, and accounts for a great deal of disability. *Anticipatory anxiety* also occurs, with the person becoming anxious just at the thought of doing something that might bring them into contact with the cause of their fear.

There are three phobic anxiety disorders: agoraphobia, social phobia and specific phobia.

#### Agoraphobia

In agoraphobia, anxiety occurs in a wide range of situations, most commonly crowded places, particularly busy supermarkets or shopping centres, and on public transport. There is often fear of losing control in public, by fainting or collapsing, or of being unable to get out of a building. Symptoms tend to gradually escalate over time so that more and more places are avoided until eventually the patient cannot leave their own home. Some can only go out if accompanied. Home is thought of as a safe place, and symptoms of anxiety are less prominent there, although often not entirely absent, and some people with agoraphobia will also fear being alone. Depressive symptoms are common, and it is important to be alert for a coexisting depressive disorder when assessing these patients. Agoraphobia has a prevalence of 0.6% in the general population. It is more common in women, with symptoms usually begin-

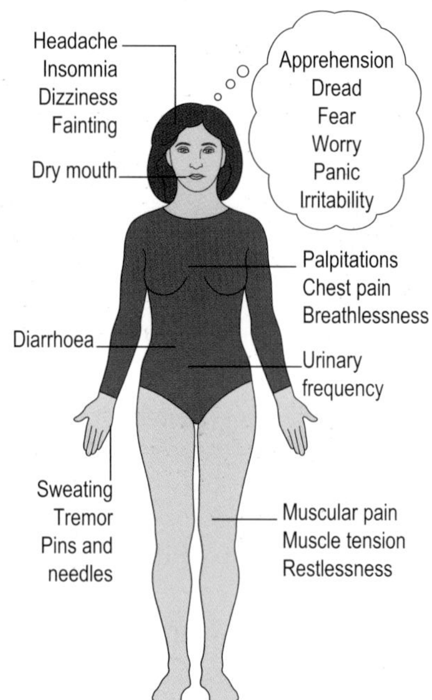


Fig. 2 **Symptoms of anxiety.**

ning in early adulthood. It tends to be a chronic disorder that fluctuates in severity.

### Social phobia

In social phobia, anxiety is provoked by social situations in which one feels on display in some way, such as meeting new people or speaking in social groups or during meetings at work. The impact of the phobia depends upon the job and lifestyle of the individual. For example, a teacher who is unable to speak in public will be severely disabled, whereas a farmer may not be greatly affected. Unlike the other phobias it occurs as frequently in men as women and usually begins in childhood or early adult life. Alcohol is often used by people with social phobia to reduce the anxiety they develop in social settings and this can become a problem in itself.

### Specific phobia

In specific phobias, anxiety is aroused by a particular object. The object can be virtually anything, although thunderstorms and animals are most often implicated. This is the commonest, and generally the least serious or disabling of the phobic anxiety disorders. However, the degree of disability depends upon the ease with which the phobic object can be avoided.

### *Panic disorder*

Panic disorder is characterised by recurrent panic attacks. The diagnosis is made if several panic attacks occur within a period of one month, but it is not uncommon for people to experience several attacks each day. Anxiety is less severe between attacks and in many cases resolves completely. Some people develop a persistent fear of having further panic attacks. Unlike the panic attacks that can occur in phobic anxiety disorders, they are not predictable or a response to a particular stressor. Panic disorder occurs in about 0.8% of the population and is slightly more common in women than men. It is most likely to begin in early adulthood.

### *Generalised anxiety disorder*

In generalised anxiety disorder (GAD), symptoms of anxiety are present most of the time over a period of at least two weeks, and often considerably longer. There does not seem to be a direct cause for the anxiety, which is often as severe when the patient is at home as when they are out. The focus of the anxiety is variable, moving from one topic to another, but the affected person will often worry that they, or someone close to them, will be involved in an accident or become unwell. GAD occurs in about 2% of the population and is more common in women than men, with onset usually in early adult life.

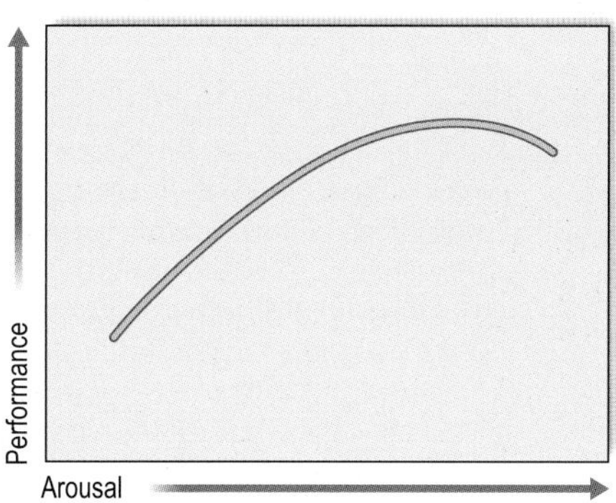


Fig. 3 **Yerkes Dodson curve.**

## Aetiology

Twin studies have shown that genetic factors play a small but significant role in predisposing individuals to anxiety disorders, particularly panic disorder. Environmental stress, such as adverse life events or chronic social problems, is the most important aetiological factor and may precipitate episodes of anxiety disorder, and perpetuate them once established. Psychological theories of anxiety disorders suggest they may arise as a result of learned behaviour, or cognitive processes. These theories and the treatments that have been developed from them are described on the following pages.

## Mixed depression and anxiety

There is considerable overlap between depressive disorders and anxiety disorders. People who have had an episode of one condition have a raised risk of developing the other sometime in the future. During episodes, symptoms of anxiety are common in depressive disorder and vice versa. Sometimes, it will be obvious which is the more severe or primary condition but if both sets of symptoms seem equally important and diagnostic criteria for a depressive episode and anxiety disorder are met at the same time, then both conditions should be diagnosed and treatment should address both sets of symptoms. Many patients, particularly in primary care, have symptoms of both depression and anxiety without meeting full diagnostic criteria for either. In these cases 'mixed anxiety and depressive disorder' is diagnosed.

### *Case history 18*

Anton is a 36-year-old business man who presents as an emergency to Casualty complaining of shortness of breath and chest pain. He has no previous medical or psychiatric history of note. He is accompanied by work colleagues who report that he collapsed just before an important presentation that he had been preparing for over several weeks.

a. What questions would you ask in order to establish whether Anton's symptoms are due to anxiety?
b. If anxiety is the principal cause of his symptoms, what is the most likely diagnosis?

### Anxiety disorders

- Anxiety is a normal reaction to stress
- Anxiety is abnormal if it is excessive, severe or prolonged, or adversely effects functioning
- Anxiety symptoms include fear, arousal, muscle tension and autonomic overactivity

# Anxiety disorders – management

## Assessment

Assessment of a person presenting with anxiety begins with a full psychiatric history. The history of the presenting complaint should establish whether the symptoms of generalised anxiety or panic attacks are present. It is often helpful to ask about a recent time when symptoms were severe and then enquire about the events leading up to it, the environment in which it occurred, who was present, what thoughts accompanied the anxiety and how it was resolved. This can help establish whether there is a phobic element or other triggers and maintaining factors for the anxiety, which will be relevant when considering psychological treatment.

The differential diagnosis of anxiety disorders is shown in Figure 1. It is important to exclude depressive disorder in every case by asking questions about mood, suicidal thoughts, sleep, appetite and energy. Alcohol and substance misuse often occurs as a result of 'self-medication' for anxiety disorder and withdrawal states are often accompanied by anxiety. A full blood count and liver function test may reveal covert alcohol problems. Schizophrenia should also be considered. A person with agoraphobia may be unable to go to a supermarket because of the fear of having a panic attack there. In contrast, a patient with schizophrenia may avoid the supermarket because of the delusional belief that their movements in shops are monitored on video cameras by terrorists.

As anxiety can present with symptoms in virtually any system of the body, the potential list of physical differential diagnoses is long. The majority can be excluded by the history and physical examination alone. There is a tendency to over-investigate these patients, and it is important to limit the investigations to those needed to exclude a real diagnostic possibility based upon positive findings on history and examination.

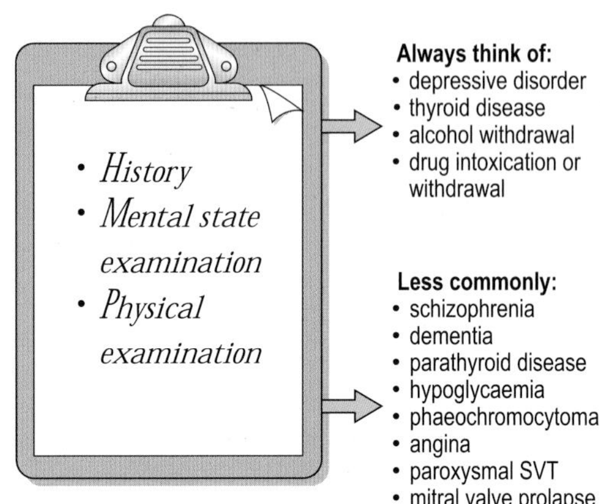


Fig. 1 **Differential diagnosis of anxiety disorders.**

## Treatment

Drug, psychological and social treatments should be discussed with the patient. The anxiety disorder in itself can place limitations on the treatment options – people with severe social phobia will avoid group treatments and asking someone with agoraphobia to attend a clinic two bus rides away from their home is unlikely to be successful! A collaborative approach to treatment is therefore vital.

### Drug treatment

Drug treatments are generally reserved for patients with chronic and severe anxiety disorders. The most useful drugs are the antidepressants, which are effective in reducing symptoms of anxiety, even in the absence of depressive disorder. SSRIs should usually be the first drug offered and there is also evidence to support the use of tricyclics, particularly in panic disorder. There is a two-week delay between the start of antidepressant drug treatment and clinical improvement, and the full therapeutic effect can take between 6 and 12 weeks to develop.

Beta-blockers can relieve the symptoms associated with autonomic arousal, such as palpitations and tremor. Benzodiazepines are effective in relieving symptoms of anxiety, but may lead to development of tolerance and dependency. They should not be routinely prescribed for anxiety disorders and treatment should usually be for no more than 2–4 weeks.

### Psychological treatment

There are a number of psychological interventions that may be helpful. An important first step for all patients is explanation and reassurance. Many believe that their symptoms indicate that something is terribly wrong with their body, and it is therefore helpful to explain why these symptoms occur and reassure them that anxiety is not a life-threatening condition. Written information about anxiety disorders and self-help groups are often helpful. Exercise is a component of good general health and some people find it helpful for anxiety. Techniques such as learning to control breathing when beginning to hyperventilate are beneficial, but non-specific relaxation training is of uncertain benefit and in some cases may increase anxiety. The 'Mindfulness' techniques discussed on page 55 have begun to be applied to anxiety disorders and appear to be effective.

Cognitive behavioural therapy (CBT) for anxiety disorders is the treatment most likely to produce a lasting improvement. Behavioural and cognitive approaches are discussed separately here and elements of each are used in CBT, depending on the needs and preferences of the patient.

#### *Behavioural therapy*

Behavioural therapies developed from the theory that phobias are learned behaviours. Two types of learning (also called conditioning) are thought to be important: classical conditioning and operant conditioning. Classical conditioning was first described by Pavlov following his famous experiment in which a bell was rung as dogs were fed meat (Fig. 2). Operant conditioning is described on page 32. Figure 3 imagines a person who feels faint, perhaps because they are hot and dehydrated, or have a viral infection, or drunk too much alcohol the previous night, and become anxious because they think they might lose consciousness. If these feelings of faintness occurred when they were shopping, they might link them to being in a crowded place, as a result of classical conditioning, and phobic avoidance would then become established as a result of operant conditioning.

Explanation of these processes helps patients understand and confront their anxiety. Operant conditioning can be used in a therapeutic way, for example in 'systematic desensitisation' for phobic anxiety disorders. The patient begins by working with the therapist to produce a list of situations that arouse anxiety, which can then be arranged according to the

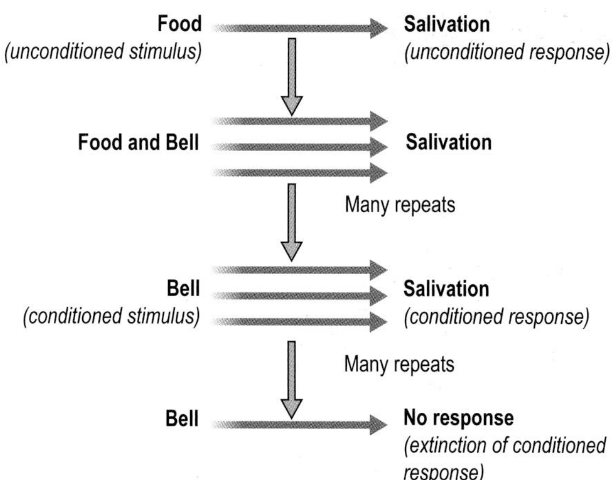


Fig. 2 **Classical conditioning.**

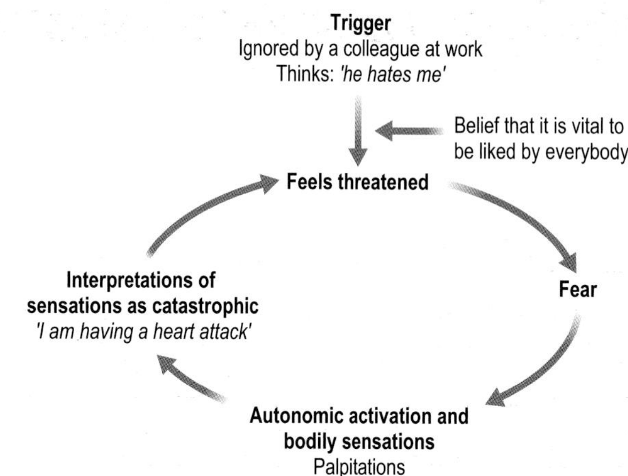


Fig. 4 **Cognitive theory in the development of panic.**

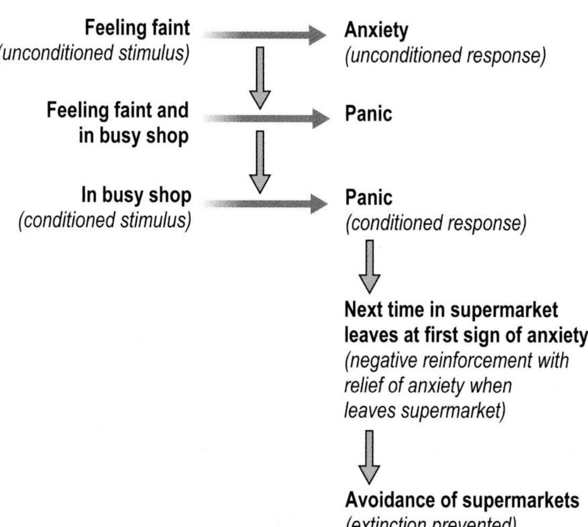


Fig. 3 **Classical and operant conditioning in the development of agoraphobia.**

fear they generate, with the most feared situation at the top of the list (a 'hierarchy'). Thus a person with a fear of dogs might place 'thinking about a dog' at the bottom of the list and 'patting a dog' at the top. The therapist then explains the psychological process of 'extinction', by which anxiety eventually wanes if the sufferer manages to remain in the feared situation for long enough. The patient will then expose themselves to feared situations until they no longer become anxious, starting at the bottom of the list and gradually working their way to the top. Each time they stay in a feared situation long enough for extinction of anxiety to occur, negative reinforcement occurs, which increases the chances of them sticking to this therapeutic approach.

### *Cognitive therapy*

Cognitive therapy depends upon the theory that anxiety occurs when the individual thinks they are unable to cope with a situation. It is the thought process that is important rather than the real threat associated with the situation. Such thoughts arise for a variety of reasons. Some people view the world in a way that makes it likely that they will overestimate the danger in any situation. Experiences in early life can give rise to cognitive schemata, such as 'it is vital to be in control all the time' or 'any mistake means failure', that will result in people feeling anxious in many situations. Once anxiety begins, a vicious cycle can be established in which symptoms escalate, as shown in Figure 4.

As discussed on pages 32–33, in cognitive therapy patients are helped to recognise links between their thoughts, feelings and behaviour. They learn to monitor the thoughts associated with episodes of anxiety, recognise thinking biases and challenge unrealistic assumptions and conclusions.

## *Case history 19*

Anton is a 36-year-old business man who has a social phobia and for the first time is doing a job that involves public speaking. He suffers severe palpitations and hyperventilation in these circumstances. This is proving to be a significant problem and he is threatened with redundancy.

a. How would you manage Anton's social phobia?

## Assessment and management of anxiety disorders

- Antidepressant drugs are effective in the treatment of anxiety disorders
- Support, reassurance and explanation of symptoms is important for all anxious patients
- Systematic desensitisation is a form of behaviour therapy that is effective in treatment of phobic anxiety disorders
- Cognitive therapy for anxiety disorders helps patients make links between their thoughts, mood and behaviour

# Obsessive–compulsive disorder

The characteristic features of obsessive–compulsive disorder (OCD) are obsessions and compulsions which interfere with a person's ability to cope with their daily life.

**Obsessions**, also known as obsessional ruminations, are unpleasant or distressing thoughts, impulses or images that come to mind over and over again, despite conscious efforts to stop them (Fig. 1). They dominate the person's mind and the sufferer is unable to distract themselves, leading to impairment of social and occupational function. Common themes for obsessional thoughts include violence, sex, contamination and blasphemy. Obsessional images may be of violent or gory scenes that come vividly to mind again and again, and cannot be ignored or suppressed. An obsessional impulse might be a recurrent impulse to hurt someone, usually someone the sufferer would not consciously wish to hurt. Such impulses are distressing and it is uncommon for people to act on them. It is important to distinguish obsessional thoughts from thought insertion, a first rank symptom of schizophrenia, in which the patient believes they are experiencing thoughts that are not their own. In contrast, obsessional thoughts are always recognised as arising from the patient's own mind.

**Compulsions** consist of a strong urge to perform an action or complex series of actions repeatedly, even though they are recognised as unnecessary. Compulsions can often be resisted for short periods, but this is usually associated with increasing levels of anxiety that can only be relieved by performing the compulsive act. Compulsions can take very many forms (Fig. 2), but the commonest are:

- hand washing and other cleaning behaviours
- counting, e.g. repeatedly counting objects in a room or avoiding particular numbers
- checking, e.g. returning home again and again to check the oven has been turned off or the door is locked
- touching, e.g. feeling compelled to touch each wall of every room entered
- arranging objects in lines, patterns, numbers, etc.

Complex rituals incorporating many of these compulsive acts may be developed and can cause substantial functional impairment.

The clinical picture in OCD is very variable. Patients may have obsessions only, compulsions only, or a combination of both. There is a very close relationship with depressive disorder. About 70% of cases have at least one episode of depressive disorder at some time in their life, and the two disorders can coexist. Patients with depressive episodes can develop obsessional symptoms without having full-blown OCD and in these cases treatment of the depressive disorder is usually enough to resolve the obsessional symptoms completely without other more specific treatments.

Impulse
' Smash the plate '
Thought
' The plate is filthy '
Image

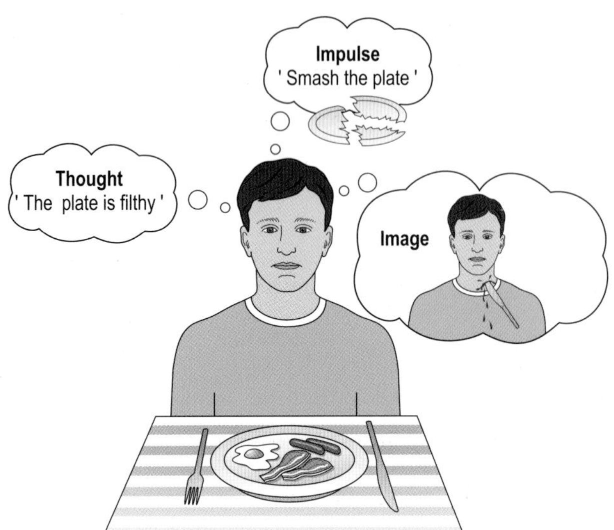

Fig. 1 **Obsessions – repeated and unpleasant thoughts, impulses or images.**

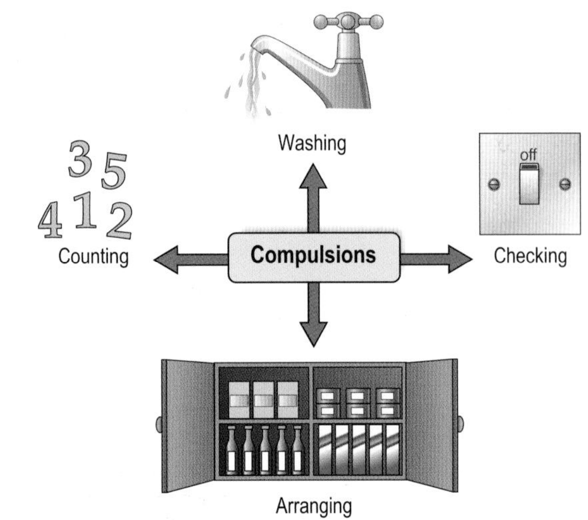


Fig. 2 **Compulsions.**

## Epidemiology

OCD is relatively common, with a lifetime prevalence of 2–3%. Unusually for the neurotic disorders it is equally common in men and women. It tends to begin in adolescence and occasionally in childhood but it takes more than 10 years on average for sufferers to seek help.

## Aetiology

There is greater concordance for OCD between monozygotic than dizygotic twins and one-third of the relatives of people who developed OCD in childhood have the condition themselves, suggesting a genetic aetiology, at least in some cases. Functional brain imaging studies have shown increased activity in the prefrontal cortex and basal ganglia, and structural scans have found a decrease in the average size of the caudate nucleus among groups of people with OCD. The effectiveness of SSRIs and clomipramine in OCD implies that serotonin transmission may be disrupted and the high rate of OCD symptoms in tic disorders and Tourette's syndrome suggests the involvement of dopamine.

Behavioural theories propose that classical and operant conditioning cause the person to associate certain objects with fear and use rituals to neutralise anxiety. Cognitive theory derives from the observation that many people occasionally have intrusive and unwanted thoughts, images and impulses and suggests that people prone to OCD exaggerate the importance of these experiences and dwell upon them.

## Management

A full psychiatric history, mental state examination and physical examination are required in all cases. The differential diagnosis of OCD is illustrated in Figure 3. Drug, psychological and social treatments should be considered and negotiated with the patient. Many patients will require a combination of all three.

### *Drug treatment*

Antidepressants which act on serotonin, such as SSRIs and the tricyclic clomipramine, are effective in some cases, even if there is no depression present. High doses are often needed and the therapeutic effect can take up to 12 weeks to develop. The combination of antidepressants and psychological treatment is the most effective.

### *Psychological treatment*

All patients with OCD should be offered cognitive behavioural therapy (CBT). Treatment sessions usually take place in clinic settings, but can involve going into patients' homes and are sometimes supported by co-therapists, who could be a nurse or a member of the patient's family. Inpatient treatment in specialist units is sometimes needed for severe cases. CBT will usually involve the following components:

- **Exposure and response prevention (ERP).** This technique is used in the prevention of rituals. The patient is exposed to an anxiety inducing situation and prevented from acting on the compulsive urge with the support of the therapist. For example, someone with an obsessional fear of contamination might be asked to touch a door handle and then resist the urge to wash their hands. The principles underlying this treatment are similar to those described for the treatment of phobic disorders on pages 58–59. ERP is the treatment for OCD with the strongest evidence base.
- **Cognitive techniques.** It is not usually the obsessional thought itself that is most problematic for the sufferer, but the anxiety and negative thoughts evoked. A patient who had recurrent thoughts about killing their child would find these repugnant and highly distressing. They might think of themselves as a terrible person and be frightened of acting on the thoughts. A cognitive approach would help them realise that the thought is merely a product of an illness, OCD, and is harmless. People with obsessional rituals often fear that something dreadful will happen if they don't follow their compulsive urge and such thoughts can be challenged using cognitive techniques. Similarly, patients can learn to question the obsessional doubt that causes their compulsion to engage in checking rituals.

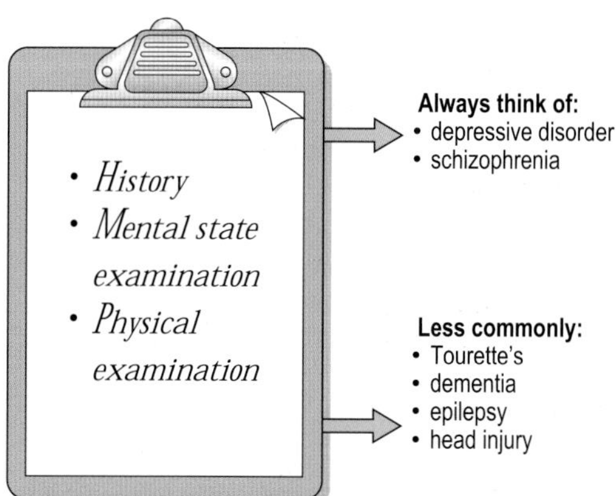


Fig. 3 **Differential diagnosis of OCD.**

### *Social treatment*

OCD can be a chronic and very disabling condition that can result in social isolation, unemployment and financial problems. The urge to carry out rituals can lead to self-neglect and the person's accommodation can become run down. Certain compulsions can cause damage, for example washing rituals can result in bathroom floors becoming damp and starting to rot. All these issues may need addressing. A person's rituals can come to dominate their home and family members can sometimes go along with the compulsive behaviours, rather than add to the person's anxiety. It is therefore important to provide support and education to families of people with OCD.

## Course and prognosis

OCD tends to be a chronic illness, with fluctuations in severity. If treatment is effective it is important to consider the long-term prevention of relapse. Education of the patient and their family about the disorder, and identification of the early signs of relapse with rapid reintroduction of treatment is helpful.

### *Case history 20*

Mary is a 42-year-old single woman who lives with her mother and works as an accountant. For most of her adult life she has been preoccupied by thoughts about dirt. She worries that things may be contaminated and has developed elaborate rituals to avoid contact with anything others may have touched. She washes her hands 50–60 times a day. She works alone in an office, and generally can limit her rituals to home, but at times her symptoms become worse and she is unable to touch paperwork that has been handled by other people.

a. What is Mary's differential diagnosis?
b. Devise a treatment plan considering drug, psychological and social treatments.

### Obsessive–compulsive disorder

- Obsessions are repeated unpleasant thoughts that persist despite attempts to resist them
- Compulsions are irresistible urges to repeatedly perform an action or ritual
- Depressive disorder is common in patients with OCD

# Reactions to stress

Many psychiatric conditions can be precipitated by 'stress' or adverse 'life events', but usually the individuals affected have some vulnerability to the mental illness as a result of genetic factors or childhood experiences, and there are many cases in which the condition develops in the absence of a precipitating factor. In contrast, the reactions to stress described here are a direct consequence of the stressful event, and would not arise without it. Two types of disorder will be described: post-traumatic stress disorder, which occurs in response to exceptionally severe stress, and adjustment disorders, which occur at the time of a life change or following a stressful event.

It is normal to react to stress in an emotional way. The disorders described here are considered to be abnormal reactions to stress either because the reaction is extreme or prolonged, or because it prevents the individual from functioning at home or work in their usual way. An abnormal reaction to stress may occur because of the nature of the stressor, or the way the individual copes with it, and often a combination of the two (Fig. 1). The stressor may be unusually intense, such as a combat situation or a natural disaster. Less intense events may be made more stressful by a long duration, or by a lack of control over events. Individual coping abilities are influenced by personality characteristics and previous experiences of stress and coping strategies. Stressful events are generally more difficult to cope with if they arise against a background of chronic social difficulties and lack of social supports.

## Acute stress reaction

This disorder is rarely seen by psychiatrists, but may present to GPs. It is short-lived, with symptoms settling within hours or at most a couple of days. The symptoms are severe, often with an initially dazed state, followed by a variety of reactions from stupor to marked agitation and overactivity. Panic attacks are common. The stress that precipitates an acute stress reaction is often an overwhelmingly traumatic physical or psychological experience, such as an assault, accident or bereavement. In most cases no treatment is required as the symptoms settle spontaneously. If medical help is sought, a short course of a benzodiazepine is an appropriate treatment, with further assessment and offer of support when the acute episode has passed.

## Post-traumatic stress disorder (PTSD)

PTSD occurs in response to an extremely stressful event, beyond the realms of usual experience, that would be distressing to anybody. This might include a serious accident or assault in which the life of the individual or their family is threatened, or a man-made or natural disaster. There is often a delay of days or weeks before the symptoms begin, although generally the disorder is established within six months of the stressor and runs a chronic, fluctuating course. The range of symptoms that may be found are shown in Figure 2 and, of the three groups of symptoms, it is recurrent thoughts about the traumatic event that differentiate PTSD from other anxiety and mood disorders. Vivid memories come to mind repeatedly despite attempts to block them out, either during waking hours or as nightmares during sleep, and these are often accompanied by the emotions that were experienced at the time of the trauma. Very intense and distressing flashbacks can occur, during which it feels to the affected person that the trauma is happening or about to happen again. Depressive disorder is a common complication, and alcohol or illicit drugs may be abused in an effort to cope with the symptoms.

The presence of the extreme stress is the key aetiological factor in PTSD. The greater the stress, the more likely it is that PTSD will develop. There is some evidence that it is more likely to develop in the aftermath of man-made as opposed to natural disasters, and if there are long-term stressful consequences to deal with, such as bereavement, disability, a court case, and loss of home or job. Those with a history of mental illness, poor coping skills or lack of social supports appear to be particularly vulnerable to PTSD.

Treatment of PTSD depends largely upon psychological therapies. Techniques used include debriefing, in which the patient is supported in recalling the traumatic event in great detail, and cognitive behavioural therapy. Considerable social support is likely to be required in most cases, as the sequelae of the trauma may have a direct impact on the patient's finances, work, accommodation and support network. SSRI antidepressants are effective in some cases, even if there is not a comorbid depressive disorder.

## Adjustment disorders

Adjustment disorders are abnormal responses to significant life changes, such as bereavement (see below), marital separation, redundancy or starting a new job. The abnormal response takes the form of an emotional disturbance, with symptoms of anxiety, depressed mood or feeling unable to cope. The symptoms are not severe enough to merit a diagnosis of depressive disorder or anxiety disorder, but interfere with the patient's ability to function normally at home, work or in social situations. Adjustment disorders usually begin within a month of the precipitating event, and in most cases resolve within six months. Simple psychological and social treatments, such as providing the patient with support, an opportunity to talk about their feelings and a practical problem-solving approach are often all that is required.

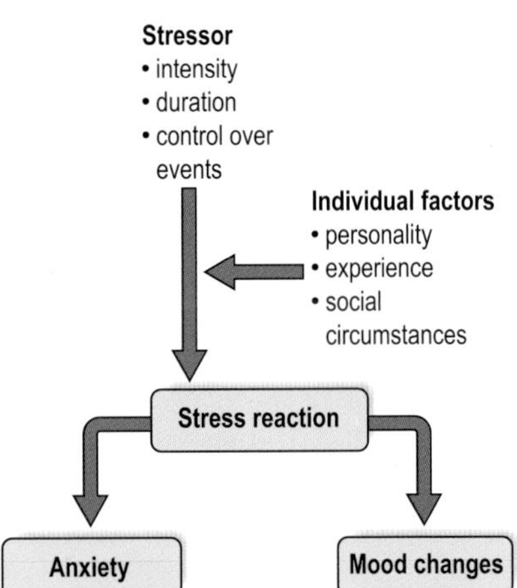


Fig. 1 **Stress reaction.**

## Bereavement

Loss of a close relative or friend is always an extremely stressful event that will inevitably provoke a marked emotional response. This is, of course, entirely normal, and the majority cope with their grief without any professional help. The normal grieving process is shown in Figure 3. It can closely resemble depressive illness with persistent low mood, insomnia, loss of appetite and thoughts of hopelessness and guilt. The only treatment required, however, is support, an opportunity to talk, and reassurance that it is part of a normal process of adjustment that will gradually improve.

### *Abnormal grief*

Grief is considered to be abnormal if:

- **There is a considerable delay before it begins.** For example, a mother of two young children felt unable to grieve after the death of her mother because she did not want

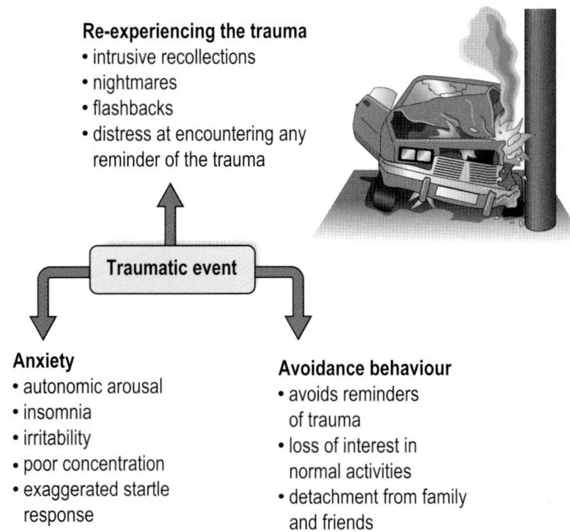


Fig. 2 **Symptoms of PTSD.**

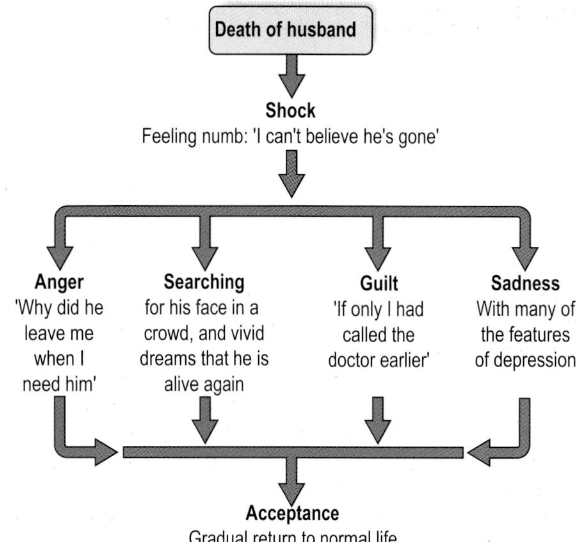


Fig. 3 **Normal grief.**

to distress her children. She put all thoughts of her mother to the back of her mind, and got on with life until 18 months later she became extremely depressed, tearful and felt life was no longer worth living after the death of her dog. The suppressed grief for her mother was finally expressed, but at an inappropriate time.

- **Symptoms are very intense.** For example, an elderly man, distressed after the sudden death of his wife, became increasingly concerned with his own health. He began to believe that his insides were rotting away and that he would die soon. These nihilistic delusions required inpatient psychiatric treatment.
- **Symptoms are very prolonged.** It is difficult to apply fixed time limits on normal grief, as it will vary depending upon the individual and the circumstances of the bereavement. Generally, however, the most intense feelings of grief will begin to resolve, with resumption of normal activities, within six months. Grief may become 'stuck' at one stage of the process, for example there may be prolonged feelings of numbness and shock, or an inability to accept the reality of the loss.

An abnormal grief reaction is more likely to arise if the death was sudden, or if the relationship with the dead person was overly dependent or difficult in some way. Treatment is often with bereavement therapy, in which the individual is encouraged to talk in detail about events leading up to the death and following it, and guided through the normal grief process, for example by being encouraged to ventilate unresolved feelings of anger and guilt. Cruse is a UK charity that provides bereavement counselling and other support for bereaved people.

## *Case history 21*

John is a 52-year-old man. He was involved in an incident 6 months ago in which he was trapped in a lift with no lights and no means of calling help. He suffered angina prior to this, and while trapped had severe chest pain, and believed that he would die. He was rescued after 4 hours, and was found to have had a myocardial infarction. Subsequently, he has been unable to return to work. He has frequent nightmares in which the incident is rerun, and during the day is preoccupied by thoughts of the incident, with high levels of anxiety and panic attacks in which he becomes breathless with chest pain and fears he will die.

a. What is the likely diagnosis?
b. What treatment options are available to him?

## Reactions to stress

- Abnormal reactions to stress occur because of the unusual severity of the stress or because the individual lacks the resources to cope with the stress
- PTSD occurs after extreme stress and is characterised by re-experiencing the stressful event, anxiety symptoms and avoidance of reminders of the stress
- Adjustment disorders are abnormal responses to significant life changes and are characterised by low mood and anxiety

# Dissociative and somatoform disorders

## Dissociative (conversion) disorders

Dissociative disorders present with physical or cognitive signs that have no organic cause. They have a sudden onset and are triggered by a traumatic event, insoluble or intolerable problems, or disturbed relationships. ICD10 describes various types of dissociative disorders.

**Dissociative amnesia** presents with loss of all memory for personal information and events. Patients present saying that they do not know who they are, where they are from or what has happened to them. They have no evidence of organic brain disorder and retain the ability to learn new information. The pattern of memory loss is therefore very different from a typical organic amnesia, where new information is not recalled but long-term memory for personal details is usually retained. **Dissociative fugue** presents with dissociative amnesia and, in addition, the affected person travels away from their usual environment, sometimes ending up many miles from home with no memory for the period of travel.

**Dissociative stupor** presents with reduced or absent movement and responsiveness, but it is clear that the patient is neither asleep or unconscious and physical examination and investigations are normal. **Dissociative disorders of movement and sensation** present with physical signs that do not conform to recognised neurological syndromes and often vary in severity, depending on whether the person is being observed and their emotional state. A variant is **Dissociative convulsions**, also known as pseudoseizures, in which there are generalised tonic–clonic movements, usually without tongue biting, incontinence of urine or true loss of consciousness.

### *Aetiology*

Dissociative disorders are said to develop as a result of two psychological defence mechanisms, dissociation and conversion, that are used to cope with trauma or emotional conflict that is so painful or distressing it cannot be allowed into the conscious mind. Dissociation results in a loss of integration between mental functions. In conversion, distressing thoughts are transformed ('converted') into physical symptoms, sometimes in a way that symbolises the trauma or conflict that caused them. For example, a boy who witnessed the murder of his mother developed dissociative sensory loss that presented with blindness.

Dissociation and conversion can lead to primary and secondary gain, as shown in Figure 1. In chronic cases, secondary gain is often a maintaining factor.

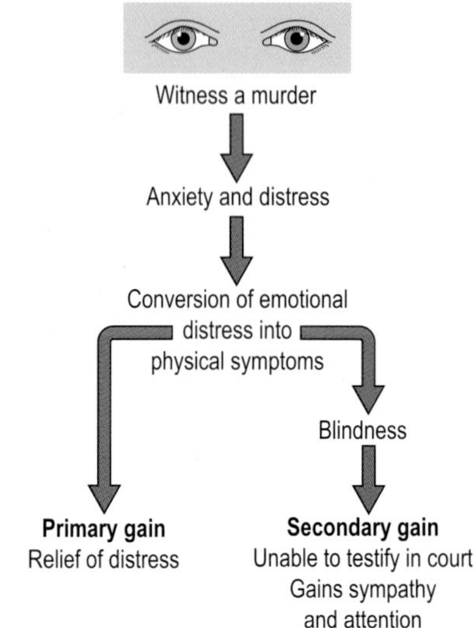


Fig. 1 **Primary and secondary gain in dissociative disorder.**

'I can't see'
'I can't see'
Dissociative disorder
• Usually neurological symptoms
• Unconcious psychological mechanisms
• Relief from distress and primary gain
'I want to come into hospital to be looked after'
'I'm in terrible pain'
Factitious disorder
• Acute physical illness
• Deliberate deception of medical staff
• Care in hospital
'If they admit me into hospital I won't be able to go to court tomorrow'
'I'm in terrible pain'
Malingering
• Acute physical illness
• Deliberate deception of medical staff
• Personal gain

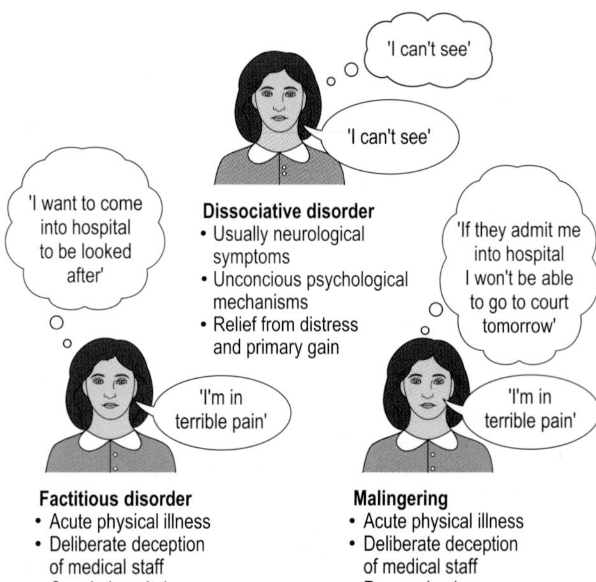

Fig. 2 **Comparison of dissociative disorder, factitious disorder and malingering.**

### *Management*

Dissociative disorder must always be a positive diagnosis, based upon a history that provides some reasonable psychological explanation of how and why the problem developed. The patient may deny recent stressful events and problems or disturbed relationships, so it is important to seek information from others. Great care must be taken to exclude organic pathology and it should be remembered that follow-up studies of people diagnosed with dissociative disorders have found that many turned out to have an underlying physical condition. Catatonic schizophrenia and severe depressive episodes should be considered in cases of stupor. Two further differential diagnoses are factitious disorder, also known as Munchausen's syndrome, and malingering, the major features of which are shown in Figure 2.

Treatment for dissociative disorder is psychological and social. Stressful events and problems should be gently explored and discussed. Practical sources of distress and interpersonal problems should be addressed. Sources of secondary gain should be reduced as much as possible.

Dissociative disorders usually remit within a few weeks, particularly if their onset was associated with a traumatic event. Chronic forms are less common and tend to be associated with insoluble problems and interpersonal difficulties.

## Somatoform disorders

Somatoform disorders present with physical symptoms that have no physical cause and do not have the abrupt onset associated with dissociative disorders. The sufferer repeatedly seeks medical treatment or investigations, even when these have consistently failed to be of benefit to them. ICD10 describes several different types.

**Somatisation disorder** is a condition in which the patient presents recurrent, frequently changing physical symptoms that cannot be explained by organic pathology. Symptoms may involve any part of the body, but most often are gastrointestinal (pain, nausea, vomiting), and abnormal skin sensations (burning, itching, tingling). Consultations with doctors tend to focus on the patient's demands that some treatment be found

The symptoms you've told me about sound a real problem. Do they cause you to worry or feel down sometimes?
I think if we work on the other problems in your life, you'll feel better in yourself and that might make it easier to deal with your physical problems. Shall we give it a try?
Most physical illnesses get worse if the person is feeling tense or depressed. Asthma is a good example – it's a physical problem like yours but it gets worse if the person is feeling bad emotionally.
Some people have physical illnesses that we never find a reason for. The good news is that there are still ways I can help you.

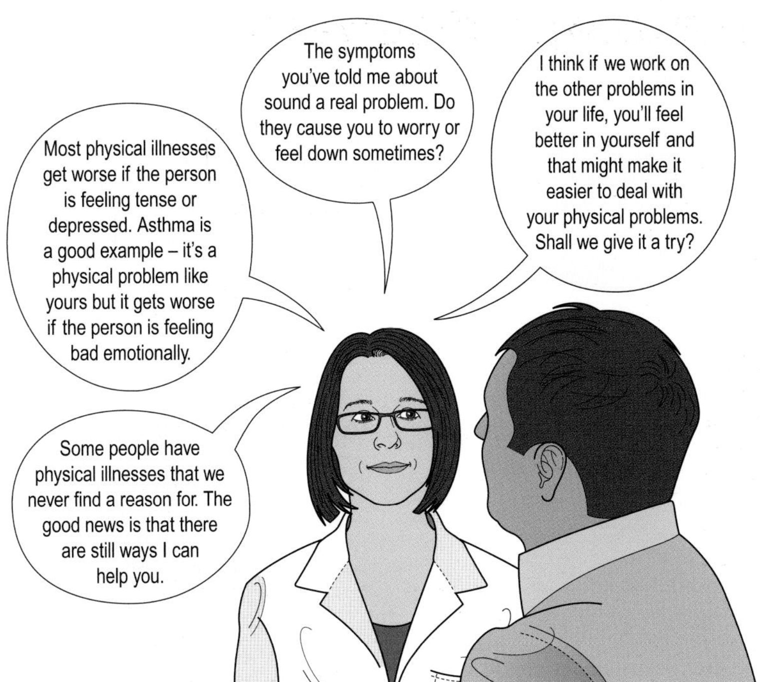

Fig. 3 **Engaging a patient with somatisation disorder in treatment.**

to relieve their symptoms. They angrily seek explanations for their symptoms, and are not satisfied with reassurances about negative investigations.

Somatisation disorder is more common in women, and usually begins in early adult life. In primary care, many cases will resolve within a year but chronic severe cases occur and are often associated with long-standing disruption of social, interpersonal and family life.

**Hypochondriacal disorder** is characterised by a persistent preoccupation with the possibility of having one or more serious and progressive physical disorders. Patients have physical symptoms but, in contrast to somatisation disorder, their main concern is what might be causing these symptoms. Sometimes their anxiety is focused on their physical appearance, which they consider to be deformed or disfigured in some way, and this variant is sometimes given the separate diagnosis of **body dysmorphic disorder**. Hypochondriasis is as common in men as women.

**Somatoform autonomic dysfunction** is similar to hypochondriasis, but presents with symptoms of autonomic arousal, such as palpitations, sweating, tremor and flushing, which are persistent and troubling. The patient is preoccupied by the possibility of a serious physical disorder, usually of the heart, respiratory system or gastrointestinal tract. **Persistent somatoform pain disorder** presents with persistent, severe and distressing pain for which no physical cause can be found.

### *Aetiology*

Most medically unexplained physical symptoms arise from people interpreting normal or commonplace bodily sensations as evidence of illness. They then dwell on these symptoms, which results in emotional disturbance, physiological arousal, and changes in interpersonal relationships, all of which can maintain the problem. A variety of factors affect the way people interpret their bodily sensations, such as personal or family experience of illness in childhood or adult life and media coverage of health issues. There are often pre-existing emotional and relationship problems and social difficulties.

### *Management*

Ideally one doctor, usually the GP, should take a lead role offering regular, planned appointments and limiting the involvement of others. Physical causes must be excluded, but the pressure to investigate excessively should be resisted, as it will compound the patient's problems. They will often resent any explanation of their condition that implies a psychological cause and some suggestions about how to broach this subject are given in Figure 3. The aim of the appointments should be to encourage the patient to look at other aspects of their life, and where appropriate make a link between physical symptoms, emotions and life events. Pain management programmes are often helpful. Depression and anxiety are frequently present and may justify specific treatment.

## *Case history 22*

Mike is a 24-year-old man who presented to hospital with paralysis of his right arm. He was brought up in a children's home and has a tendency to think other people don't care about him. On the day of admission he met his girlfriend's family for the first time and was keen to make a good impression. His girlfriend's brother was rude and abusive towards him, and Mike had a very strong impulse to hit him.

a. What precipitated this disorder?
b. What psychological mechanism underlies it?
c. Can you identify possible primary and secondary gains for Mike?

## Dissociative and somatoform disorders

- Dissociative disorders present with physical and cognitive signs, somatoform disorders with physical symptoms
- The disorders are not due to organic pathology
- Initial presentation is to GPs and general hospital doctors
- The patient does not recognise the psychological factors underlying the symptoms

# Liaison psychiatry

Very few disorders can be considered to wholly affect the body but not the mind, and vice versa. The majority of psychiatric disorders have some impact upon the patient's physical wellbeing. For example, depression can result in weight loss, constipation and tiredness, in addition to having an impact on the individual's ability to cope with any existing physical illness. Pain from arthritis is often worse during a depressive episode. Similarly, physical disorders will often affect the emotional state of the patient. Feelings of anxiety, depressed mood, anger and frustration are common accompaniments to physical illness. They will impact upon the recovery process (Fig. 1), and mental illness may be precipitated.

High rates of mental illness have been found in general hospitals, even when those patients being treated for overdose and other forms of deliberate self harm are excluded from the figures. Up to 60% of medical inpatients have a mental disorder, and up to half of all medical outpatients. A quarter of male medical inpatients have problems associated with alcohol abuse. The reasons for these high rates are illustrated in Figure 2.

## Liaison psychiatry

Liaison psychiatry is a sub-specialty of psychiatry in which a service is offered to patients of a general hospital. A liaison psychiatry team in a general hospital would usually include a psychiatrist, a psychologist, psychiatric nurses and social workers, and sometimes other mental health professionals. They provide input to patients in the hospital in two ways:

- **consultation**, in which patients are assessed by members of the liaison psychiatrist at the request of the physician or surgeon caring for them
- **liaison**, in which members of the liaison psychiatry team have a broader role and become integrated into the work of their general hospital colleagues. They may attend ward rounds or take part in assessment or follow-up of patients attending outpatient clinics. This approach is time-consuming but improves joint working between general hospital and mental health staff. It also reduces the stigma of a psychiatric referral, which can be a problem with the consultation model, particularly for patients with conditions such as somatisation disorder, in which psychological explanations for symptoms are actively resisted.

The consultation model of service is the most widely practised, and at the most basic level psychiatrists may provide consultations for patients admitted following deliberate self harm and psychiatric emergencies only. The integrated liaison model of service, where it exists, is usually focused on specific areas where psychiatric morbidity is highest and has most impact on the management of the physical illness. This may include pain clinics, oncology wards, paediatric and geriatric departments.

## Psychological causes of physical illness

There is good evidence that stress plays an important role in the aetiology of many physical disorders. For example, studies have demonstrated an increase in stressful life events in the weeks prior to myocardial infarction, acute abdominal pain and acute subarachnoid haemorrhage.

Mental illness is also associated with increased morbidity and mortality from a wide range of physical disorders. This continues to be true even when disorders directly associated with the mental illness are not included in the figures, such as deliberate self harm and the effects of alcohol abuse. This is likely to be due to a combination of factors, including the effects of stress, increased tendency to smoke and take illicit drugs, harmful effects of prescribed drugs and failure to seek medical help.

Mental illness may present with physical symptoms, thereby obscuring the primary diagnosis, and in some cases

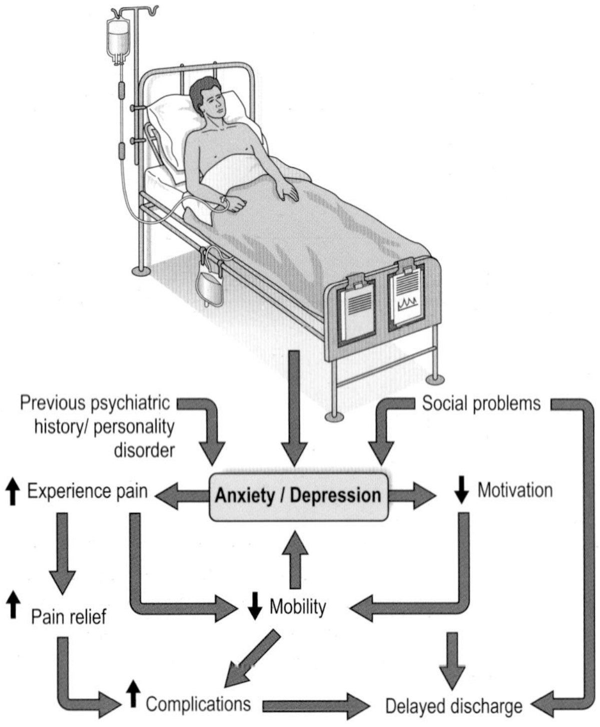


Fig. 1 **Impact of psychological symptoms on recovery from physical illness.**

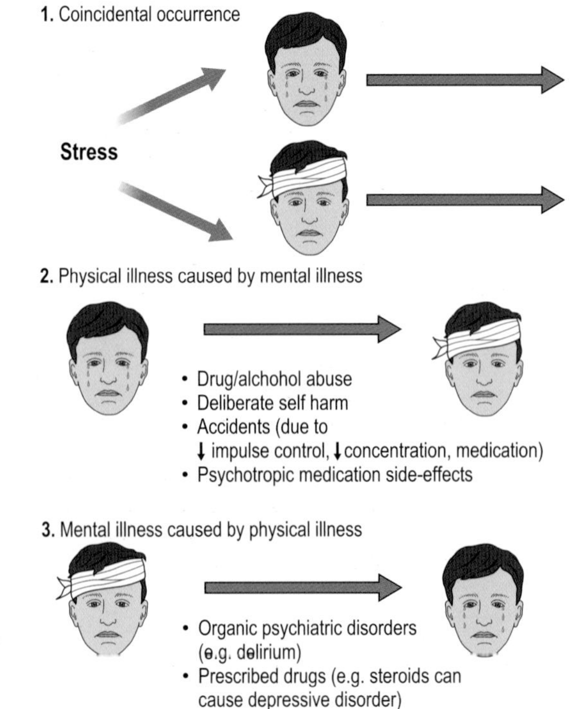


Fig. 2 **Factors determining the coexistence of physical and mental illness.**

resulting in unnecessary and potentially harmful investigations and treatment. For example:

- **Depressive disorder** may present with biological symptoms including sleep disturbance, loss of energy and lethargy, sexual dysfunction, loss of appetite and weight loss and loss of concentration with apparent memory loss resulting in a misdiagnosis of dementia (known as pseudodementia).
- **Anxiety disorders** frequently present with predominantly physical symptoms. They include sweating, palpitations, tremor, urinary frequency, diarrhoea, hyperventilation, muscular pain, dry mouth, muscle tension, restlessness, dizziness, syncope, chest pain, chest tightness, shortness of breath, paraesthesia and headache. Anxiety symptoms may occur in other mental illnesses such as depression, schizophrenia and obsessive–compulsive disorder.
- **Eating disorders** may present with weight loss and its consequences, which include bradycardia, hypotension, constipation, amenorrhoea, muscle weakness, peripheral oedema, osteoporosis and fractures (p. 76).
- **Dependence on alcohol** can have an impact on virtually any body system. Effects on the cardiovascular system include hypertension and atrial fibrillation. The gastrointestinal system is often profoundly affected, with increased risk of carcinomas of the gastrointestinal tract, gastritis, pancreatitis, nutritional deficiencies and hepatic disorders including cirrhosis, cancer and hepatitis. Infertility, impotence and loss of secondary sexual characteristics are common. Alcoholics are prone to accidents, including those involving road traffic. Problems also arise as a result of withdrawal, with convulsions and acute confusional states. All patients, whether they are seen in medical, surgical or psychiatric settings, should be asked about alcohol consumption.
- **Dissociative disorders** present with physical signs that have no organic cause, but instead are due to psychological factors of which the patient has no conscious awareness (see p. 64).
- **Somatoform disorders** present with physical symptoms that have no organic cause. People with the condition often end up being seen in specialist clinics, in the hope that an underlying physical illness will be found and some will end up being admitted to general hospitals because of their demands that something be done about their symptoms. They are very difficult to engage in treatment, because they are convinced there is a physical cause of their problems, and liaison psychiatry teams develop expertise in their management.
- **Factitious disorder (Munchausen's syndrome)** is a condition in which the person manufactures symptoms and sometimes signs of physical illness, so that they are admitted to hospital. Their underlying problem is a need to be cared for and many have emotionally unstable personality disorder, borderline type.

## Psychological consequences of physical illness

Almost all physical illnesses evoke some form of psychological reaction, but in most cases this is not distressing, and has minimal impact on the patient's life. More severe reactions usually manifest themselves as depressive symptoms, anxiety or anger, and in most cases are transient. Mental illness may occur, most often adjustment disorders or depression. They are more likely to occur in patients with a personal or family history of mental illness, personality disorder or chronic social problems. Factors such as previous negative experience of illness, lack of social support, compensation claims or other forms of litigation can have a significant impact on the patient's ability to cope with their illness, and their emotional response.

The majority of emotional reactions to illness can be managed without referral to a psychiatrist. Good communication between staff and patient is essential. Anxieties often respond to open discussion about the illness, investigations, treatment and prognosis. Patients and their carers need to have information presented in a meaningful way, and an opportunity to ask questions and talk about their worries.

Some physical illnesses can present with psychological symptoms, and cause diagnostic difficulties (see Table 1).

Table 1 **Physical illness may present with psychological symptoms**

| Symptom | Physical disorder |
|---|---|
| Depressed mood | Drugs<br>Carcinoma<br>Infections<br>Neurological disorders<br>Diabetes<br>Thyroid disorders<br>Cushing disease |
| Anxiety | Hyperthyroidism<br>Hyperventilation<br>Phaeochromocytoma<br>Hypoglycaemia<br>Drug withdrawal |
| Disturbed behaviour | Epilepsy<br>Hypoglycaemia<br>Toxic states |

### *Case history 23*

Mary is a 46-year-old woman who is married with no children. She consults her GP often, sometimes several times a week, and at least monthly over many years. Her complaints have varied, and include abdominal pain, dysuria, dysmenorrhoea, menorrhagia, and tiredness. Over the years she has been referred to gynaecologists, urologists and general surgeons. Extensive investigations have revealed no organic cause for her symptoms. Despite this she remains convinced that she has a serious physical illness that is undiagnosed, and demands further referrals, investigations, and pain relief. She angrily refuses psychiatric referral. She is disabled by her symptoms to the extent that her husband has recently given up work to become her full-time carer.

a. What is the likely diagnosis?
b. How would you advise the GP to manage her care?

### Liaison psychiatry

- Physical and mental illness frequently coexist
- Mental illness is associated with high morbidity and mortality from a wide range of physical disorders
- Primary mental illness may present with physical symptoms and vice versa
- Emotional reactions to physical illness are common and should be managed by providing information and giving the patient an opportunity to talk

# Psychiatry in primary care

The majority of people who are diagnosed with a mental illness have no contact with the psychiatric services; instead they are treated by their general practitioner (GP) and other members of the primary healthcare team. The most common mental illnesses treated by GPs are depressive disorder, generalised anxiety disorder and mixed depression and anxiety. Many more patients have emotional problems, such as low mood, and worries that do not amount to a mental illness. Many will also have a coexisting physical illness and will not complain directly about their psychological symptoms. Recognising mental illness in these circumstances poses a special challenge and is described in more detail below.

## Psychiatric disorders in primary care

### Mood disorders

Depressive disorder is the most common psychiatric disorder treated in primary care and is present in about 10% of all GP attenders, with a further 10% having depressive symptoms. In comparison with depressed patients seen by psychiatric services those in primary care tend to be less severely ill and have more anxiety symptoms. The presentation is often with physical symptoms rather than depressed mood. The treatment should be with antidepressant drugs in moderate or severe cases. Mild cases will often resolve with support and help to address social problems. Psychological treatments that are known to be effective in depression, such as cognitive therapy, are rarely available in primary care. The effectiveness of non-specific 'counselling' in depression is not known. GPs can expect one of their patients to commit suicide every 4 years. Up to 40% of patients who die by suicide have seen their GP in the month before death, and half of these in the week before death.

### Anxiety disorders

There is a great overlap between depression and anxiety disorders in primary care, and patients presenting with anxiety symptoms should be asked about mood symptoms. Many cases are mild and will respond to advice, reassurance and support.

### Alcohol abuse

There is evidence that patients act on advice from their GP to reduce their alcohol consumption, and reductions of up to 20% of the number of problem drinkers can be achieved by the GP routinely asking about alcohol consumption and giving appropriate advice.

## Recognising mental illness in primary care

Only half of the patients presenting with the most common conditions found in primary care, depression and anxiety, are recognised as mentally ill by their GP. The reasons and some possible ways of addressing them are summarised in Figure 1. In part this is because patients frequently present with physical rather than psychological complaints. Patients come to psychiatric outpatient clinics expecting to talk about their feelings, and will often have had an opportunity to think about their emotional state in preparation for this. The expectations of a GP consultation are quite different. Patients often believe that the doctor will be interested in physical symptoms only and may not consider their emotions to be relevant to any diagnosis, and so omit to mention them. Instead, the complaint may be of the biological symptoms of depression (insomnia, anorexia, weight loss) or health concerns due to hypochondriacal preoccupations, or of an exacerbation of an existing physical illness. Pain, discomfort and disability may be more difficult to bear when depressed. In these circumstances it is up to the doctor to be alert to any indications of emotional distress demonstrated during the consultation (see Fig. 2), and to ask direct questions about psychological symptoms, for example:

- 'You seem tense (angry, unhappy, worried …), can you tell me about that?'
- 'How have you been feeling in yourself recently?'
- 'Have you been worried about anything in particular?'

Some doctors are more sensitive to patients' emotions and are more comfortable talking about feelings than others. It has been shown that the doctor's behaviour has a great effect on the likelihood of a patient revealing any feelings of distress. Patients disclose more to doctors who:

- appear to be unhurried, with time to talk about problems
- make eye contact as the patient enters the room and maintain regular eye contact

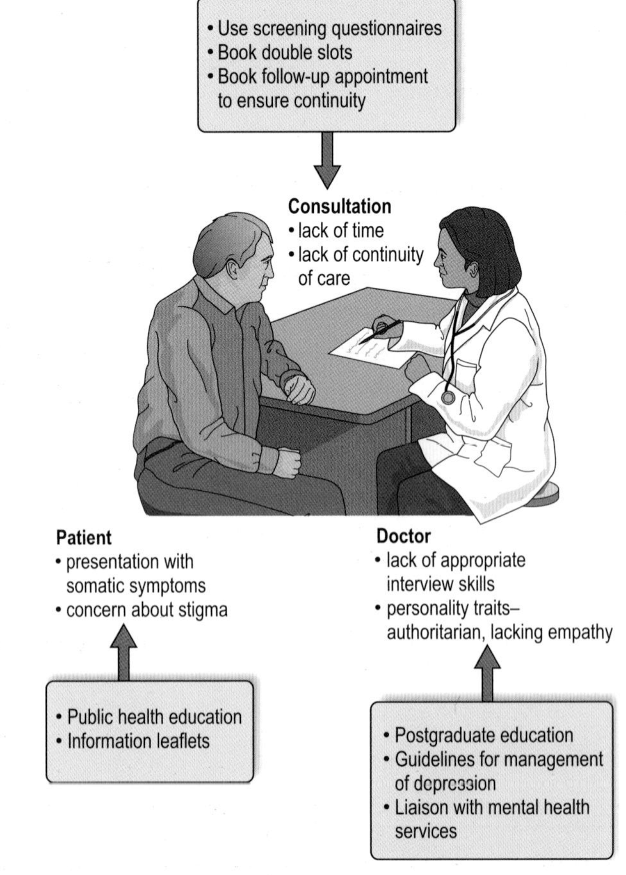


Fig. 1 **Reasons and potential solutions for non-recognition of mental illness in primary care.**

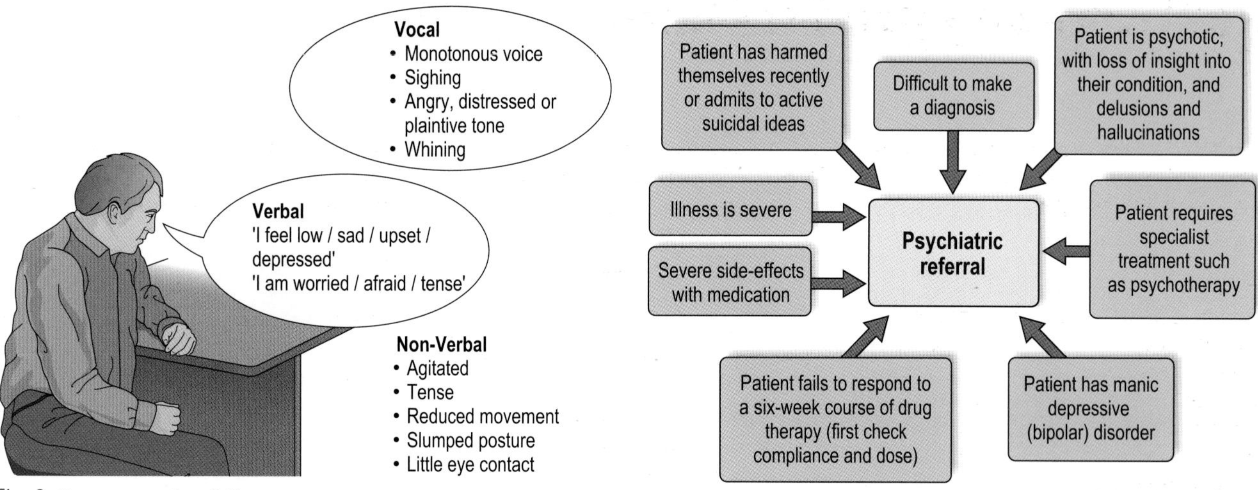


Fig. 2 **Cues to emotional distress.**

Fig. 3 **Referral to psychiatric services.**

- talk less and listen more
- ask open questions about psychological and social issues
- demonstrate empathy
- notice and comment on verbal and non-verbal signs of distress.

Time constraints are a great problem in primary care. Consultations last 5–10 minutes on average, and it is difficult to manage an unhurried, open and empathic interview in this time. Patients with mental illness are likely to need longer than average consultations, and it is often helpful to book them into a double slot to avoid holding everyone else up. Assessments may also be done over several visits, and this may be supplemented with information leaflets for patients to read between visits that will provide a useful focus for discussion of symptoms at later consultations.

## Management of mental illness in primary care

The GP's role in the management of mental illness includes assessment, diagnosis and development of a management plan with the patient. Some patients are reluctant to accept a diagnosis of mental illness, and it is worth spending some time with them to explain the reasons for making the diagnosis and the opportunities for treatment. Information leaflets and videotapes are often useful in reinforcing this message. It is important to avoid the situation where a patient who talks about worries feels he has not been heard and simply sent away with a prescription of antidepressants. The patient may not realise that the doctor has recognised evidence of an illness that if treated may allow him to cope more effectively with the problem. The prescription is likely to be thrown away in these circumstances. Patients with depressive disorder and generalised anxiety disorder are likely to benefit from antidepressant drug prescription. Compliance with these drugs is known to be very poor in primary care. Up to two-thirds of patients will no longer be taking the tablets one month after the initial prescription.

Many psychological treatments for mental illness are now provided by practitioners working in primary care. The stepped care of depression, described on pages 54–55, is an example of this. The practitioners who provide psychological treatments for depression in primary care also work with people with anxiety disorders, OCD, PTSD and adjustment disorders.

Other members of the primary healthcare team have important roles in the detection and treatment of mental illness. Practice nurses are often actively involved in health promotion, screening new patients and the elderly for early signs of preventable or treatable conditions, and providing information and advice. Screening for depressive illness, anxiety disorders and alcohol abuse should be a part of this work. They may also monitor patient compliance and progress with drug treatment. Health visitors are ideally placed to detect postnatal depression, and district nurses work with the elderly and chronically physically ill and disabled patients, who also have an increased risk of depressive illness.

## Referral to secondary mental health services

There is an increasing trend towards secondary mental health services moving out to the community and in some cases locating outpatient clinics in primary care surgeries. Community psychiatric nurses may also use the surgeries as a base. There are therefore increasing opportunities for face to face liaison between psychiatrists, CPNs and GPs. The common reasons for referral to psychiatric services are shown in Figure 3.

### *Case history 24*

Jane is a 26-year-old single mother of two children aged 3 years and 6 months. The children's father left her before the birth of the baby and has had no contact with them and provided no financial support. Jane attends her GP very frequently, usually with concerns about the children's health and complaints that she feels run down and tired all the time. Her GP thinks she has postnatal depression.

a. How should the GP manage her depression?
b. Which other members of the primary healthcare team may have a role in managing Jane's problems?

### Psychiatry in primary care

- 90% of patients diagnosed with mental illness are managed exclusively in primary care
- 20% of all patients consulting in primary care are depressed
- About half of these patients are not recognised as mentally ill by their GP
- The commonest disorders are depressive disorder, generalised anxiety disorder and alcohol abuse

# Syndromes of cognitive impairment

As described on page 7, organic disorders are 'diseases of the body' which present with psychiatric symptoms. In contrast, functional psychiatric disorders are considered to be 'diseases of the mind'. Classifying psychiatric disorders in this way is becoming outdated now that more is known about the 'organic' basis of functional illnesses, such as abnormal brain structure in schizophrenia. However, the term organic is still commonly used and is included in ICD10. Organic disorders will be described in this section, starting with syndromes of cognitive impairment.

## Delirium and dementia

In both dementia and delirium, there is a generalised impairment of brain function which causes global impairment in cognitive function and altered mood and behaviour. The difference between the two is that delirium is an acute syndrome characterised by fluctuating levels of consciousness and attention whereas dementia is a chronic syndrome which occurs in clear consciousness without rapid fluctuations. Both conditions are more common in older people, but the diagnoses need to be considered in any patient who presents with a generalised impairment of brain function.

### *Delirium*

In delirium a group of characteristic symptoms occur as a result of an acute, generalised impairment of brain function. The most common causes are shown in Table 1. Delirium is more likely to occur in children, when the brain is still developing, and in the elderly, when the brain is starting to degenerate. People with dementia are particularly at risk and so it is always important to rule out a superimposed delirium if the cognitive function of people with dementia deteriorates acutely. Another high risk group is people admitted to elderly medicine wards – studies have found 15–50% show evidence of delirium.

The patient's level of consciousness and attention fluctuates, often with a diurnal pattern, usually being worse at night. They are drowsy with a reduced response to external stimuli at times, and at other times are hypervigilant and distractable. Other common features are disorientation, impaired recall, disturbances of the sleep–wake cycle, persecutory delusions, perceptual disturbance and emotional disturbance. These features are summarised and contrasted with typical symptoms of dementia in Table 2.

The primary goal in the management of delirium is investigation and treatment of the underlying cause. While this is taking place, it will be necessary to manage the patient symptomatically. They should be nursed in a well-lit room by as few people as possible, in order to reduce their confusion. Sedation with low doses of antipsychotic drugs may be required. Confusion can be exacerbated by anticholinergic drugs; haloperidol is often used because it has little effect on cholinergic receptors. Benzodiazepines are an alternative but can exacerbate delerium.

### *Dementia*

Dementia is a chronic generalised impairment of brain function. It is usually progressive but does not have to be for the diagnosis to be made. The risk increases with age with 5% of people over 65 years and 20% of people over 80 years being affected. An easily remembered definition of dementia is that it is a global **IMP**airment of **I**ntellect, **M**emory and **P**ersonality. However, it will be seen from the following list of typical symptoms that other aspects of brain function are also affected:

- **Memory** is virtually always affected, with short-term memory and memory for recent events being lost first. Memory of events from the distant past is usually preserved until the late stages of the illness.
- **Orientation in time and place** are lost relatively early in the illness which may result in the person becoming lost and wandering aimlessly. In the later stages of the illness, orientation in person may be lost with the person not recognising familiar people or themselves.
- **Praxis**, the ability to co-ordinate complex motor acts, is affected. The person may not be able to perform acts on command but still perform them spontaneously (ideomotor apraxia), or may be unable to carry out a sequence of tasks despite being able to perform each task individually (ideational apraxia).
- **Language function** is impaired, initially with difficulty finding words (nominal dysphasia), progressing to difficulties generating speech (expressive dysphasia), comprehending speech (receptive dysphasia) or a combination of the two (mixed dysphasia).
- **Thinking** is often impoverished with a reduced flow of ideas and difficulty attending to more than one

Table 1 **Causes of delirium**

| | |
|---|---|
| Intoxication with drugs | Anticholinergics<br>Anticonvulsants<br>Anxiolytics/hypnotics<br>Digoxin<br>L-dopa<br>Corticosteroids<br>Alcohol<br>Solvents<br>Illicit drugs |
| Drug withdrawal | Alcohol<br>Benzodiazepines |
| Systemic | Infection<br>Endocrine<br>■ hypoglycaemia<br>■ hyperparathyroidism<br>■ Addison's disease<br>Metabolic<br>■ electrolyte imbalance<br>■ hypoxia<br>■ renal failure<br>■ liver failure<br>■ thiamine deficiency<br>■ porphyria |
| Neurological | Infections<br>■ meningitis<br>■ encephalitis<br>Raised intracranial pressure<br>Space occupying lesions<br>Head injury<br>Epilepsy<br>■ epileptic status<br>■ post-ictal states |

Table 2 **Features of delirium and dementia**

| | Delirium | Dementia |
|---|---|---|
| **Onset** | Acute, usually within hours or days | Gradual, usually at least 6 months |
| **Diurnal variation** | Yes, usually worse at night | May be worse at night |
| **Duration** | Days or weeks, usually less than 6 months | Months or years |
| **Consciousness/Alertness** | Drowsy or hypervigilant | Normal |
| **Attention** | Usually poor | Usually maintained |
| **Orientation** | Disorientated in time, often in place and person | Similar changes but later in course of illness |
| **Instant recall** | Impaired | Only impaired in late stages |
| **Memory** | Impaired | Impaired |
| **Thinking** | Increased, reduced or muddled | Reduced |
| **Delusions** | Common | Occur, but less common |
| **Illusions/Hallucinations** | Common, usually visual | Only occur in late stages |
| **Sleep** | Reversal of sleep–wake cycle common | Insomnia in some cases |

thing at a time. Persecutory ideas may develop, often as a consequence of poor memory and disorientation.

- **Abstract thinking and judgement** are impaired, leaving the person unable to deal with problems or unfamiliar situations.
- **Personality changes** are common, often involving a coarsening of pre-existing personality traits.
- **Social behaviour** deteriorates, often becoming shallow or inappropriate.
- **Mood changes** are common with depression, irritability and anxiety all occurring in some cases.

For a diagnosis of dementia to be made with certainty, there must be evidence of deficits in several of these areas. Once the diagnosis is made, it is important to try to establish the cause of the dementia as this will influence treatment and prognosis. As with delirium, dementia is a syndrome with a variety of causes, as shown in Table 3. The three commonest causes (Alzheimer's disease, vascular dementia and Lewy body dementia) are discussed on page 90. Less common neurological causes of dementia are described on pages 72–73.

## Syndromes caused by focal brain damage

### *Amnesic syndrome*

Amnesic syndrome is a disorder of memory in which other aspects of cognitive function remain relatively unaffected. This distinguishes it from dementia, in which there is a global impairment of cognitive function. Patients with amnesic syndrome have normal instant recall but cannot learn new information and have marked impairment of 5 minute recall. There is poor memory of recent and past events, with memory for more recent events being worse than distant memory. Social skills and other aspects of cognitive function are relatively well preserved. Confabulation, in which the patient makes up plausible answers to questions, is sometimes said to be a specific feature of amnesic syndrome but also occurs in delirium and other forms of memory loss.

In developed countries, amnesic syndrome is most commonly caused by the thiamine deficiency associated with alcohol dependence and this variant of the condition was formerly known as Korsakoff's syndrome. When caused by thiamine deficiency, the syndrome is usually preceded by a form of delirium known as Wernicke's encephalopathy; if treatment with parenteral thiamine is given at this point, the development of amnesic syndrome may be prevented. The pathology of Wernicke's encephalopathy and amnesic syndrome caused by thiamine deficiency is similar, with small haemorrhagic lesions in the mamillary bodies, thalamic nuclei and the floor of the third ventricle. Other conditions that cause localised lesions in this part of the brain can also present with amnesic syndrome, as summarised in Figure 1.

### *Other syndromes caused by focal brain damage*

Common signs of damage to the frontal, parietal, temporal and occipital lobes are shown in Figure 2.

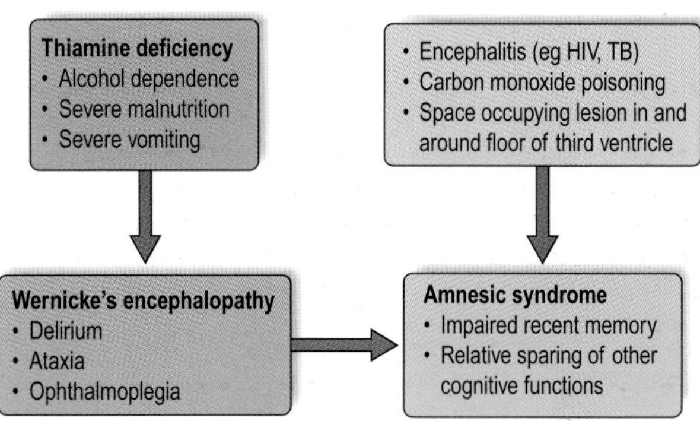


Fig. 1 **Wernicke's encephalopathy and amnesic syndrome.**

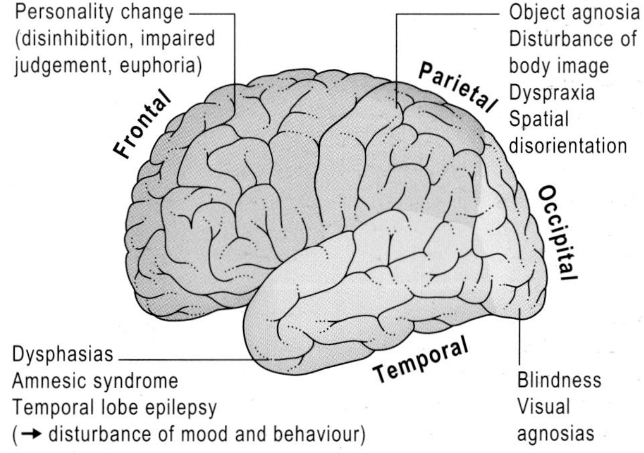


Fig. 2 **Common signs of damage to the frontal, parietal, temporal and occipital lobes.**

Table 3 **Causes of dementia**

| Neurological | Systemic |
|---|---|
| **Degenerative** | **Endocrine** |
| ■ Alzheimer's disease | ■ Hypothyroidism |
| ■ Lewy body dementia | ■ Cushing's disease |
| ■ Parkinson's disease | ■ Hypopituitarism |
| ■ Huntington's disease | **Metabolic** |
| ■ Pick's disease | ■ Anaemia |
| ■ Normal pressure hydrocephalus | ■ Hypoxia |
| **Vascular** | ■ Renal failure |
| ■ Vascular dementia (sudden onset suggests arteritis or carotid artery occlusion) | ■ Liver failure |
| | ■ Deficiency of vitamin B |
| ■ Vitamins and folate | ■ Carcinomatosis |
| **Infections** | **Toxic** |
| ■ Creutzfeldt–Jakob disease | ■ Chronic alcohol abuse |
| ■ Neurosyphilis | ■ Heavy metal poisoning |
| ■ HIV | **Other** |
| ■ Cerebral abscess | ■ SLE |
| **Space-occupying lesion** | ■ Sarcoidosis |
| ■ Tumour | |
| ■ Subdural haematoma | |
| **Traumatic** | |
| ■ Severe or repeated head injury | |

### Syndromes of cognitive impairment

- In delirium there is a fluctuating level of consciousness and attention, with global impairment of cognitive function
- Dementia is a global impairment of intellect, memory and personality, occurring in clear consciousness
- Amnesic syndrome is usually due to thiamine deficiency and is characterised by an inability to learn new information

# Neurology and psychiatry

Many neurological conditions may present with cognitive impairment or psychiatric symptoms. Those conditions which are usually dealt with by neurologists or neuropsychiatrists are discussed below. Those which are usually dealt with by old age psychiatrists (i.e. Alzheimer's disease, vascular dementia, Lewy body disease and Pick's disease) are discussed on pages 90–91, along with a description of the management of dementia. The principles of management discussed on page 91 are just as applicable to the causes of dementia described below

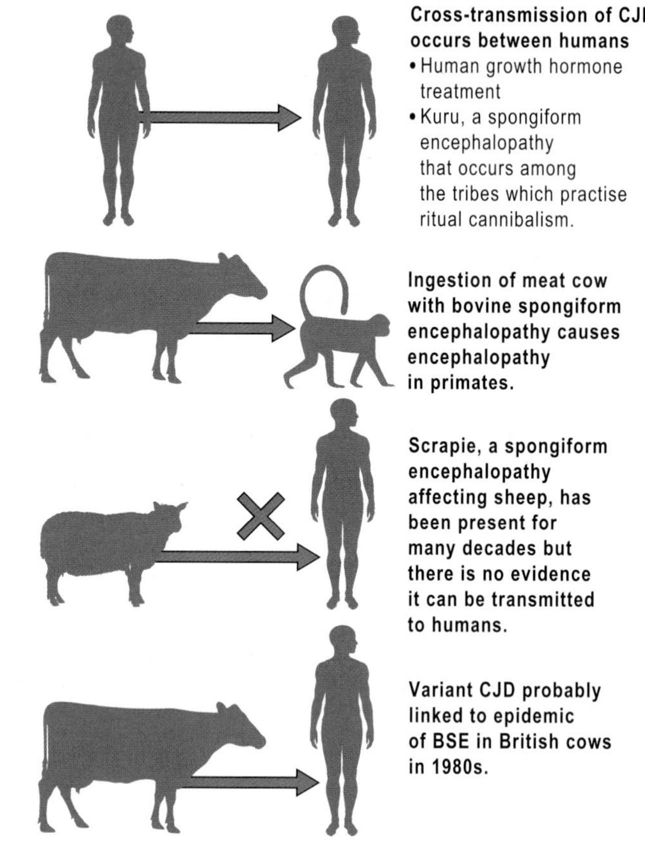


Fig. 1 **Transmission of spongiform encephalopathies.**

## Creutzfeldt–Jakob disease (CJD)

This rare infective form of dementia is the most common human form of the spongiform encephalopathies, so-called because of the sponge-like appearance of the brain at postmortem. It is caused by transmission of an abnormal prion protein that is found in plaques in the brain of affected cases. The risk of contracting CJD is thought to depend on the extent of exposure to the abnormal prion protein and genetic susceptibility factors in the exposed person. Following infection, it may be several decades before dementia develops, as evidenced by the adult-onset of dementia in people who had been treated with contaminated human growth hormone during childhood. Variant CJD (vCJD) is a new disorder, first described in 1996, and is strongly linked to exposure to beef products that have been infected with bovine spongiform encephalopathy (BSE). Some of the issues concerning transmission of CJD and other spongiform encephalopathies are summarised in Figure 1.

CJD can present initially with psychiatric symptoms, especially depression and anxiety, but rapidly progresses to a severe dementia associated with neurological deficits that include pyramidal, extrapyramidal and cerebellar signs. There is a characteristic triphasic pattern on EEG.

## Huntington's disease

This condition is also known as Huntington's chorea. It is caused by an abnormal trinucleide repeat on chromosome 4 which is inherited in an autosomal dominant fashion. The mean age of onset is in the fifth decade, with age of onset being inversely correlated with the length of the abnormal trinucleide repeat. There is marked neuronal degeneration in the frontal lobes and basal ganglia, especially the caudate nucleus. The mechanism by which the genetic abnormality causes this neuropathology is unknown.

The three main groups of symptoms are choreiform movements, dementia and psychiatric symptoms. The onset of these different symptoms can be several years apart and diagnosis may be difficult if choreiform movements are not the first symptoms to appear. The choreiform movements are sudden, involuntary movements which initially affect the face and shoulders, appearing like a mild twitch or shrug. They progress into severe writhing movements associated with ataxia. Dementia usually occurs late in the course of illness and memory and insight are relatively well preserved compared with other cognitive functions. Psychiatric symptoms occur at an early stage and are often the first to present. Depressive symptoms are most common and mania and paranoid psychosis also occur.

### *Genetic testing*

Children of patients with Huntington's disease have a 50% chance of developing the condition themselves. Using genetic probes, it is now possible to determine whether family members carry genetic markers on chromosome 4 which are associated with the disease. However, as nothing can be done to stop the disease developing, many relatives choose not to be tested. Prenatal testing is also possible, though it is important to remember that a positive test in a fetus implies that the parent at risk will go on to develop the disease.

## Parkinson's disease

Depression occurs in up to 40% of cases of Parkinson's disease. This is a higher rate than in conditions that cause a similar amount of disability, suggesting that changes in brain structure or function contribute to the depression. There is also a raised risk of dementia in patients with Parkinson's disease, with many cases probably caused by Lewy body disease (p. 90).

## Multiple sclerosis

Cognitive impairment may develop at any stage of the illness. Dementia is usually a late complication but eventually develops in up to 50% of patients. Psychiatric symptoms are even more common, with one-third of patients developing depressive episodes and nearly all patients experiencing depressive and anxiety symptoms at times. This is not surprising considering the enormous psychosocial impact of having multiple sclerosis. Lesions in the brain may also contribute to depressive mood changes, and are nearly always the cause of the euphoric mood which occurs in up to 10% of patients.

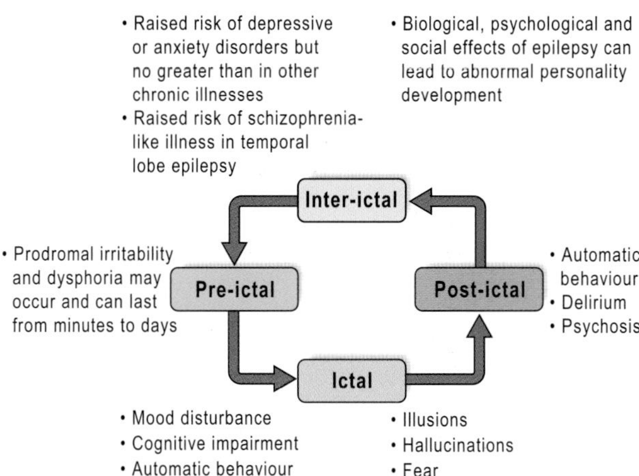

Fig. 2 **Psychiatric consequences of epilepsy.**

Table 1 **CNS infections and psychiatric symptoms**

| | |
|---|---|
| HIV | ■ See text |
| Syphilis | ■ Presents 5–25 years after primary infection<br>■ May present with mood symptoms (depressive or manic)<br>■ Progresses to dementia<br>■ Argyll–Robertson pupils in 50% of cases |
| Tuberculous meningitis | ■ Typical signs of meningitis late to develop<br>■ May be preceded by apathy, irritability and personality change<br>■ Tuberculosis increasingly common among homeless people |
| Encephalitis | ■ May present with delirium or, very rarely, with cognitive impairment in clear consciousness or psychosis<br>■ Medium- to long-term complications of infection include dementia, personality change, anxiety and depression |
| Cerebral abscess | ■ May present with depressive symptoms and cognitive impairment<br>■ Patient pyrexial and appears physically unwell |

## HIV disease and other infections

Mild cognitive impairment is common in HIV infection. Typical symptoms include apathy, reduced spontaneity, mental slowness, poor concentration and forgetfulness. Dementia is an uncommon complication and can occur in patients with or without AIDS. A rare presentation of HIV infection is with affective or psychotic symptoms. It is important to distinguish this from the depressive and anxiety symptoms which commonly occur in patients being tested for HIV infection.

Infections of the central nervous system which may present with cognitive impairment and psychiatric symptoms are summarised in Table 1. They are all uncommon but are worth keeping in mind as potentially treatable causes of cognitive impairment and psychiatric symptoms.

## Brain tumours

Brain tumours commonly cause cognitive impairment and psychiatric symptoms, but neurological symptoms are usually the most prominent feature. Delirium may be an early feature of fast-growing tumours. Slow-growing tumours, especially of the frontal lobes, may rarely present with personality change and cognitive impairment before the onset of neurological signs. Psychiatric symptoms alone, such as depression or psychosis, are an even rarer form of presentation.

## Head injury

Delirium often occurs following head injury. The risk of long-term psychiatric consequences is closely related to the duration of post-traumatic amnesia, which is the time taken to regain the ability to learn new information following the injury. Cognitive impairment is common and any of the features of dementia described on page 70 may occur, depending on the extent and location of brain damage. Cognitive function improves gradually but runs a chronic course in some cases. Depression and anxiety are also common and mania and schizophrenia-like illnesses are more likely than in the general population. Social and family treatments are often required for patients with psychiatric complications of head injury. Behavioural and cognitive therapy may be useful for symptoms of personality change such as apathy or aggression. Anticonvulsants are needed in patients who develop seizures and are sometimes helpful in reducing aggression. Standard treatments for psychiatric symptoms should be used.

## Epilepsy

There are four types of epilepsy that are likely to present to psychiatrists:

- **Absence seizures** are characterised by sudden loss of consciousness, making the patient seem unresponsive to others. Automatisms may occur and there is a sudden recovery with no post-ictal phase. Absence seizures usually last only a few seconds but absence status may be confused with mental illness, especially dissociative fugue.
- **Generalised motor seizures** can feature psychiatric symptoms in the post-ictal phase.
- **Simple partial seizures** consist of involuntary movements or abnormal sensory experiences that occur in clear consciousness.
- **Complex partial seizures** are the form of epilepsy most commonly associated with the ictal phenomena listed in Figure 2. Therefore, they constitute the form of epilepsy most likely to be misdiagnosed as a psychiatric disorder. Temporal lobe epilepsy is the most common type of complex partial seizure but seizure activity can arise anywhere in the brain. Complex partial seizures are often preceded by a simple partial seizure (most commonly a churning sensation spreading upwards from the epigastrium) which are sometimes called an 'aura'. Impaired consciousness and a variety of partial seizures then develop.

Epilepsy can present to psychiatrists in a number of different ways, as shown in Figure 2. The diagnosis is usually suggested by the history and if it is suspected, an EEG should be performed. Treatment depends on the relationship of the psychiatric disturbance to the seizures:

- **Pre-ictal, ictal and post-ictal disorders** are a direct consequence of seizure activity and so anticonvulsant treatment should be reviewed in an attempt to reduce further seizure activity. If acute control of symptoms is required, benzodiazepines should be used. Antipsychotic drugs lower seizure threshold and so they should only be used to control severe behavioural disturbance, and then only in combination with benzodiazepines.
- **Inter-ictal psychiatric problems** are not caused by seizure activity, so standard psychiatric treatments should be used. If medication is required, it is important to remember that some antidepressants, especially tricyclics, and antipsychotics lower seizure threshold. There are also many interactions between psychiatric drugs and anticonvulsants. It is important to ensure that patients receive good care for their epilepsy as poor seizure control is likely to exacerbate any psychiatric problems.

**Neurology and psychiatry**

- Psychiatric symptoms are common in some neurological illnesses
- Psychiatric symptoms can occur alone, but usually neurological symptoms are also present

# Organic causes of psychiatric symptoms

On pages 72 and 73, we discussed how organic disease can present with cognitive impairment. Patients with organic disease can also present with psychiatric symptoms such as mood disturbance, anxiety and psychosis. There are several ways in which this may occur, as illustrated in Figure 1. There is often some overlap between these four groups but it is easier to consider them separately.

## Psychiatric symptoms of organic disorders

Table 1 shows some of the organic illnesses in which psychiatric symptoms occur as a direct result of the organic disease process. ICD10 classifies such episodes as 'other mental disorders due to brain damage and dysfunction and physical disease'. By 'other mental disorders', it means disorders other than dementia, amnesic syndrome and delirium which are also due to brain damage and dysfunction or physical disease. It splits these other mental disorders into subgroups, depending on the nature of the psychiatric symptoms caused by the organic disorder. Examples of these subgroups include:

- organic hallucinosis
- organic delusional disorder
- organic mood disorder
- organic anxiety disorder.

The possibility of an organic cause should always be kept in mind when assessing patients with psychiatric symptoms. There may be clues that the patient has an organic disorder, as summarised in Figure 2. As an example, think of the differential diagnosis of a patient with episodes of anxiety and breathlessness. These symptoms are often caused by panic disorder. However, it would be important to look for symptoms and signs of organic disorders known to cause anxiety. For instance, the patient might also show evidence of heat intolerance and brisk deep tendon reflexes, in which case hyperthyroidism should be considered. An unusual description of symptoms might also suggest a medical cause. For instance, if their anxiety was mild and seemed to be secondary to their breathlessness, a cardiac or respiratory cause should be considered. An unusual presentation should also lead you to suspect a medical cause. For instance, first onset of panic disorder would be very unusual in a 50-year-old man with no previous psychiatric history and no recent stresses or adverse life events. With such a presentation, organic causes should be investigated fully.

Recognition of medical disorders presenting with psychiatric symptoms is clearly important as the patient will not usually recover until the underlying medical condition has been treated. Symptomatic treatment with psychotropic drugs may be required before the medical disorder has been treated. Psychotropics may also be needed if the medical disorder is untreatable, or if psychiatric symptoms persist after successful treatment of the medical condition.

## Psychiatric illness occurring as an indirect result of organic illness

Medical illness is often distressing and can affect all aspects of a patient's life. It is not surprising therefore that psychiatric illness often occurs as a result. The consequences of medical illness most likely to cause this are shown in Figure 1.

Patients at risk of psychiatric illness, such as those with a family history or past history of psychiatric illness, are more likely to develop a psychiatric illness when medically ill, just as they are more likely to develop a psychiatric illness when faced with any adverse life event. It is also important to remember that medical illnesses will have different consequences for different patients, thereby altering their risk of psychiatric illness. For instance, myocardial infarction in a heavy goods vehicle driver will leave them unable to return to their pre-

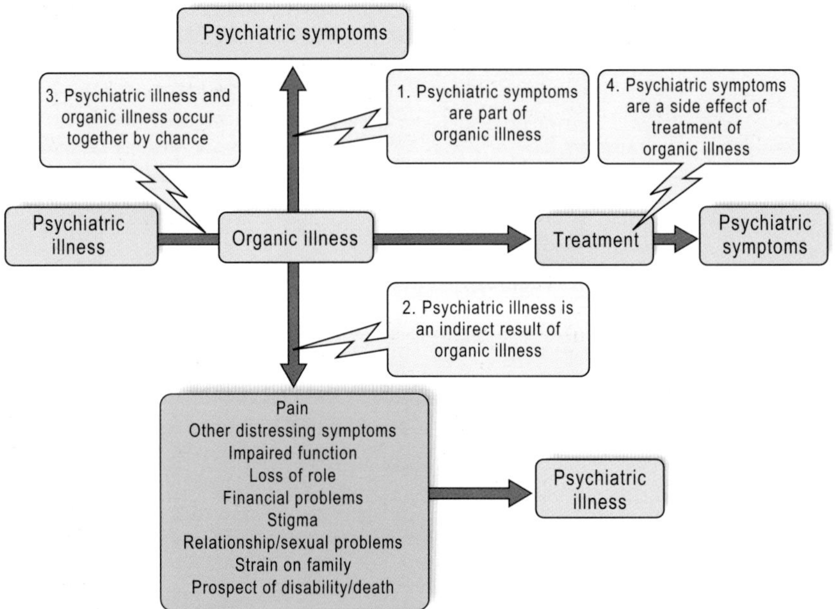


Fig. 1 **Four ways in which psychiatric symptoms can occur in patients with organic illness.**

Table 1 **Organic causes of psychiatric symptoms**

| | Neurological | Endocrine | Other | Prescribed drugs |
|---|---|---|---|---|
| Depression | Most dementias | Hypothyroidism | Anaemia | Corticosteroids |
| | (especially vascular and Huntington's) | Cushing's syndrome | Infections | Beta-blockers |
| | Parkinson's disease | Addison's disease | Carcinomatosis | Calcium channel blockers |
| | Multiple sclerosis | Hypopituitarism | SLE | Anticonvulsants |
| | Neurosyphilis | Hyperparathyroidism | Acute porphyria | L-dopa |
| | | | | Oral contraceptive pill |
| Elation | Multiple sclerosis | Cushing's syndrome | | Corticosteroids |
| | Neurosyphilis | | | Antidepressants |
| Anxiety | | Hyperthyroidism | | SSRI antidepressants |
| | | Hypoglycaemia | | |
| | | Phaeochromocytoma | | |
| Psychosis | Huntington's disease | | SLE | Corticosteroids |
| | Multiple sclerosis | | Acute porphyria | Beta-blockers |
| | Space occupying lesion | | | L-dopa |
| | CNS infections | | | Sympathomimetics |

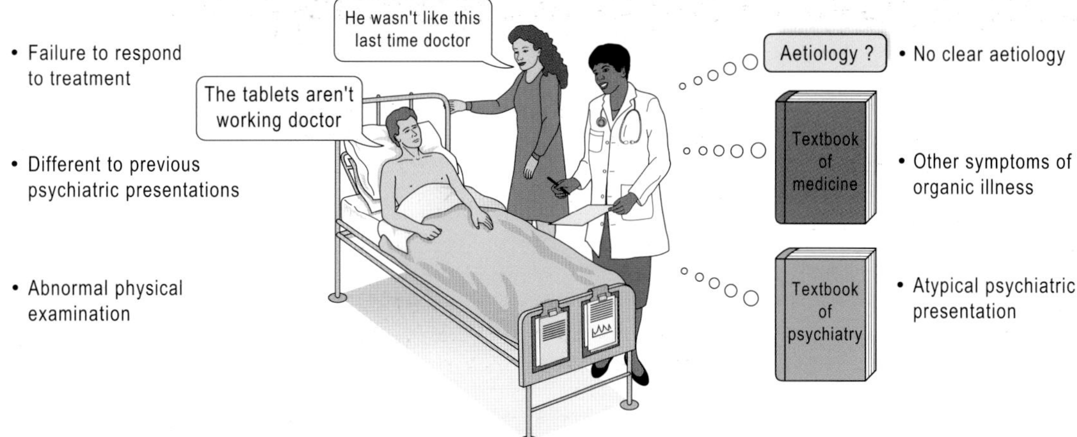


Fig. 2 **Six factors which suggest an organic cause of psychiatric symptoms.**

vious job, raising the risk of depression. A stomach ulcer in a patient whose father died of gastric cancer might leave him terrified of suffering a similar fate, with consequent panic attacks.

Once a psychiatric illness has developed, it can often exacerbate symptoms of the physical illness which precipitated it. For instance, depression often results in an exacerbation of pain. Patients' general level of function, which is often reduced as a result of their medical illness, may be reduced further as a result of psychiatric symptoms such as lethargy, anxiety or loss of confidence.

The risk of psychiatric consequences of medical illness is reduced by giving patients a full explanation of the illness and what can be done to help them, paying particular attention to any specific fears the patient may have. Practical advice about how they can cope with the consequences of the illness is also useful. Involving patients' families in this process will clarify the support they need to give the patient and allow them to voice any concerns of their own. All this is best carried out by members of the medical team dealing with the patient and some specialist services, such as breast clinics or diabetic clinics, have designated members of staff to do this.

In addition to these general measures, specific treatments for the psychiatric disorder will be required in some cases. Standard treatments should be used, provided they are not contraindicated by the medical illness. This is most likely to be the case for drug treatments and a list of medical conditions which can be exacerbated by psychiatric drugs is given in Table 2. It is also important to be aware of the potential for drug interactions in patients receiving treatment for physical and psychiatric illness.

### *Case history 25*

A 45-year-old woman with multiple sclerosis is admitted to a neurological ward following an acute relapse. During this admission, she is referred to a liaison psychiatrist after developing symptoms of depression and anxiety.

a. What are the possible causes of these symptoms?
b. How should they be managed?

## Organic and psychiatric illness occurring together by chance

Organic and psychiatric illness are both common and so it is not surprising that they often occur together by chance. When they do occur together, each can make the other worse, as described above. The physical and psychiatric conditions should be treated separately in the usual way, bearing in mind the medical side effects of psychiatric drugs, the psychiatric side effects of drugs used to treat organic illness, and the risk of drug interactions.

Table 2 **Organic conditions exacerbated by psychotropic drugs**

Drugs with antimuscarinic effects (tricyclic and MAOI antidepressants, some antipsychotics)
- cardiovascular disease
- glaucoma
- constipation
- prostatism
- dementia

Drugs with antiadrenergic effects (tricyclic and MAOI antidepressants, some antipsychotics)
- postural hypotension (older patients, patients on antihypertensive drugs)

Antipsychotic drugs
- Parkinson's disease
- Lewy body dementia

Drugs which lower seizure threshold (most antidepressants and antipsychotics)
- epilepsy

## Psychiatric side effects of medication

Drugs which cause psychiatric side effects are shown in Table 1. If such side effects occur, the dose should be reduced or an alternative drug should be used. Occasionally, the risks of doing this outweigh the benefits and in such cases the psychiatric symptoms may require separate treatment.

### Organic causes of psychiatric symptoms

- Psychiatric symptoms are a direct consequence of some organic diseases
- Organic disease can have an enormous impact on patients' lives and so may precipitate functional psychiatric illness
- Psychotropic drugs should be prescribed cautiously in patients with organic illness, because of side effects and interactions

# Eating disorders

Anorexia nervosa was first described by William Gull in 1868 and is characterised by deliberate and extreme weight loss. In bulimia nervosa, episodes of overeating are followed by self-induced purging, usually in the form of vomiting. There is considerable overlap between these two eating disorders.

## Anorexia nervosa

Concerns about weight, and dieting in order to lose weight are extremely common in the general population, particularly among young women. Anorexia nervosa represents an extreme form of this behaviour. Fear of being fat leads to the adoption of a starvation diet. Weight falls to at least 15% below normal, so that the body mass index (BMI) is 17.5 or less (Fig. 1). Despite this, anorexics continue to believe they are overweight, even when faced with their emaciated reflection in the mirror. This distorted body image drives them to continue to lose weight, and they may adopt other methods such as excessive exercise, self-induced vomiting or abuse of laxatives, diuretics or appetite suppressants such as amphetamine. They may become preoccupied with food, hoarding it, or becoming very interested in cookery, creating elaborate meals for their family while still refusing to eat. Amenorrhoea occurs in the early stages of weight loss and is an indication of a widespread endocrine disorder. Figure 2 shows the signs and symptoms found in anorexia nervosa.

## Bulimia nervosa

In bulimia nervosa there is also a fear of fatness, but the characteristic symptom is binge eating. 'Binges' are the consumption of huge quantities of food at a single sitting, particularly carbohydrate-rich items such as biscuits, cakes and bread. They often take place in secret, and away from meal times. Some bulimics will eat normally at other times, although calorie-controlled diets are common. A small number also have anorexia nervosa. In bulimia nervosa, binges provoke feelings of guilt and disgust and a sense of being out of control. These feelings lead to a desire to get rid of the food, usually achieved by putting fingers down the throat to induce vomiting. Many bulimics are eventually able to spontaneously vomit. As in anorexia, laxative and diuretic abuse may be further threats to health. Despite a dread of weight gain, many maintain a normal weight and may even be overweight. Menstruation is often normal.

## Epidemiology

Bulimia is more common than anorexia nervosa. Anorexia nervosa usually starts in adolescence, and bulimia a few years later. Surveys of young women have found a prevalence of 3–4% for bulimia and 1–2% for anorexia nervosa. Both are more common in women than men. Occupations that depend upon keeping a low body weight, such as ballet dancing and modelling, have a particularly high risk of anorexia.

## Aetiology

The aetiology for both anorexia nervosa and bulimia nervosa is similar. There are many factors thought to be important and most cases will be due to a combination of causes.

### *Predisposing factors*

- **Cultural factors**. Anorexia nervosa and bulimia nervosa are disorders of the food-rich developed world. Western society has developed a stereotyped view of physical attractiveness which equates 'thin' with 'beautiful', and promotes negative attitudes about obesity. The media bombard us with idealised images of underweight models alongside advertisements for confectionery. Adolescents are particularly vulnerable to these cultural pressures to conform and to be attractive.
- **Genetic factors**. Twin studies have shown that genetic factors do play a role, probably by creating a vulnerability to weight loss so that in the presence of environmental pressures an eating disorder may develop.
- **Hypothalamic dysfunction**. The hypothalamic area of the brain controls feeding behaviour, temperature regulation and fluid balance. There are marked changes in the functioning of the endocrine system in anorexia (Fig. 2). In the main these changes are secondary to the weight loss, but the early onset of amenorrhoea in some anorexic women suggests that some changes may be primary.

### *Precipitating and maintaining factors*

- **Family issues**. Preparing and sharing food plays an important role in family relationships. The conflicts that often arise between adolescents and their parents can be acted out at meal times, with refusal to eat becoming an act of rebellion. There is often some abnormality in family relationships, although the problems may be a result of the eating disorder, rather than the cause of it.

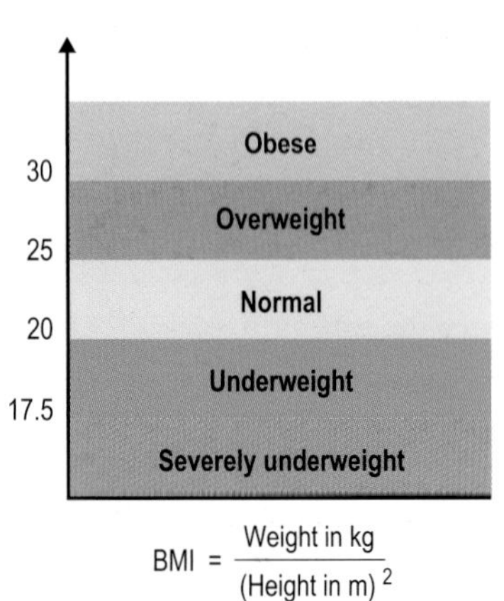


Fig. 1 **Body mass index (BMI).**

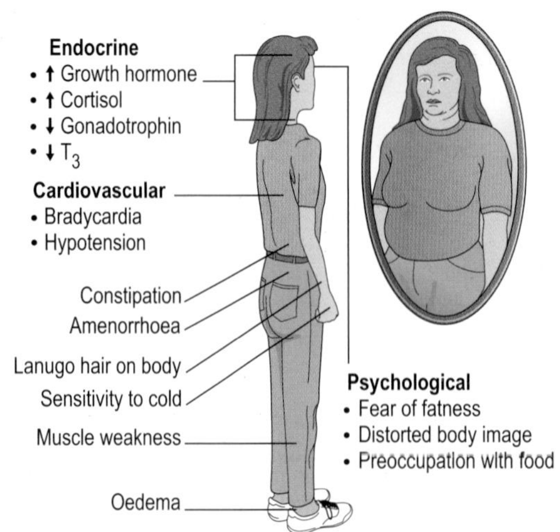


Fig. 2 **Signs and symptoms of anorexia nervosa.**

It is common for the mother to have some concerns about weight and dieting, and in some cases to also have an eating disorder.

- **Psychological issues**. Adolescence may be a time of conflict with parents and others. Feelings of having little control over events, lack of confidence and poor self image are common. In some cases anorexia nervosa can be a way of coping with some of these psychological pressures, by creating an illusion of being in control. Another theory is that the amenorrhoea and arrested physical development of anorexia nervosa fulfils a wish to escape the problems of adolescence and avoid adulthood. Parents who do not want their little girl to grow into a woman and leave home may collude in this illusion of prolonged childhood.

## Management

Patients with eating disorders are often very reluctant to accept that they are ill, and have the realistic fear that the main aim of treatment will be weight gain. Therefore the first challenge in managing eating disorders is engaging the patient in treatment. It may take many hours over several appointments to gain the patient's trust, complete an assessment and build a therapeutic relationship that will allow change to begin to happen.

Assessment begins with a full psychiatric history and mental state examination and an informant from the family can often provide valuable information. The main psychiatric differential diagnosis to consider is depressive disorder. A detailed physical examination is important, looking for evidence of malnutrition and effects of repeated vomiting. Physical illnesses that present with weight loss must be excluded, in particular chronic debilitating diseases, malabsorption syndromes and thyrotoxicosis. Investigations may include full blood count, urea and electrolytes, creatinine, liver function tests, ECG and chest X-ray.

The aim of a treatment programme must be to achieve a healthy weight, at a weekly rate of about 0.5kg, and reduce behaviour that puts health at risk. It is helpful to work towards a realistic target weight that is reached through negotiation with the patient. Psychological, physical and social treatments should be considered.

### *Psychological treatment*

- **Cognitive therapy**. This has been shown to be successful in research studies. It aims to examine and change thought processes underlying the abnormal behaviour. Therapy may include keeping a diary, for example recording binges or vomiting and the thoughts and feelings that occur before, during and after this behaviour. The diary is used in therapy sessions for the patient and therapist to work together to find a strategy to change the behaviour.
- **Self-help programmes**. There are a number of structured self-help programmes available that can be very effective in the treatment of bulimia nervosa. The role of the professional is to provide support and encouragement, and for many patients this will be all that is required. Provision of information to the patient and their carers is very helpful in managing all eating disorders.
- **Family therapy**. This may be the treatment of choice if abnormal family relationships are thought to have a role in the eating disorder. There are many different models of family therapy. In most cases two therapists work together with the family. The family as a whole is seen as the source of the problems rather than the individual with the eating disorder, and it is acknowledged all members of the family will be affected in some way. Family relationships are examined, and conflicts may be acted out in the therapy sessions, giving the family an opportunity to understand the way the family functions and make changes.

### *Physical treatment*

There is only a limited role for drug treatment in the management of eating disorders. Fluoxetine, a specific serotonin reuptake inhibitor (SSRI) which is usually used in the treatment of depression, is also used in bulimia to suppress the appetite and limit bingeing. It is not an adequate treatment for bulimia in itself and must be used alongside psychological therapies.

### *Social treatment*

Some patients will require social interventions, in particular help to gain confidence and independence. Social and self-help groups, advice about housing and finances and occupational therapy may be useful.

### *Hospital treatment*

The majority of anorexic and bulimic patients can be managed as outpatients. However, if the weight falls to a dangerously low level, admission may become necessary, ideally to the shared care of both a psychiatrist and physician. Weight gain is achieved with a diet of regular meals, supplemented if necessary with high calorie drinks and snacks. The nursing staff has an important but difficult role in management. They must strike a balance between building a trusting relationship with the patient and adopting a monitoring role, supervising meal times, ensuring there is no self-induced vomiting, and recording weight gain.

## Course and prognosis

The course of eating disorders tends to be variable and fluctuating. In general about 65% have a good outcome and maintain normal weight, 20% remain moderately underweight long term and 15% have a poor outcome, with persisting seriously low weight. Poor outcome is associated with very early or late onset of illness, a chronic course, severe weight loss, coexisting anorexia and bulimia and persisting relationship difficulties. Men generally have a worse prognosis.

### *Case history 26*

Sarah is a 17-year-old school girl with a 2-year history of weight loss. She is 1.7m tall and 48kg in weight. She has set a target weight of 40kg and in order to achieve this more rapidly has limited her diet to raw vegetables and water for several months, and works out in the gym twice a day. Sarah believes that she is currently overweight, and is disgusted by her reflection in the mirror.

a. What is her body mass index (BMI)?
b. What would be a normal weight for her height?
c. What is the diagnosis?
d. What impact is the weight loss likely to have on her physical health?

### Eating disorders

Anorexia nervosa is characterised by:

- deliberate weight loss, with BMI of 17.5 or less
- distorted body image
- fear of fatness
- amenorrhoea

Bulimia nervosa is characterised by:

- episodes of binge eating
- self-induced vomiting
- fear of fatness

# Perinatal psychiatry

## Case history 27

Bronwyn is 32 years old. She has two children and is in the tenth week of pregnancy. She has a history of recurrent depression, including an episode following the birth of her second child. She stopped sertraline four months ago, prior to conception. She now presents with low mood, tearfulness, poor sleep, fatigue and impaired concentration that has caused her to make uncharacteristic mistakes at work.

a. What additional information is needed?
b. Should she restart sertraline?

Perinatal psychiatry involves the recognition, assessment and management of mental disorders during pregnancy and the postnatal period. Traditionally, the focus has been on the period following delivery, during which there is a raised risk of depression and psychosis, and it is the postnatal conditions, outlined in Figure 1, that will be discussed in detail here. However, mental illness also occurs during pregnancy and, when present, will often persist postnatally.

## Postnatal depression

There is a high rate of depression among women in the 12 months following childbirth. Community surveys have shown a prevalence of up to 20% and around 5% of women will consult their GP regarding depression during the postnatal period. These findings have given rise to the concept of postnatal depression as a discrete disorder, somehow different to other depressive illnesses, perhaps as a result of hormonal changes occurring after childbirth. This has been helpful in promoting the acceptance of depression in the postnatal period and reducing the feelings of shame felt by women who are not experiencing the happiness babies are expected to bring.

The epidemiology of depression in the postnatal period suggests the condition is not distinct from other depressive disorders. While the **baby blues**, consisting of a brief period of tearfulness, anxiety, irritability and fatigue, occurring in mothers typically around four days after delivery, may well be linked to hormonal changes, this does not seem to be the case with depression. There is no peak of new cases of depression in the first few weeks of the postnatal period, and the period of raised risk extends throughout the first year. Hormonal treatments, such as progesterone, do not appear to be effective. There is also no difference between the symptoms of depression in the postnatal period and those occurring at other times of life, and risk factors are also similar.

It seems more likely that raised rate of depression in the postnatal period is the result of psychological and social factors. Looking after a baby is challenging and the risk of depression is increased in cases of neonatal illness. The arrival of a new child has a great effect on relationships and family finances, and social isolation may occur. Notably, postnatal depression is more common following the birth of a first child and unwanted pregnancies, which suggests that adjustment to motherhood is an important factor.

Standard treatments for depression should be offered. Specific interventions, such as mother and baby groups, may be particularly helpful for women struggling to adjust to motherhood and those who have become socially isolated. Consideration of drug treatments should take into account the problems that may be encountered during breast-feeding, which are summarised below. Drugs with sedative effects should be prescribed with caution if there are not other people available to care for the baby.

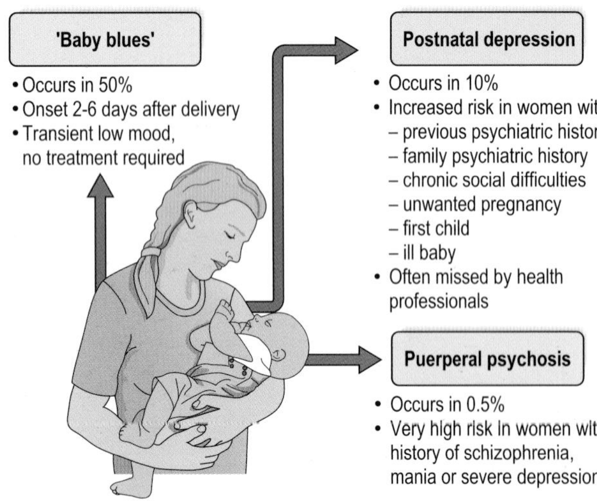


Fig. 1 **Postnatal mood changes.**

## Puerperal psychosis

In contrast to postnatal depression, it seems likely that the psychotic illnesses that occur following childbirth have a biological cause. There is a dramatic increase in the risk of severe mental illness following childbirth, with different studies showing a 10–30-fold increase in the risk of psychiatric admission in the early postnatal period. Onset is usually within two weeks of delivery.

Although schizophrenia-like illnesses can occur, puerperal psychosis is typically affective in nature, presenting with mania or severe depression. Symptoms are often florid and changeable. A common feature is confusion and so delirium needs to be excluded. Women with a history or family history of bipolar disorder are at greatest risk and most women who develop puerperal psychosis will experience puerperal and non-puerperal episodes of mania and depression in the future.

Drug treatments are usually required, with prescribing following guidelines for the type of psychosis with which the woman presents. Lithium is often advocated for the prevention of affective episodes in women at high risk. Electroconvulsive therapy (ECT) is usually effective for puerperal mania and depression and has a relatively rapid onset of action.

## Organisation of services

Women encounter a variety of services and professionals during pregnancy and the postnatal period. Good communication and interdisciplinary working is essential. All professionals involved in routine antenatal and postnatal care should be able to screen for depression and be alert for signs of other mental disorders. Suggested screening questions for depression are shown in Figure 2.

The treatment of mild to moderate depression will usually be provided in primary care, with health visitors, who by the nature of their work become very experienced in dealing with the condition, often taking a lead role. For more severe conditions, mental health teams will collaborate with health visitors, colleagues in primary care and, when necessary, Child and Family Social Services teams. In some areas, specialised perina-

During the past month, have you often been bothered by having little interest or pleasure in doing things?
During the past month, have you often been bothered by feeling down, depressed or hopeless?
(IF YES TO EITHER OF ABOVE) Is this something you feel you need or want help with?
SCREEN FOR DEPRESSION
• At booking into antenatal clinic
• 4-6 weeks postpartum
• 3-4 months postpartum

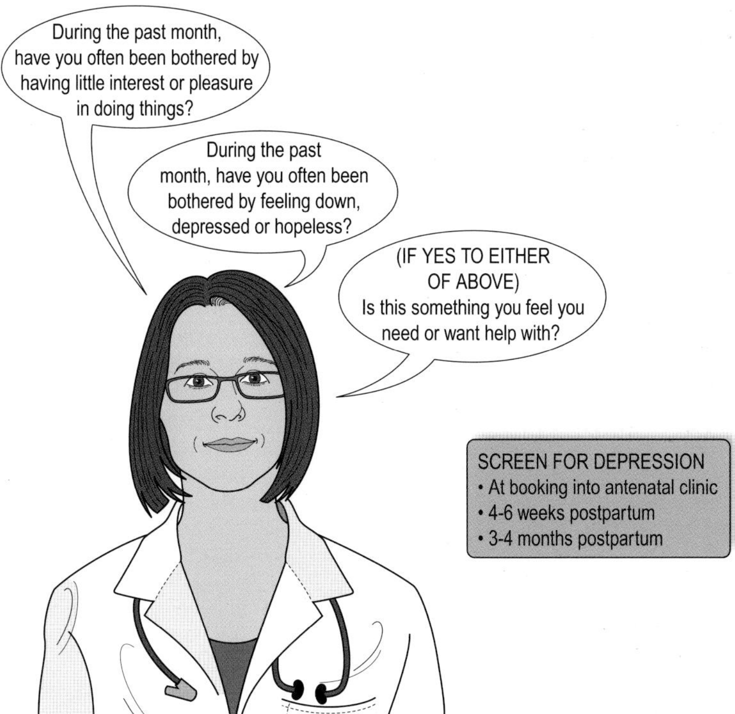

Fig. 2 **Screening for depression in the perinatal period.**

tal mental health teams have been set up. For women who develop mental illnesses so severe that hospital treatment is required, mother and baby units should be available.

## Identification of women at risk

At a woman's first contact with antenatal and postnatal services, she should be asked about:

- past or present severe mental illness including schizophrenia, bipolar disorder, psychosis in the postnatal period and severe depression
- previous contact with psychiatrists or mental health services
- a family history of perinatal mental illness.

Women answering yes to any of these questions should at least be discussed with mental health services and in many cases referred.

Some women will be vulnerable to depression but unlikely to become so unwell that they require input from mental health services. Factors such as lack of family support, social isolation, financial and social problems, caring for other young children and a history of depression increase the risk of depression in the perinatal period. In such cases, it is worth considering measures such as increased input from community midwives and health visitors, attendance of mother and baby groups, improved childcare arrangements for older children and advice and advocacy regarding issues such as finances and accommodation.

## Drug treatment during pregnancy

The evidence regarding psychiatric drugs with teratogenic effects is summarised in Table 1. A particular point to note from this table is the relatively high risk of neural tube defects with valproate and carbamazepine. This risk is associated with drug exposure in very early pregnancy and damage may be done before the woman concerned realises she is pregnant. For this reason, the prescription of valproate and carbamazepine to women of childbearing age should be avoided.

Concerns about teratogenicity mean that psychological and social interventions are preferred in cases where drug treatment is not essential. However, in situations where drug treatment is likely to be of substantial benefit, women may come to the conclusion that the risk of harm to their baby is outweighed by the benefits of good mental health during the perinatal period.

The discontinuation syndrome that occurs following cessation of antidepressants can also affect neonates whose mother has been taking these drugs. In most cases, this causes no more than mild jitteriness, tremor and myoclonus in the baby, for a few days at most.

## Drug treatment during breast-feeding

Exposure to antidepressants in breast milk is not known to be harmful, but should be avoided if possible. Only small amounts of imipramine and sertraline pass into breast milk and these drugs are viewed as relatively safe. Levels of fluoxetine and citalopram in breast milk are relatively high.

Antipsychotics pass into breast milk in small amounts that are unlikely to be harmful but sedation of babies has been reported and animal studies suggest possible adverse effects on the developing nervous system, so use of these drugs when breast-feeding is not usually advised. Women should not breast-feed when taking lithium, because of the risk of toxicity in the baby. Benzodiazepines pass into breast milk and should be avoided.

Table 1 **Psychiatric drugs with teratogenic effects. (E) Risk associated with exposure in early pregnancy. (L) Risk associated with exposure in late pregnancy**

| Drug | Problem | Rate | |
|---|---|---|---|
| | | **Exposed** | **Unexposed** |
| Valproate(E) | Neural tube defects | 100–200 per 10,000 | 6 per 10,000 |
| Carbamazepine (E) | Neural tube defects | 50 per 10,000 | 6 per 10,000 |
| Lamotrigine (E) | Oral cleft | 9 per 1000 | 1 per 600 |
| Lithium (E) | Heart defects (Epstein's anomaly) | 60 per 1000 (10 per 20,000) | 8 per 1000 (1 per 20,000) |
| Clozapine | Agranulocytosis | Unknown – risk in adults taking clozapine is 0.5% | |
| SSRIs (E) | Heart defects | 9 per 1000 | 5 per 1000 |
| SSRIs (L) | Persistent pulmonary hypertension | 6–10 per 1000 | 1–2 per 1000 |
| Benzodiazepines (E) | Oral cleft & other major malformations | Risk demonstrated in case-control but not cohort studies | |

## Perinatal psychiatry

- Postnatal depression is common and is often missed by health professionals
- Puerperal psychosis is uncommon but women with a history of mania or psychosis are at high risk

# Personality disorders – introduction and classification

## Personality and its assessment

Personality determines the way people behave and feel in response to things that happen to them. It has a strong genetic basis and is also influenced by childhood environment. In most cases, personality is fully formed by adolescence or earlier and then remains relatively stable over time, manifesting itself in different environments and situations. Descriptions of personality are usually confined to emotions and behaviours that are observable by others. Personality is considered to be disordered if it persistently causes dysfunctional relationships or distress to the person or those around them. These features are summarised in Figure 1.

## Classification of abnormal personality

### *Personality disorders: the type model*

The type model of personality states that there are different categories of abnormal personality. Not surprisingly, it has been developed mainly by psychiatrists who are used to using standardised diagnoses to categorise patient's problems. The term used for these different types of abnormal personality is personality disorders. ICD10 gives the following description of personality disorders:

> *These types of condition comprise deeply ingrained and enduring behaviour patterns, manifesting themselves as inflexible responses to a broad range of personal and social situations ... they are frequently, but not always, associated with various degrees of subjective distress and problems in social functioning and performance.*

The personality disorders included in ICD10 are summarised in Table 1.

The type model is widely used clinically although, as discussed below, it does have limitations. It is certainly helpful for research into personality disorders. For instance, dysthymia and cyclothymia used to be classified as personality disorders but are now considered to be mood disorders after epidemiological research and treatment studies showed that they were closely related to other mood disorders. Similarly, schizotypal disorder was previously considered to be a personality disorder but is now grouped with schizophrenia and delusional disorders. Of the remaining personality disorders, research using the type model has provided clinically valuable information about epidemiology, treatment and prognosis.

One problem with the type model is that most patients with abnormal personalities do not fit conveniently into a single category of personality disorder. ICD10 deals with this by having a category of mixed personality disorder for patients with features of different personality disorders without a predominant set of symptoms that would allow a more specific diagnosis. It also allows more than one diagnosis to be made if a patient meets criteria for more than one personality disorder.

Another way of dealing with the limitations of the type model is suggested by the observation that certain personality disorders are more likely to overlap with each other – in other words, some personality disorders tend to cluster together. There appear to be three main clusters which are shown in Table 1. Because the clusters are broad, most patients with abnormalities of personality will fit fairly well into one of them. This means that if you diagnose a mixed personality disorder you will usually be able to identify which cluster the abnormalities of personality fall into. Saying that someone has a mixed personality disorder with, for example, a predominance of cluster B characteristics is more informative than just saying they have a mixed personality disorder. However, it is still a crude method of description.

### *Other models of abnormal personality*

There are several alternatives to the type model. The **trait model** assumes there are different aspects of personality, known as traits. Examples of abnormal personality traits include neuroticism, obsessionality, impulsivity, aggression and suspiciousness. If a patient has abnormal personality traits that cause distress to themselves or others, these traits can be described individually. This model is very flexible as it can be used to describe any combination of abnormal personality traits. If you are having trouble understanding the differences between the type and trait models, consider the following. We might describe someone as having blond hair, pale skin, an angular facial appearance and a tall, muscular build, which would be a trait model. Alternatively, we might use a type model and say they had a typical Scandinavian appearance.

The **situationist model** considers that the most important determinant of how someone feels or behaves is the situation they are in. Using this model, personality assessment would involve finding out whether particular situations consistently caused distressing behaviour or emotion.

The **interactionist model** is a combination of the trait and situationist model and involves a description of abnormal personality traits and the situations most likely to provoke them.

The trait and interactionist models are often used in clinical practice because they usually provide a more accurate description of patients' problems than the type model. Patients also find it more useful to talk about aspects of their personality that lead to problems in particular situations, rather than just being told they have a personality disorder. Another advantage of these more descriptive methods of classification is that they make clear which aspects of personality need to be worked on.

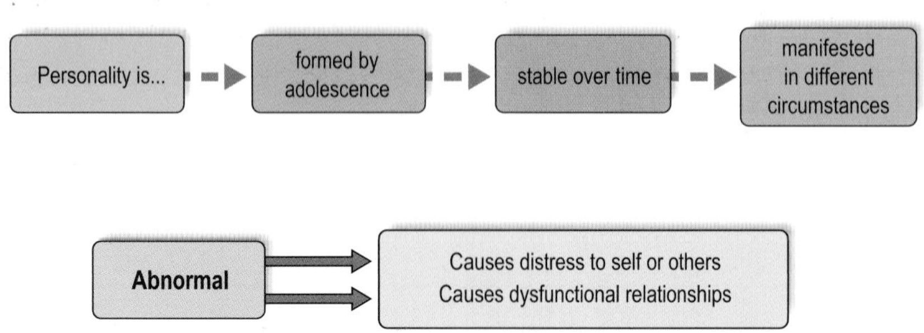


Fig. 1 **Characteristics of personality.**

Table 1 **ICD10 personality disorders**

| |
|---|
| **Cluster A** |
| Paranoid personality disorder |
| ■ Easily upset when things go wrong, blaming others and holding persistent grudges |
| ■ Mistrust others and suspect that events in their own life or in the world at large are the result of a conspiracy |
| ■ Have an excessive sense of their own importance and their personal rights |
| Schizoid personality disorder |
| ■ Emotionally cold and detached, deriving pleasure from few, if any, activities |
| ■ Solitary and introspective with little interest in sexual or other close relationships |
| ■ Indifferent to expectations of others and society |
| **Cluster B** |
| Dissocial personality disorder |
| ■ Persistent disregard for the feelings of others and for social rules and norms |
| ■ Failure to feel guilt or learn from experience |
| ■ Easily frustrated with low threshold for aggression and violence |
| Histrionic personality disorder |
| ■ Dramatic, exaggerated expression of emotions |
| ■ Craves attention and excitement |
| ■ Shallow personality, easily influenced by others or circumstances |
| Emotionally unstable personality disorder, borderline type |
| ■ Chronic dysphoria and feelings of emptiness |
| ■ Form intense, unstable relationships, with marked distress if feeling rejected |
| ■ Recurrent suicidal threats and acts of self-harm |
| Emotionally unstable personality disorder, impulsive type |
| ■ Impulsive and lack self control |
| ■ Sudden outbursts of anger leading to suicidal gestures or violence |
| **Cluster C** |
| Anankastic (obsessional) personality disorder |
| ■ Rigid, stubborn, pedantic and excessively organised |
| ■ Perfectionism that makes it difficult to complete tasks |
| ■ Insist others do things their way or not at all |
| Anxious (avoidant) personality disorder |
| ■ Persistent feelings of tension and apprehension |
| ■ Feel inept, unlikeable and inferior to others |
| ■ Avoid situations where may feel criticised, rejected or disapproved of |
| Dependent personality disorder |
| ■ Feel unable to cope and make decisions alone |
| ■ Fear being left alone and so put the needs of those they are dependent on ahead of their own |

## Epidemiology and aetiology

Prevalence studies of abnormal personality usually use the type model. Prevalence in the general population is 2–13% depending on how personality disorder is defined. Among psychiatric patients, prevalence is around 20%. Dissocial personality disorder is particularly common in prison populations, affecting around 70% of all prisoners. Some personality disorders are more common in men (e.g. dissocial, anankastic) and others more common in women (e.g. paranoid, dependent). There may be gender bias in the diagnosis of personality disorder by psychiatrists – for example, 75% of people treated for borderline personality disorder are female, but in community studies the gender ratio is much narrower. More general associations of personality disorder include an increased risk of social, employment and medical problems.

Genetic factors play a substantial role in determining personality. Siblings usually have very different personalities despite receiving similar upbringings, and twin studies have confirmed a genetic effect. The role of childhood environment has been most studied in dissocial personality disorder. Risk factors include social deprivation and parental disharmony and violence, whereas protective factors include having at least one positive relationship with an adult. Borderline personality disorder is often associated with childhood sexual abuse.

There is some evidence that brain function is abnormal in some personality disorders. Personality changes including aggression and impulsivity are often seen following head injury. Increased slow wave activity on EEGs has been demonstrated in dissocial personality disorder, leading to the theory that the disorder is caused by the failure of the brain to mature normally, and there is also evidence of impaired serotonin function among people with impulsive or aggressive personality traits, but neither of these findings have been consistently replicated.

### *Case history 28*

David is a 32-year-old man who has always felt inferior to others. He feels tense much of the time. He avoids situations where he might be judged by others. He often makes rash decisions and can become violent if people try to stop him acting on these (see Fig. 2).

a. What type of personality disorder (ICD10) do you think he has?

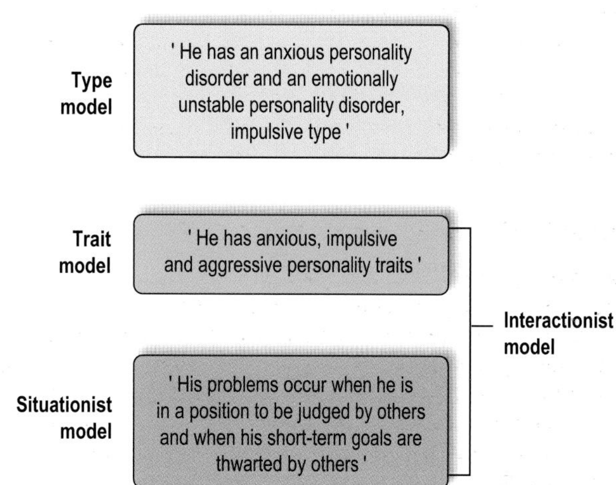


Fig. 2 **Examples of how the problems in the case history can be described using the four models of abnormal personality.**

### Personality disorders – introduction and classification

- Personality determines the way people respond to different situations
- Personality remains fairly constant throughout adulthood
- Personality is considered to be disordered if it consistently causes distress or dysfunctional relationships

# Personality disorders – management

The management of patients with personality disorders can be enormously challenging. They may be extremely distressed and demanding, and often disagree with the treatment plan offered. Patients who repeatedly threaten or carry out harm to themselves or others are particularly draining to those involved in their care. One way to deal with these challenges is to refuse to take them on and this approach may be justified in cases where psychiatric care has been ineffective or even made things worse. However, if specific treatments are combined with some basic principles of management, it is often possible to help what may seem like a relentless tide of problems (Fig. 1).

## Clinical assessment

Before diagnosing a personality disorder, it is essential to establish that the abnormalities of behaviour and emotion exhibited by the patient are recurrent and long-standing. For instance, in the case history of David given in this and the previous pages, certain questions would be particularly relevant. Did he show evidence of nervousness or aggression during childhood? Was he anxious when starting new schools or new jobs? Is he someone who has always got into fights, lost jobs or failed to maintain relationships because of aggression? Does the nervousness and aggression only occur in particular situations, for instance when reprimanded by authority figures, or is there evidence of it occurring in a range of circumstances? Is this information corroborated by people who have known him a long time? Is his presentation in fact the result of another disorder – such as mental illness, alcohol and substance misuse or learning disability – all of which can all lead to abnormalities of behaviour and emotion similar to those seen in people with personality disorder?

## Treatment

### General principles

When managing patients with personality disorders, it is essential to be realistic. Treatment will only work if the patient is committed to it. So, while acknowledging that they need help in achieving change, it is important to make sure the patient realises that ultimate responsibility rests with them. If improvement occurs at all, it is likely to be slow and if patients are led to believe otherwise, they will inevitably be disappointed. It is important that professionals involved in the care of patients with personality disorders also take this long-term view, or they too will become frustrated if the patient is not making progress.

Consistency is essential in the management of this group of patients, especially as different people and teams are likely to be involved in their care, for example in primary care, Casualty departments and mental health teams. It is important to have a clear plan that states what treatment is to be offered, and by whom. Without such clarity, the interpersonal problems caused by the patient's personality disorder will undermine their relationships with people involved in their care. However, if a consistent approach can be maintained in the face of these challenges, good working relationships often develop.

### Drug treatments

Drug treatments have a small part to play in the management of personality disorders. Specific serotonin reuptake inhibitors are sometimes used to reduce impulsivity and antipsychotic drugs sometimes reduce tension and overarousal. However, there is a very limited evidence base for these forms of treatment. Given the risks of overdose in some personality disorders and of falsely raising patients' expectations, physical treatments should be used with caution. An exception to this is when the patient is thought to have developed a mental illness in addition to their personality disorder, in which case standard physical treatments should be used.

### Psychological treatments

Psychological treatments are widely used for personality disorders. The psychological defence mechanisms considered in dynamic psychotherapy, such as splitting and projection, are often helpful in understanding personality disorders and sometimes provide a useful basis for treatment. Cognitive behaviour therapy is often used, as thinking biases are a prominent feature of personality disorders, and schema work (see pp. 32–33) is often important. For example, people with paranoid personalities view the world with mistrust and those with dependent personality traits automatically assume they will not be able to cope alone. A specific form of psychological treatment, dialectic behaviour therapy (DBT), is used to treat borderline personality disorder. Patients must commit themselves to stopping self-harm and, in return, their need to be cared for is met in a structured way, through a combination of group work, in which self-management techniques are discussed, and individual therapy sessions.

### Social treatments

Personality disorder often leads to problems with relationships, accommodation, finances and work, and giving simple advice and support or using problem-solving techniques to help patients improve their social circumstances is often beneficial. People with some personality disorders fare poorly if they have nothing to do other than dwell on their circumstances and so should be helped to structure their time with a range of meaningful activities, such as education, work and leisure pursuits.

### Crisis management

The nature of personality disorders means that patients may find themselves overwhelmed by their problems and such crises are often the reason for presentation to medical services. Although it is essential that patients with personality disorders take responsibility for solving their problems, expecting too much of them in the middle of a crisis is likely to make things worse. In such situations, a crisis management approach

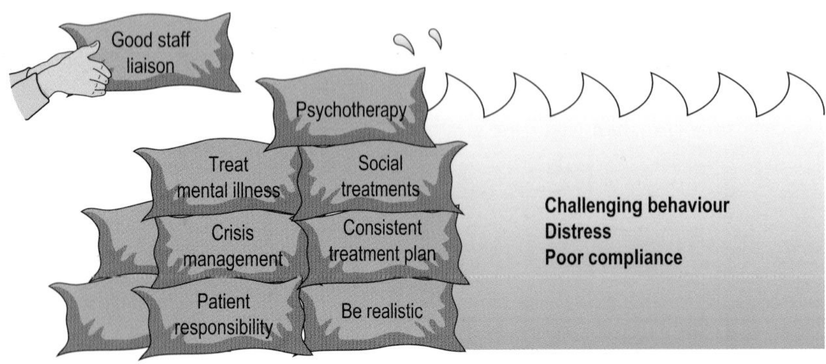


Fig. 1 **Management of personality disorder.**

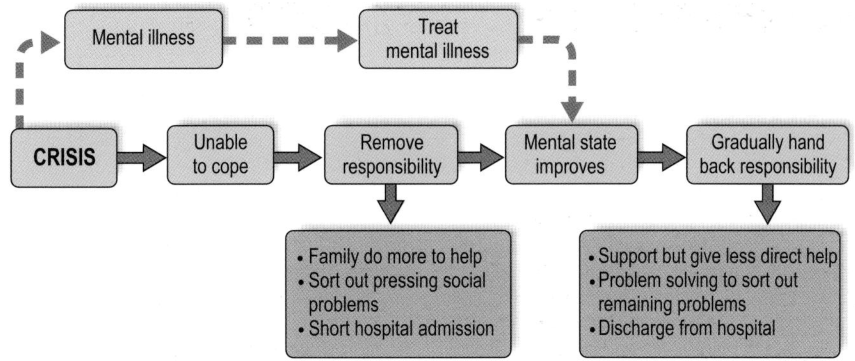


Fig. 2 **Crisis management for personality disorder without (and with) mental illness.**

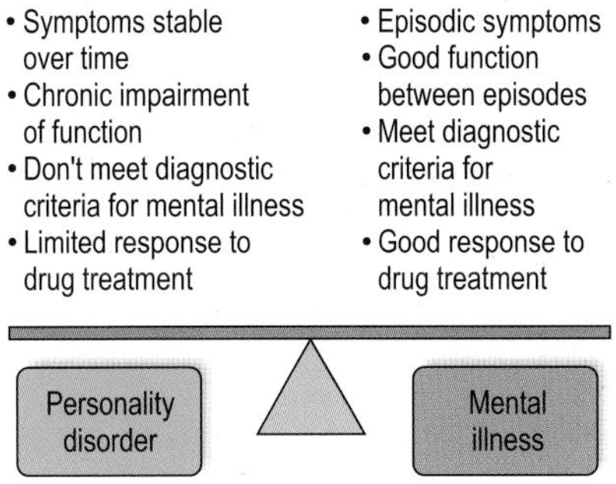

• Symptoms stable over time
• Chronic impairment of function
• Don't meet diagnostic criteria for mental illness
• Limited response to drug treatment

• Episodic symptoms
• Good function between episodes
• Meet diagnostic criteria for mental illness
• Good response to drug treatment

Personality disorder | Mental illness

Fig. 3 **Distinguishing between personality disorder and mental illness.**

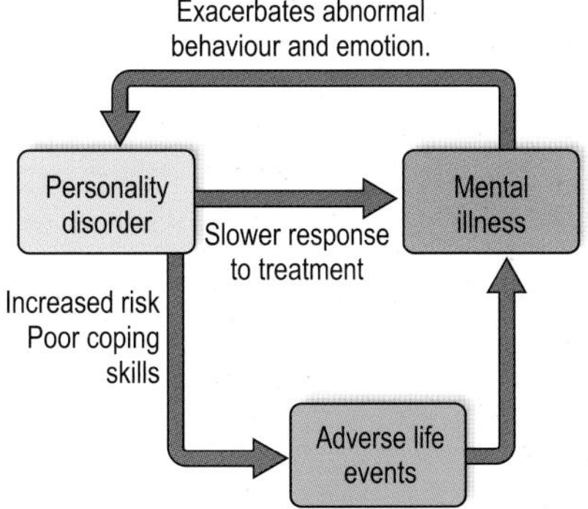


Fig. 4 **Relationship between personality disorder and mental illness.**

> ### *Case history 29*
>
> Following his presentation described in the previous pages, David is placed on the waiting list for an anxiety management group. While waiting for a place to become available, his condition deteriorates. He presents to his doctor saying that he feels like he is about to explode and that everyone looks down on him. He is facing homelessness after being asked to leave by his girlfriend and is likely to lose his job because of arguments with his boss.
>
> a. What treatment should be offered?

should be taken, as described in Figure 2.

## Personality disorder and mental illness

Patients with personality disorders are at considerably increased risk of developing mental illness, especially anxiety and depressive disorders. This is not surprising, as personality disorders by their very nature are likely to lead to an increased frequency of adverse life events. Patients with personality disorders are likely to deal less effectively with adverse life events, and to become more distressed by them, which will increase their risk of developing a mental illness.

If patients with personality disorder develop a mental illness, emotions and behaviours associated with the personality disorder usually become more pronounced. For instance, mental illness may exacerbate the rigidity and stubbornness of a patient with anankastic personality disorder, or the attention seeking behaviour of a patient with histrionic personality disorder. This may result in the patient's problems being wrongly attributed to personality disorder alone and so it is important always to look for evidence of mental illness in such cases. However, it is also important not to diagnose mental illness when it is not present, as this will result in the patient receiving unnecessary treatment and being given unrealistic expectations. It may also result in them not receiving the interventions most likely to help. The important distinction between personality disorder and mental illness can usually be made using the criteria in Figure 3.

Mental illness in patients with personality disorder should be treated in the standard way. Patients with personality disorder will often respond more slowly to treatment and risk assessment and management are often complex and demanding. As a result, referral to mental health services is often needed.

The relationship between mental illness and personality disorder is summarised in Figure 4.

> ### Personality disorders – management
>
> - Management of personality disorder needs to be consistent and realistic: change will be slow and requires commitment from the patient
> - Short-term interventions are often required at times of crisis
> - There is an increased risk of mental illness which should be treated actively

# Learning disability

As with many other areas of psychiatry, the terminology used to describe what ICD10 classifies as mental retardation has changed regularly, to reflect changing philosophies of care and in an attempt to reduce stigma. The term 'Learning disability' is generally used in the UK and so is the one we have adopted in this book. An alternative term still used occasionally is mental handicap.

In learning disability there is impaired intellectual and social functioning that is apparent from early childhood. Intelligence is a broad concept that includes the ability to reason, comprehend and make judgements. It is measured with standardised tests such as the Wechsler Intelligence Scale, which has both performance and verbal sub-scales that can be reported separately or combined to produce a single IQ (intelligence quotient) score. An IQ of 70 and over is considered to be normal. Some 2–3% of the population have an IQ below 70, although half of these have a reasonable level of social functioning and can live independently without extra support. About 0.4% of adolescents have an IQ of less than 50.

## Classification

Learning disability is classified as mild (IQ 50–69), moderate (IQ 35–49), severe (IQ 20–34) or profound (IQ under 20). The division into these four groups is fairly arbitrary and there is a great deal of overlap between them. The spectrum of disability for the key areas of language skills, self care, mobility, academic achievement and ability to work are shown in Table 1.

## Aetiology

The cause of mild learning disability is unknown in about half of cases. Many of these simply represent the lower end of the normal distribution of intelligence. With increasing severity of learning disability, the likelihood of finding a cause increases, with at least 80% of severe cases having some evidence of organic brain damage or disease. Some of the aetiological factors are listed in Figure 1.

It is clear that social factors also play a role in causing learning disability. It has been estimated that up to 5% of cases are due to child abuse, with many being a consequence of brain damage, occurring as a direct result of physical assaults, usually by the parents. Other forms of abuse also appear to have an impact on intellectual performance. Emotional abuse by cruel and neglectful parents who fail to provide a stimulating and nurturing environment for their child results in impaired psychological and physical development. Institutional care can have a similar effect.

Two of the more common clinical syndromes that cause learning disability are described below.

### *Down's syndrome*

Down's syndrome occurs in about 0.2% of all births and 1% of children born to women over 40 years. It is caused by a chromosomal abnormality, trisomy 21, in which there is an extra chromosome 21. People with Down's syndrome have a characteristic facial appearance (Fig. 2). Congenital cardiac abnormalities are found in 40%. Nearly all have moderate or severe learning disability. It used to be thought that Down's syndrome was associated with a particularly compliant and cheerful personality, but this is no longer considered to be the case and it is possible that these characteristics were due to the style of institutional care provided. In fact, children with Down's syndrome have more behavioural problems than children of normal intelligence, although generally less than others with a comparable IQ.

### *Fragile X syndrome*

Fragile X syndrome was first discovered in 1991 and is now thought to be the most common hereditary cause of learning disability. Affected individuals have an abnormal X chromosome which has a fragile site, visible as a constriction near one end of the chromosome. Males are more severely affected by Fragile X because females have a second normal X chromosome. The syndrome is characterised by learning disability and language impairment. Girls may be of normal intelligence. Up to 20% of autistic boys have Fragile X.

Table 1 **Intellectual and social functioning in learning disability**

| | Profound → | Severe → | Moderate → | Mild |
|---|---|---|---|---|
| **IQ** | Under 20 | 20–34 | 35–49 | 50–69 |
| **Language** | Severely limited | → | → | Delayed |
| **Self care** | Totally dependent on others | → | → | Independent |
| **Mobility** | Immobile | → | → | Usually full mobility |
| **Academic** | Unable to read, write or count | → | → | Able to read, write and count with special education |
| **Work** | Unable to work | → | → | Unskilled and semi-skilled manual labour |

**Genetic**
- **Chromosome abnormalities:** Down's syndrome, Fragile X, Klinefelter's syndrome, Turner's syndrome
  **Metabolic disorders:** phenylketonuria, Tay–Sachs, Gaucher's, Lesch–Nyhan syndrome
- **Tuberous sclerosis**
- **Neurofibromatosis**
- **Hydrocephaly**
- **Microcephaly**

**Intra–uterine**
- **Infections:** rubella, lysteria, CMV, syphilis
- **Toxins:** alcohol, lead
- **Physical damage:** injury, radiation, hypoxia
- **Placental dysfunction:** toxaemia

**Perinatal**
- Birth trauma
- Complications of prematurity

**Postnatal**
- **Brain injury:** accidental, child abuse
- **Infections:** encephalitis, meningitis

**MENTAL RETARDATION**

Fig. 1 **Aetiology of learning disability.**

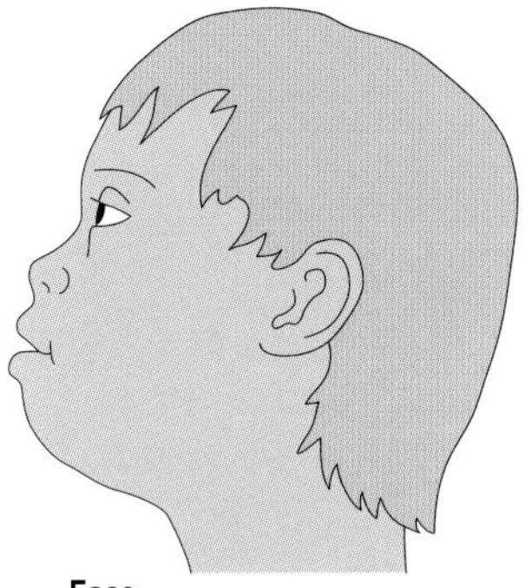


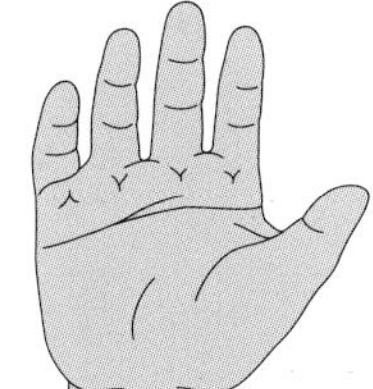


Fig. 2 **Features of Down's syndrome.**

## Mental illness and learning disability

About 40% of all children and adults with learning disability have a mental illness. The risk increases with the severity of the learning impairment. The presence of organic brain disease increases vulnerability to mental illness, but emotional factors also play an important role and must not be overlooked. Children with learning disability often have a sense of being a disappointment to their parents and different from other people. They may be isolated from their family and the community, stigmatised, bullied or abused. They may lack the skills to express their feelings of sadness or anger, and so these feelings will go unrecognised.

The commonest forms of mental illness found in children with learning disability are hyperkinetic disorder and conduct disorders. They are also at increased risk of exploitation and abuse.

In adults, schizophrenia, affective disorders, neurotic disorders and personality disorders are all found more frequently than in the general population. Diagnosis can present a challenge as they may not be able to describe their feelings and experiences, and when making a diagnosis it is often necessary to rely on behavioural changes such as psychomotor retardation, agitation or possible responses to hallucinations. It is sometimes worth giving a trial of medication if the diagnosis is uncertain. Treatment of mental illness is the same as for other patients, although psychological treatments will need to be delivered in a way that takes into account the patient's intellectual and social abilities.

## Management of learning disability

Assessment begins with taking a full psychiatric and medical history from informants, usually the parents or other carers. The family history, achievement of developmental milestones and problem behaviours are particularly important. Mental state examination will rely largely upon observation of the patient's behaviour during the interview, although some will be able to participate in the interview. A thorough physical examination is required, remembering to assess vision and hearing. Finally, a developmental assessment is needed, including standardised measures of intelligence, language, motor performance and social skills. Other sources of information should be approached to complete the picture, including other doctors involved (GP, neurologist, paediatrician, etc.), the school and social services.

A treatment package might include the following:

- *Education in special schools.* Assessment of needs should be completed by an educational psychologist.
- *Support for families.* The birth of a child with learning disability can have a devastating effect on a family. The parents often experience grief over the loss of the anticipated perfect child and may have prolonged feelings of depression, guilt, shame or anger. The majority of families adjust well with support, although a few reject the child or become over-involved, and this can be associated with marital disharmony.
- *Recognition of emotional needs.* As mentioned above, a person with learning disability may have powerful feelings of sadness or anger that they find difficult to express. Creative therapies, such as art or music, can allow communication through media other than words.
- *Employment opportunities.* Many people with mild to moderate learning disability have practical skills that can be developed in sheltered workshops and supported work placements.
- *Institutional care is only needed for a minority.* It is usually provided in small well-staffed community units near the child's family.

### *Case history 30*

Jane is a 34-year-old woman with Down's syndrome and moderate learning disability. She has lived in a staffed hostel with four other residents for the past year since her elderly mother has been unwell and unable to care for her. Her mother died a month ago. She was told of this and went to the funeral but has not spoken of it again. Since then staff report she has been difficult to manage – eating little, irritable and lashing out at times and refusing to take part in her usual activities.

a. What is the cause of Jane's change of behaviour?
b. What could be done to help her?

### Learning disability

- In learning disability (mental retardation in ICD10) both intellectual and social functioning is impaired from early childhood
- 2–3% of the population have an IQ below 70 and half of these require input from specialist services
- Brain disease or damage may occur as a result of genetic, intra-uterine, perinatal, postnatal and social factors
- About 40% of all children and adults with learning disability have a mental illness

# Child psychiatry I

The psychiatric disorders that present in childhood are distinct from those in adults because they arise within complex and intimate family relationships, and are influenced by the developmental stage of the child. Children also present special challenges for assessment and treatment. The psychiatric disorders that present in childhood or adolescence are listed in Table 1.

## Normal childhood development

Some of the features of normal child development are shown in Figure 1. It is essential to consider the developmental stage of the child during a psychiatric assessment, as what is accepted as normal at one stage would be abnormal at another.

Early childhood experiences play an important role in determining what type of person we become in adulthood. The role of parents in this is central. The child with parents (or parent) who are loving and tolerant, yet able to set and enforce clear and reasonable limits is likely to develop a high self esteem, and secure attachment to the parents that will provide a template for secure attachments to others in later life. The theory of 'attachment' was first described by John Bowlby in the 1950s. It derived from his study of young children separated from their mother in hospital. Attachment behaviour begins at around 7 months and consists of clinginess and unwillingness to be separated from the main carer, usually mother. It serves to strengthen the bond between mother and child and has the evolutionary function of ensuring the child is protected from predators. A securely attached child is able to use the mother as a safe base from which exploration of the outside world can begin, and will also be able to cope well with brief separations. If the attachment is insecure, because the parent fails to respond to the child's need for attention or holding, or is inconsistent, the child will have difficulty exploring and separating. This pattern of insecure attachment may persist throughout life, affecting adult relationships.

## Assessment of children

The way in which a psychiatric history is taken and the child is examined will depend upon the age, confidence and language skills of the child. Much of the history will come from the parents, and children who are prepared to separate from their parents can then be seen alone. It is usually best to see adolescents alone and before their parents in order to establish a trusting relationship with them. The interview should take place in a relaxed and friendly atmosphere, with toys and drawing materials provided for children less than 10 years.

The history should include the following:

- **Presenting complaint** – described by both the parent and child. It is important to lead up to asking the child about the presenting complaint gently, after gaining their confidence and talking about neutral topics.
- **Recent behaviour or emotional difficulties** – including general health, mood, sleep, appetite, elimination, relationships, antisocial behaviours, fantasy life and play, and school behaviour.

Table 1 **Classification of psychiatric disorders of childhood and adolescence**

- Pervasive developmental disorders
- Specific developmental disorders
- Hyperkinetic disorders
- Conduct disorders
- Emotional disorders
- Psychiatric aspects of child abuse
- Disorders of elimination

- **Personal history** – pregnancy, birth, milestones (motor, speech, feeding, toilet training, social behaviour), medical history, separations from parents, schools attended and progress in them.
- **Family structure and function** – construction of a genogram is often useful (see Fig. 2 for the genogram constructed for the Case history, Liam). Relationships between family members should be asked about, and the interactions during the interview observed.
- **Temperamental traits** – traits such as activity level, regularity of functions (sleep, bowels, eating), adaptability to new circumstances, willingness to approach new people or situations, quality and intensity of mood, quality of relationships within and outside the family, attention and persistence can be observed from a very young age.

A mental state examination of the child should be completed, although this will often rely on watching behaviour and play. The following should be considered:

- **Appearance** – looking for any abnormality, bruises, cuts, or grazes and appropriateness of dress.
- **Behaviour** – activity level, interactions with parents, motor function, attention and persistence with tasks.
- **Talk** – articulation, vocabulary and use of language.
- **Mood** – happy, elated, unhappy, depressed, anxious, hostile or resentful.
- **Thoughts** – content of speech and fantasy life, for example by asking for three magic wishes.

The assessment should be completed with a physical examination and by speaking to other informants involved with the child or family, such as the family doctor, school teacher, educational psychologist, or social services. Investigations may be performed, most commonly intelligence tests and tests of academic attainment, such as standardised reading tests.

## Pervasive developmental disorder (autism)

Autism is a severe disorder that begins early in life and is apparent by the third birthday. It is characterised by a failure to make social relationships, poor language development and resistance to change with limited and repetitive behaviours and interests. These children fail to notice or respond to other people's emotions or social signals. They do not adapt their behaviour appropriately to new environments, and are very restricted in their play, rarely engaging in make-believe play. Some will have very limited language skills, and those skills that are present will generally not be used in social conversation with others. Three-quarters have significant mental retardation. The outcome is generally poor, with only 15% ever achieving independent functioning.

Autism is at the severe end of a spectrum of disorders, which merges into Asperger's syndrome at the milder end. The autistic spectrum disorders have a prevalence of about 1 in 100 and are four times more common in boys than girls. Genetic factors, and in some cases brain damage, are thought to play an important role in aetiology. Families require a great deal of support and counselling. Social skills and communication training, packages aimed at improving recognition of other people's emotions and behavioural therapy can help.

## Specific developmental disorders

In these disorders, specific skills such as reading, spelling, arithmetical skills, and language are disturbed. The problems are present from early childhood. In order to make a diagnosis of specific developmental disorder, acquired brain trauma or disease must be excluded and the child must have had reasonable opportunities to acquire these skills at home or school.

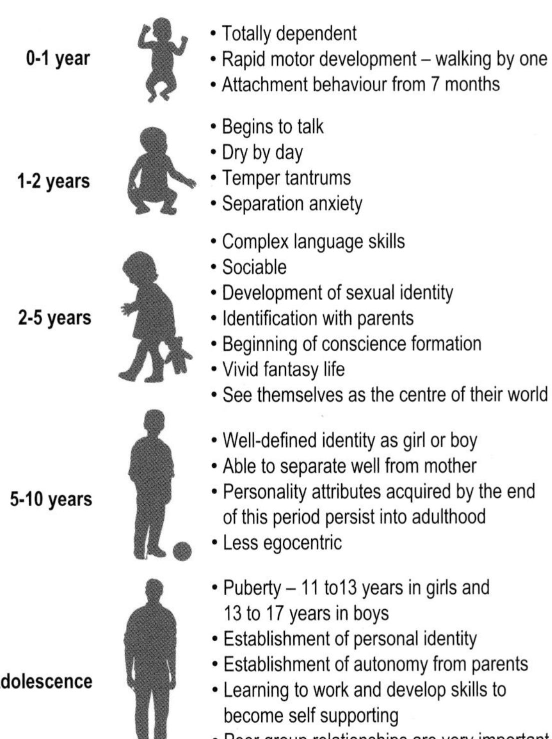


Fig. 1 **Normal childhood development.**

The causes of the specific developmental disorders are not known for sure but are thought to stem from abnormalities in cognitive processing. They are all much more common in boys than girls.

**Specific reading disorder** is particularly common, with a prevalence of 5–10%. Typical reading problems include distortions or additions of words or parts of words, slow reading rate and loss of place in the text. Although specific reading disorder is not due to inadequate schooling, truancy is a common consequence of the academic difficulties. Conduct disorders and specific reading disorder frequently coexist.

## Hyperkinetic disorder

In America this is known as attention deficit hyperactivity disorder (ADHD). The main features of the disorder are overactivity, restlessness, short attention span, distractibility and impulsive behaviour. These children are often clumsy, accident prone and get into trouble with parents and teachers because they act without thinking. Other children will often avoid them and they can become socially isolated.

Symptoms are usually present from an early age, but it is most commonly diagnosed in 6–9-year-olds in whom there is a prevalence of about 8%. It is three times more common in boys than girls. Many causes have been suggested, from genetic factors to allergies and poor parenting. This is one of the very few childhood psychiatric conditions that can be treated with medication. Amphetamine-like stimulants are used, such as methylphenidate, which have the paradoxical effect of reducing activity levels and improving attention in the short term. This can result in improvements in academic and social performance. Behavioural therapy, using a system of rewards for good behaviour, is also useful for these children.

### *Case history 31*

Liam is a 6-year-old boy who lives with his mother, step-father, older brother and baby sister. He has always been a noisy, active and demanding child, difficult to engage in any activity for more than a few minutes. He is having great difficulty at school, finding it almost impossible to sit still and frequently disrupting the class. He has temper tantrums if frustrated and has to be carefully monitored with his sister as he has been aggressive towards her at times. He has no friends at school because he is unable to settle to play with them. His mother feels unable to cope, she thinks her husband is too strict with Liam and she tries to compensate for this and avoid confrontations. Liam's family tree (genogram) is shown in Figure 2.

a. What is the most likely diagnosis?
b. What factors may be contributing to Liam's problems?
c. What practical advice could you give his mother about handling his difficult behaviour?

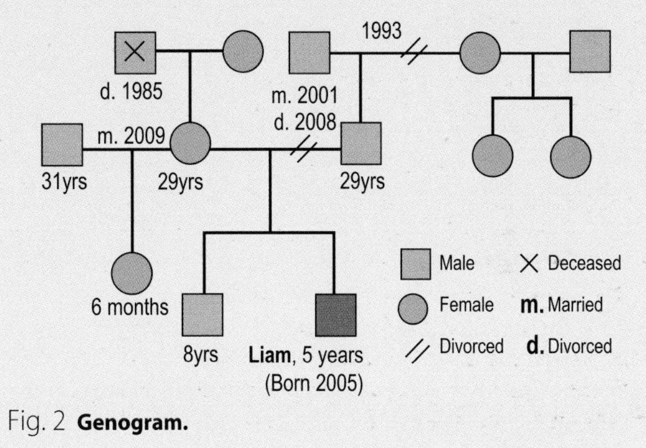


Fig. 2 **Genogram.**

Hyperactivity disorder tends to improve with age, with only one-quarter having persisting problems in adolescence. About half of these will continue to exhibit some features of the hyperactivity into adulthood, and this often expresses itself as dissocial behaviour.

### Child psychiatry 1

- In assessing children it is essential to consider their family relationships and developmental stage
- Pervasive developmental disorder (autism) is more common in boys than girls, and is characterised by a failure to make social relationships, poor language development, resistance to change, and mental retardation in the majority
- Hyperkinetic disorder is more common in boys than girls and is characterised by overactivity, restlessness, short attention span, distractibility and impulsivity

# Child psychiatry II

## Conduct disorder

The main features of conduct disorders are persistent antisocial behaviours such as fighting, bullying, severe temper tantrums, damaging property, starting fires, stealing, truancy, and persistent and defiant disobedience. The child's age must be taken into account, and normal naughtiness should not be considered a sign of conduct disorder. A third of cases have specific reading disorder, and there is considerable overlap with hyperactivity disorder. Conduct disorders are common. Among adolescents about 8% of boys and 5% of girls have a conduct disorder. It is less common in younger children, particularly in girls.

There are two types of conduct disorder:

- **Socialised conduct disorder**. These children are able to make friends who usually also behave in an antisocial way. The bad behaviour is therefore usually most evident away from home. Relationships with adults may be good, although there are often difficulties with authority figures.
- **Unsocialised conduct disorder**. These children do not have friends, either because they have been rejected by their peers or because they deliberately choose to isolate themselves. The antisocial behaviour therefore occurs alone. Some degree of emotional disorder is often also present in these children.

The causes of conduct disorders are a complex interaction between the biological make-up of the child, family influences and environmental factors as summarised in Figure 1. The style of parenting is thought to be important. Conduct disorders are likely to develop if parents fail to give clear boundaries, monitor behaviour and administer ineffective or inconsistent discipline. Improving parenting skills is likely to improve behaviour even if other causative factors are present. Other treatment approaches include family therapy, behavioural therapy, remedial teaching and provision of alternative peer group activities. The outcome is better for the socialised group. Two-thirds of the unsocialised group will have persisting dissocial behaviour in adulthood.

## Emotional disorders

Emotional disorders of childhood are characterised by anxiety and depression. They are present in 2–3% of children and, unusually for childhood psychiatric disorders, are more common in girls. They generally have a good prognosis.

### *Separation anxiety disorder*

It is normal for toddlers and pre-school children to feel some anxiety over real or threatened separation from their parents. In separation anxiety disorder the anxiety is unusually severe or occurs in older children, and causes some problems in social functioning such as preventing the child from attending school. Symptoms include persistent worries about separation from the attachment figure (usually mother) and great distress if forced to do so. Some will refuse to go to sleep without their mother nearby and have nightmares about separation. Parental overprotection is commonly present and other causes include the child's temperament and stressful events, particularly those involving separation such as family breakdown, bereavement or illness.

### *Anxiety disorders of childhood*

Specific phobias about animals, the dark or strangers are normal in young children and rarely need treatment. Generalised anxiety disorder can occur and is frequently characterised by somatic symptoms, particularly abdominal pain.

### *Depressive illness*

The symptoms of depressive illness are much the same in children as in adults – low mood, anhedonia, altered sleep and appetite, and depressive thoughts. Fleeting suicidal thoughts are quite common, but completed suicide is rare. Moderate and severe depressive illness is uncommon in pre-pubertal children, with a steady increase in incidence over the teenage years. The causes of depression and its treatment are also similar to those in adults, although antidepressant drugs are less effective in children, and should be used with caution. Psychological treatment approaches are preferred.

### *School refusal*

In school refusal the child refuses to attend school because of specific fears about the school, the journey to it or separation anxiety. This accounts for about 1% of all school absences and is much less common than truancy in which the child conceals their absence from school from their parents. The characteristics of children with school refusal are compared to those who habitually truant in Table 1. School refusal should be treated by returning the child to school as quickly as possible as avoidance is likely to heighten the anxiety. A graded reintroduction may be necessary, with support for both child and parents.

## Child abuse

Child abuse may take the form of neglect, emotional, physical or sexual abuse. It plays a role in precipitating psychiatric disorders in children which may continue through to adulthood. It is essential that all professionals who come into contact with children are alert to the possibility of abuse playing a role in the problems presented by a child and its family.

The incidence of abuse is difficult to measure as the majority of cases go unreported, and definitions of what constitutes abuse varies. Official figures for reported cases of abuse have risen in recent years, although this is likely to be due to greater reporting rather than a true increase in abuse. A British study found that 12% of women and 8% of men reported some form of sexual abuse before the age of 16 years.

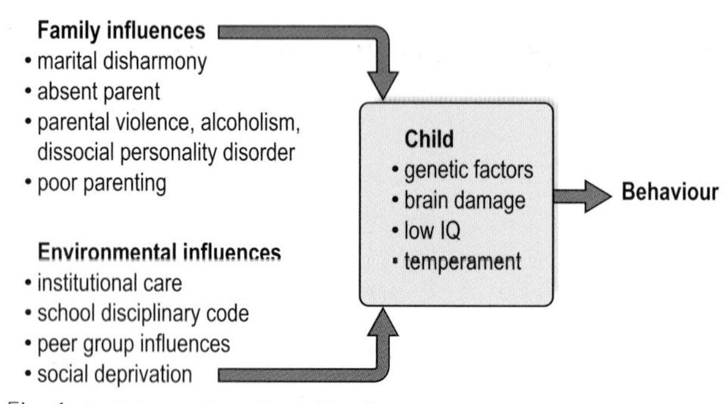


Fig. 1 **Aetiology of conduct disorder.**

Table 1 **Comparison of characteristics of children presenting with persistent truancy and school refusal**

| School refusal | Truancy |
|---|---|
| Absence from school known to parents | Absence from school concealed from parents |
| Spends day at home alone or with parent | May spend day away from home with peers |
| Peak incidence at 11 years | Increases with age |
| Fear of school or separation anxiety | No emotional disorder |
| All social classes | Increased incidence in lower social classes |
| No increase in parental marital discord | Dysfunctional family |
| Overprotective parenting | Harsh parenting |

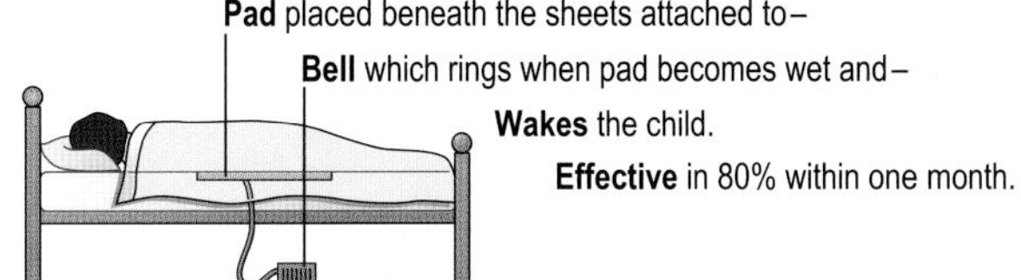


Fig. 2 **Pad and bell – a behavioural treatment for nocturnal enuresis.**

There are many contributory factors in the abuse of children. Some children are more vulnerable than others, for example those who are unwanted, have early separation from the mother, are mentally or physically handicapped, or have temperamental characteristics that make them difficult to handle. Some parents are more likely to be abusive, particularly those who have themselves been abused as children, live in poor socioeconomic circumstances and have unrealistic styles of disciplining their children.

The most common form of sexual abuse is father–daughter incest. Sexually abused children may present with a sudden change in their social behaviour or academic performance, or with conduct disorders. Some engage in repetitive sexual play and are sexually precocious. It is important to give these children an opportunity to disclose their abuse, but great care must be taken to avoid adding to their trauma. Social services must be informed of any disclosure of sexual abuse by a child and have responsibility for ensuring the safety of the child and instigating childcare proceedings. The emotional effects of childhood sexual abuse may be addressed in individual psychotherapy with the child. Adolescents and adults may also be offered group therapy which has the advantages of reducing the sense of isolation and allowing development of trust and self esteem. One-third of sexually abused children have no long-term negative effects, the rest are prone to depressive illness, low self esteem, sexual problems and have a tendency to re-victimisation in adulthood.

## Disorders of elimination

### *Enuresis*

Enuresis is involuntary emptying of the bladder occurring after the age of 5 years in the absence of an organic cause. Bedwetting (nocturnal enuresis) is common, occurring in 10% of 5-year-olds, 5% of 10-year-olds and 1% of 15-year-olds. Daytime enuresis is less common. The enuresis is considered to be primary if there has been no preceding period of bladder control, and secondary if it follows a period of continence. It is twice as common in boys than girls, and most cases are thought to be due to delayed neurological maturation which simply corrects itself with time. There is often a positive family history of the same problem. Secondary enuresis may occur as a feature of regressive behaviour at times of stress. Management consists of excluding a physical cause, particularly a urinary tract infection, reassuring the parents and encouraging them to handle the problem calmly and gently. Instituting a simple behavioural programme such as a star chart or pad and bell (see Fig. 2) can be used.

### *Encopresis*

Encopresis is defecation in inappropriate places despite having normal bowel control. Most children are fecally continent by the age of 3 years. At 8 years, 2% of boys and 1% of girls have encopresis. This may be due to inadequate toilet training or may have a psychological cause with the behaviour representing the child's feelings of anger or regression at a time of stress. Constipation with overflow incontinence is the main differential diagnosis to be excluded.

## Adolescence

Adolescents have difficult social and emotional issues to deal with. For example, there is frequently conflict over the degree of independence they wish for and are allowed to have from their parents. The peer group becomes very important and influential, and can provide valuable support for individuals to try new things away from the family. They can also arouse a great deal of anxiety about rejection from the group, and may promote delinquent behaviour. Development of sexual relationships is another potential source of confusion, anxiety and conflict.

The pattern of psychiatric disorders changes as children become adolescents. There is a marked increase in depressive disorder, particularly in girls, and schizophrenia becomes much more common in late adolescence. Problems with alcohol and drug abuse and eating disorders also tend to emerge at this time. Development disorders have usually resolved.

### *Case history 32*

Charlotte is a 7-year-old-girl who lives with her mother and two younger sisters. Her parents have recently separated and she has weekly contact with her father. She has started to wet the bed after being dry at night for 4 years. Her mother is angry with her, believing that the bed wetting is deliberate defiance.

a. What is the most likely diagnosis?
b. What other causes should be excluded?
c. How would you advise Charlotte's mother to manage this problem?

### Child psychiatry 2

- Conduct disorders are more common in boys than girls, and are most likely to occur in 12–16-year-olds
- Conduct disorders may be 'socialised', in which the problem behaviour occurs within a peer group, or 'unsocialised' in which the behaviour occurs alone
- Emotional disorders are more common in girls than boys and include separation anxiety, phobias, depression and school refusal
- It is important to be alert to the possibility of childhood neglect or abuse, which may be physical, emotional or sexual in nature

# Old age psychiatry I

## Dementia

The prevalence of dementia rises sharply in old age, with 5% of people over 65 years and 20% of people over 80 years being affected. The commonest causes of dementia in old age in the UK are Alzheimer's disease (up to 65% of cases), vascular dementia (up to 20%) and Lewy body disease (up to 10%). Alzheimer's disease is also the commonest form of presenile dementia (dementia presenting before the age of 65), but is usually managed by old age psychiatrists whatever the age of presentation. Pick's disease is included in this section for the same reason, even though the majority of cases present before the age of 65. Other causes of presenile dementia are described on pages 70–71.

### Alzheimer's disease

#### *Epidemiology and aetiology*

Women develop Alzheimer's disease slightly more often than men. There is a strong genetic component with the risk being three times higher in people with an affected first-degree relative. In the early onset form, there is sometimes an autosomal dominant pattern of inheritance. Abnormalities of the amyloid precursor gene on chromosome 21 have been established in some pedigrees which is not surprising for two reasons – amyloid peptide is found in senile plaques and Alzheimer's disease develops in up to 50% of patients with Down's syndrome who survive beyond the age of 40 years. Linkage with a site on chromosome 14 has also been established in other early onset cases and loci on other chromosomes are almost certainly involved. In contrast, late-onset Alzheimer's disease is familial but does not show a Mendelian pattern of inheritance, which suggests a polygenic aetiology, perhaps in combination with environmental factors. Association with a number of genes has been demonstrated, one example being the E4 allele of apolipoprotein E on chromosome 19 which is found in up to 50% of cases of Alzheimer's disease but in only 10% of the general population.

#### *Pathology*

The characteristic pathology of Alzheimer's disease consists of progressive atrophy of cortical and subcortical structures. Histologically, there are neurofibrillary tangles and amyloid containing senile plaques throughout the brain. While many neurotransmitters are affected, there is widespread loss of neurones containing acetylcholine which correlates well with the degree of cognitive impairment observed clinically. Both neurofibrillary tangles and senile plaques occur in normal ageing but are more numerous and widespread in Alzheimer's disease.

#### *Presenting features*

In many ways, Alzheimer's disease is a diagnosis of exclusion, being made when features of other causes of dementia are not present. Any combination of the features of dementia described on page 70 may occur, but many cases present with a characteristic clinical picture which includes:

- poor memory
- disorientation as an early sign which can lead to perplexity, fear and wandering as the illness progresses
- 'coarsening' of premorbid personality traits, e.g. a person who has always been stuck in their ways may become much more rigid and inflexible
- gradual deterioration of social skills and behaviour
- non-specific mood changes: depressed, euphoric, flattened or labile
- frontal and parietal lobe signs.

### Pick's disease

Recent claims that Pick's disease is the cause of up to 20% of cases of presenile dementia are probably exaggerated but it is certainly an important cause of dementia in younger people. It usually presents between the ages of 50 and 60 years. In the small number of cases with a family history, the inheritance appears to be autosomal dominant but in most cases there is no identifiable cause. The characteristic pathology is of cortical atrophy, known as knifeblade atrophy because of the appearance of the atrophic gyri. Within the atrophic areas are silver staining intracellular inclusions known as Pick bodies and swollen neurones known as Pick cells. This atrophy is usually confined to the frontal and temporal lobes and as a result, the clinical picture in the early stages is often dominated by apathy, disinhibition and other changes in personality and social behaviour, with abnormalities of speech developing as the disease progresses.

### Vascular dementia

This is the second most common cause of dementia. It was previously known as multi-infarct dementia but this term has been replaced by vascular dementia in ICD10. There is generalised or localised atrophy of the brain which results in enlarged ventricles. The distinctive pathological finding is areas of infarction, usually in several parts of the brain.

Reduced cholinergic function is not a cause of cognitive impairment in vascular dementia. Now that cholinergic drugs are being advocated for the treatment of Alzheimer's disease, it is important to be able to differentiate between the two conditions. Establishing the diagnosis also affects prognosis as the life expectancy of 4–5 years in vascular dementia is shorter than in Alzheimer's disease. The clinical features of Alzheimer's and vascular dementia are contrasted in Table 1.

### Lewy body dementia

This is the third most common cause of dementia. It is characterised histologically by intracellular inclusion bodies (Lewy bodies) in the cerebral cortex. Lewy bodies are also found in subcortical areas, particularly the substantia nigra – which explains why Parkinsonian signs are common in this form of dementia. This pathology also explains why there is extreme sensitivity to the side effects of antipsychotic drugs, with some patients becoming very unwell following relatively low doses. The other features that help distinguish Lewy body disease from Alzheimer's disease are a fluctuating rather than gradual course and the occurrence of hallucinations, which are usually visual and can lead to a mistaken diagnosis of delirium.

There is a considerable overlap between Lewy body dementia and Parkinson's disease in which Lewy bodies are also found, predominantly in the substantia nigra rather than in the cerebral cortex. Some patients with Parkinson's disease go on to develop dementia and in these cases there is considerable Lewy body disease in both the substantia nigra and the cerebral cortex.

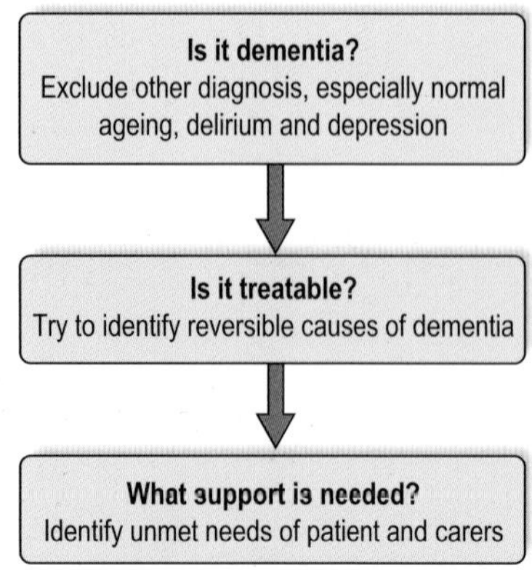


Fig. 1 **Assessment of patients with suspected dementia.**

| Table 1 **Clinical differences between vascular dementia and Alzheimer's disease** | |
|---|---|
| **Vascular dementia** | **Alzheimer's disease** |
| Step-wise course with relatively sudden onset/deterioration following infarction | Insidious onset, gradual course |
| Insight and personality deteriorate later | Insight and personality deteriorate earlier |
| Depression and anxiety common | Depression and anxiety less common |
| Patchy cognitive deficits, i.e. only a few aspects of cognitive function affected | Global cognitive deficits, i.e. many aspects of cognitive function affected |
| Hard neurological signs (e.g. old CVA, Parkinsonism) | Soft signs only |
| History of cardiovascular disease | |

## Management of dementia

### *Clinical assessment*

Assessment and management of patients with suspected dementia is a three-stage process, as shown in Figure 1. As patients with dementia are often unable to give a full account of their problems, mental state examination and history from informants are particularly important. Physical examination and investigations are essential, to exclude possible causes of delirium (p. 70) and treatable causes of dementia. Physical investigations required are shown in Table 2 and some important treatable causes of dementia are illustrated in Figure 2.

### *Person-centred care*

Any management plan must be person-centred, that is, it must take full account of the individual characteristics and perspective of the patient, their circumstances, the importance of their relationships with others, and the needs of their carers. The ability of the patient to engage in planning about their care and treatment will depend upon their capacity to make decisions (see p. 16). There are many potential non-drug interventions that may be helpful in reducing agitation, such as aromatherapy, multisensory stimulation or music therapy. Simple behavioural techniques such as use of prompts can be useful for mild memory impairment. Psychologists may have a role in developing interventions tailored to the individual to address specific behavioural problems. Psychological treatment is also widely used to support carers. Social treatments, which are outlined in Figure 3, provide structured activity and care.

### *Drug treatments*

Underlying causes should be treated in the usual way but otherwise, physical treatments have a limited role. Night sedation is helpful for sleep disturbance and nocturnal wandering. If persistent depressive symptoms occur, antidepressant drugs can be useful, bearing in mind that older patients are particularly susceptible to antimuscarinic side effects which include impaired cognitive function. Antipsychotic drugs are of very limited use, and must be used with caution as they are associated with increased risk of cerebrovascular disease and death. Patients with Lewy Body dementia are also at risk of developing severe extrapyramidal side effects.

Drug treatments for Alzheimer's disease have been developed. They are acetylcholinesterase inhibitors, and are described on page 30.

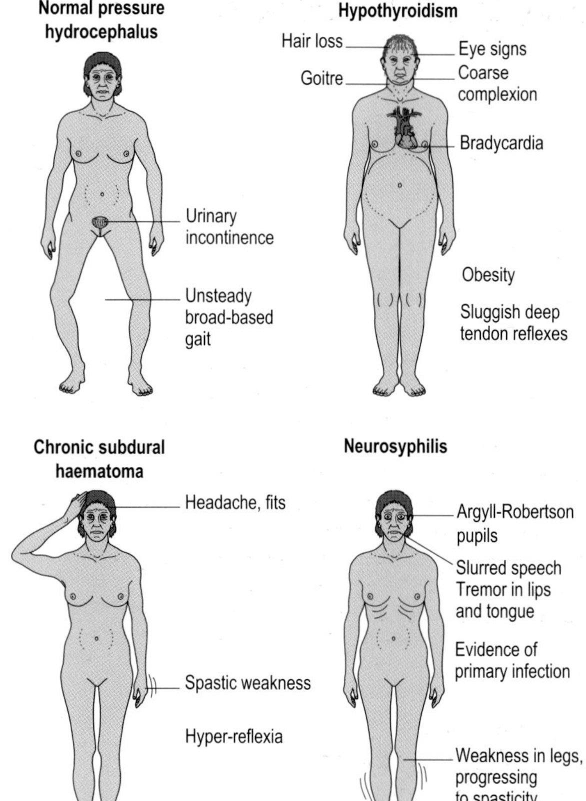


Fig. 2 **Some treatable causes of dementia.**

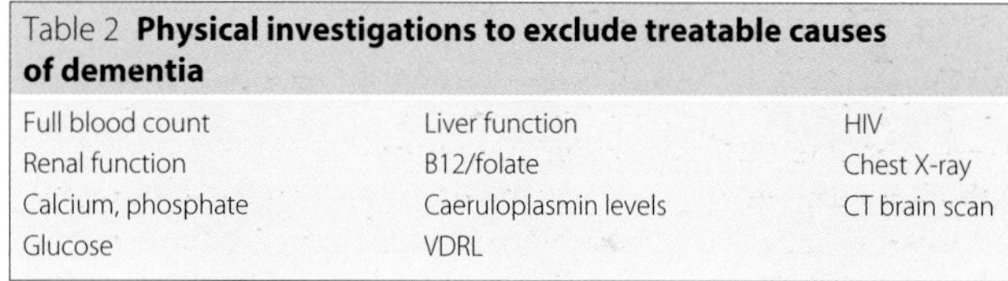

| Table 2 **Physical investigations to exclude treatable causes of dementia** | | |
|---|---|---|
| Full blood count | Liver function | HIV |
| Renal function | B12/folate | Chest X-ray |
| Calcium, phosphate | Caeruloplasmin levels | CT brain scan |
| Glucose | VDRL | |

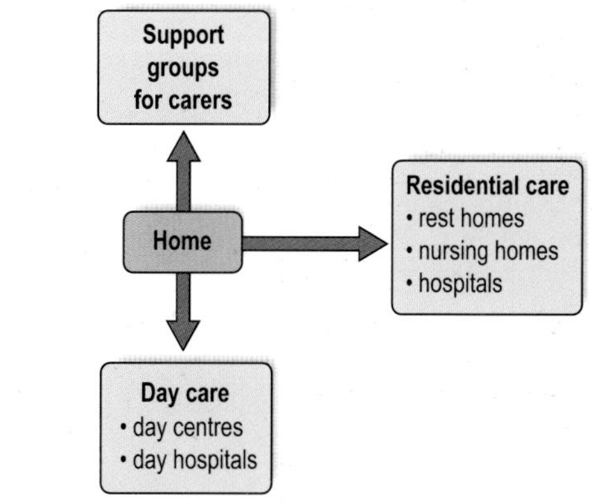


Fig. 3 **Social treatments for dementia.**

### *Case history 33*

Frank is 74 years old. He has hypertension and smokes a pipe. His daughter says that his memory has been gradually deteriorating. He struggles to think of words when talking. He is having trouble dressing himself and has become apathetic and disengaged. He is unsteady on his feet. He becomes lost when away from his home environment. He has been incontinent a few times. He seems indifferent to these problems.

a. What is the likely diagnosis?
b. Is there any treatment likely to improve his condition?

**Old age psychiatry 1**

- Dementia is a syndrome with many causes
- Some causes are treatable
- Social treatments ease the burden of dementia for patients and their carers

# Old age psychiatry II

## Other conditions common in old age

If dementia did not exist, there probably would not be a separate speciality of Old Age Psychiatry. However, there are several reasons why having a separate speciality is also an advantage when it comes to the assessment and management of other mental health problems. First, there are differences in the way functional mental illnesses present in elderly people, as will be described below. Second, it can sometimes be difficult to differentiate between the mental illnesses found most frequently among elderly people, and old age psychiatrists become skilled in making this differential diagnosis (Fig. 1). Third, prescribing psychotropic medication for elderly people is particularly challenging (Fig. 2), especially as there is a high rate of medical problems among elderly people with mental illness. Finally, social problems are an important cause of mental health problems in all age groups. The social needs of elderly patients are usually different to their younger counterparts and so are more likely to be met by teams with expertise in this area.

### Depressive disorders

It used to be thought that the prevalence of depressive disorders increased with age. However, more recent research has found the prevalence of depressive episodes to be 3–5% in people over 65 years, with a further 10% suffering from depressive symptoms which are not severe enough for a diagnosis of depressive episode to be made. These rates are similar or even slightly lower than rates in younger people. Many elderly people with depression are suffering a recurrence of a depressive disorder that started earlier in their lives and the risk of becoming depressed for the first time actually decreases from 60 years onwards. Women are affected more often than men, as is the case for all age groups. There are some differences in aetiology compared with younger patients, as described in Figure 3.

#### *Presentation*

Clinical presentation of depression in the elderly is much the same as in younger people with a few differences. Older people are less likely to complain of low mood, perhaps because discussion of emotions is a relatively recent fashion. As a result, the diagnosis often has to be based on other symptoms of depression such as loss of interest and enjoyment of life and disturbed sleep and appetite. Symptoms such as psychomotor retardation or agitation, paranoid beliefs, nihilistic delusions and hypochondriacal worries probably occur more often than in younger people, although this is controversial. Depression often has an impact on concentration and attention, which in turn can impair memory. Some patients will present with prominent cognitive impairment as a consequence of depression. This is sometimes referred to as 'pseudodementia'. Anxiety disorders usually begin earlier in life and so an underlying depressive episode should be suspected if anxiety symptoms develop for the first time in an elderly person.

#### *Treatment*

Physical treatments for depression are usually very effective, with about 85% of cases responding within a few months.

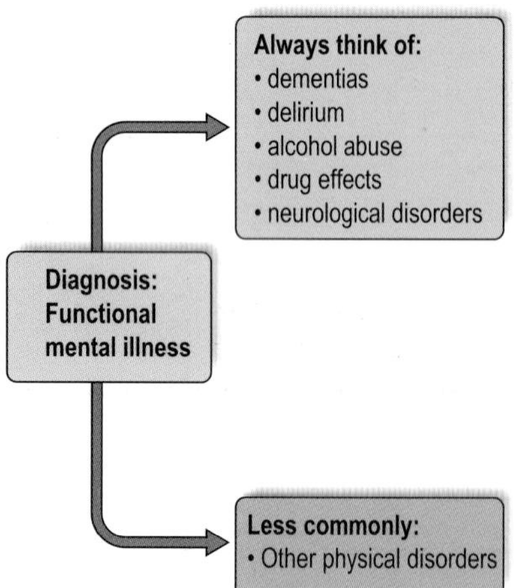


Fig. 1 **Differential diagnosis of functional illness in the elderly.**

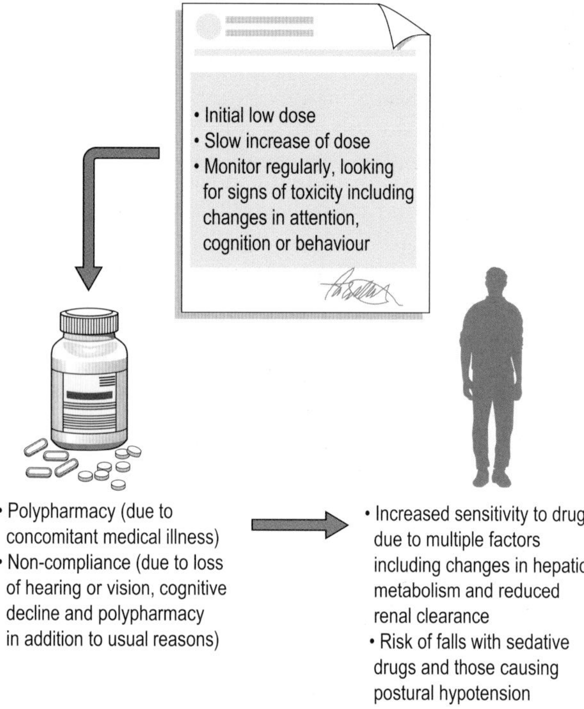


Fig. 2 **Problems associated with prescribing psychotropic medication in the elderly.**

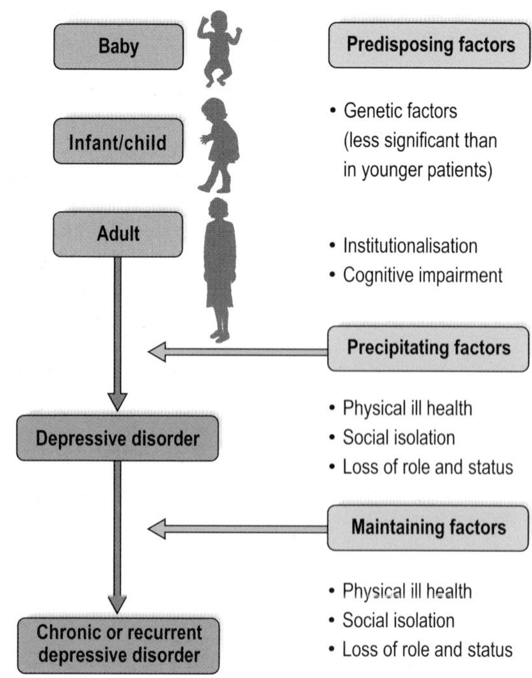


Fig. 3 **Aetiology of depression in the elderly.**

Along with these benefits, it is important to remember the problems associated with prescribing in the elderly (Fig. 2). ECT is a safe procedure in the elderly provided they are fit to receive an anaesthetic. Social treatments are important when there are social factors precipitating or perpetuating depressive episodes. Apart from supportive psychotherapy, psychological treatments are used less often than in younger patients. The exception to this is bereavement counselling, for obvious reasons. Prognosis is not as good as in younger patients, and is determined by a number of factors as summarised in Figure 4.

## Hypomania

The clinical presentation and treatment of hypomania is similar for all age groups. When it occurs in the elderly, there is nearly always a past history of bipolar affective disorder. If hypomanic symptoms occur for the first time in old age, an organic cause should be strongly suspected. Full-blown manic episodes are unusual in the elderly.

## Schizophrenia and delusional disorder

Patients with schizophrenia that starts in early adult life have a reduced life expectancy. There are a number of reasons for this, including their increased risk of suicide and their high rate of cigarette smoking. As a result, a relatively low proportion survives into old age. Those that do may still present with acute psychotic episodes but more often will have developed chronic schizophrenia with predominantly negative symptoms.

It is relatively uncommon for paranoid illnesses to present for the first time in old age. When they do, loss of vision and hearing, and social isolation often play a significant role in the aetiology. In the past, late-onset paranoid illnesses were labelled 'paraphrenia', but this term is not included in ICD10. The same diagnostic criteria are therefore used regardless of age of onset.

## Alcohol problems

Alcohol consumption tends to decrease with age. Elderly people may reduce their alcohol intake because they are less tolerant to the effects of alcohol and worry more about the consequences of intoxication, especially falls. They also spend less time in social environments where alcohol consumption takes place. Because of this, alcohol problems are less common than among younger people. However, they still occur in the elderly and so it is important to overcome the embarrassment that is often felt about asking older people about their alcohol consumption. It is also necessary to acknowledge differences in the way some elderly people view alcohol. For instance, some may drink for what they consider to be medicinal purposes and might not mention this if not directly asked. Also, some of the current generation of elderly people add alcohol to hot drinks but do not include this when asked about their alcohol consumption.

Some patients who present in old age have had lifelong alcohol problems. They may become worse following retirement because of having more time in which to drink alcohol. They may present with the medical complications of alcohol abuse, which are more likely to affect older people. Patients without a history of alcohol problems earlier in life will usually have started drinking excessively in response to adverse life events, difficult social circumstances or the pain and disability caused by physical illness. It is especially important to check for symptoms of an underlying mental illness in this late-onset group, particularly depression.

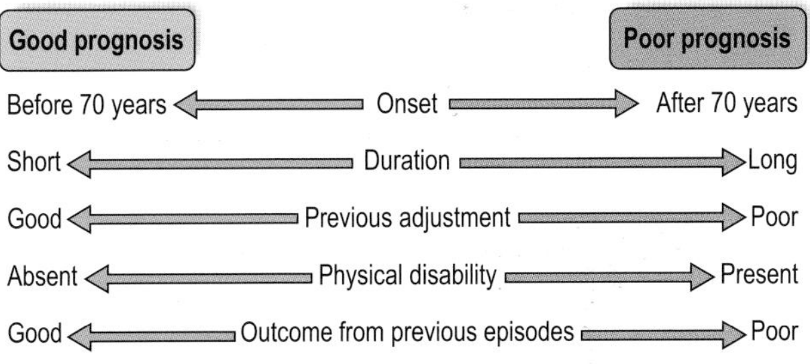

Fig. 4 **Outcome of depression in the elderly.**

## Suicide and deliberate self-harm

Suicide rates are highest among people aged 40–60 years but they are much higher among the over-60s than the under-40s. As in other age groups, depressive disorder and alcohol dependence are the disorders most commonly associated with suicide in elderly people. Concurrent physical illness is found in about 60% of deaths which highlights the fact that elderly people with both mental and physical illness are at particularly high risk of suicide. Social isolation and being widowed or separated also increase the risk.

Deliberate self harm is uncommon among the elderly. When it occurs it is considerably more likely to be a failed suicide attempt than a 'cry for help'. As a result, great care should be taken when assessing suicide risk in this group, particularly as older patients are often embarrassed to admit to suicidal motives.

### *Case history 34*

Elsie is an 82-year-old woman who lives alone and has been widowed for 8 years. She has atrial fibrillation and her mobility is limited by rheumatoid arthritis. She presents with a 2-month history of psychomotor retardation, loss of interest in her usual activities, self neglect and loss of appetite with weight loss. In the past 24 hours she has refused to eat or drink because she believes her insides have rotted away.

a. What is the diagnosis?
b. How would you treat her?

### Old age psychiatry 2

- Caution is required in prescribing for the elderly, as they are more sensitive to drug effects and suffer more side effects
- Rates of depression in the elderly are similar to those in younger people
- Schizophrenia presenting for the first time in old age is uncommon
- It is important to ask elderly patients directly and in detail about alcohol consumption
- Deliberate self harm is relatively uncommon, and suicide more common amongst the elderly as compared to young people

# Forensic psychiatry

Forensic psychiatry is a sub-speciality concerned with the assessment and treatment of mentally disordered offenders. A large part of the work of forensic psychiatrists is the assessment of people held at various stages of the criminal justice system, which is portrayed in Figure 1. They may also be asked to assess patients under the care of general psychiatric services who are thought to be at high risk of committing an offence. In some areas, there are community forensic psychiatry teams that work with psychiatric patients likely to commit criminal offences.

Forensic psychiatrists also provide inpatient care in conditions of high, medium or low security. Until 1980, the main provision for forensic inpatient treatment in England and Wales was in three Special Hospitals which provided psychiatric care in conditions of high security. A series of scandals following revelations of security breaches and abuses emerged, and led to reform of the way inpatient care was delivered, and a move towards treating mentally disordered offenders in Regional Secure Units, which provide conditions of medium security. Patients are either admitted to these directly, or are transferred there from one of the High Secure Hospitals when they no longer require this level of security. Regional Secure Units have the advantage of keeping patients closer to their family and friends and, because they are much smaller than the High Secure Hospitals, have fewer of the problems associated with large institutions. They are also able to work more closely with the local psychiatric services in their region, which makes it safer and easier to transfer the care of patients who no longer require conditions of medium security.

A minority of patients in Regional Secure Units and Special Hospitals are referred directly from district psychiatric units rather than the criminal justice system. These are patients whose risk to themselves or others cannot safely be managed within their local psychiatric hospital.

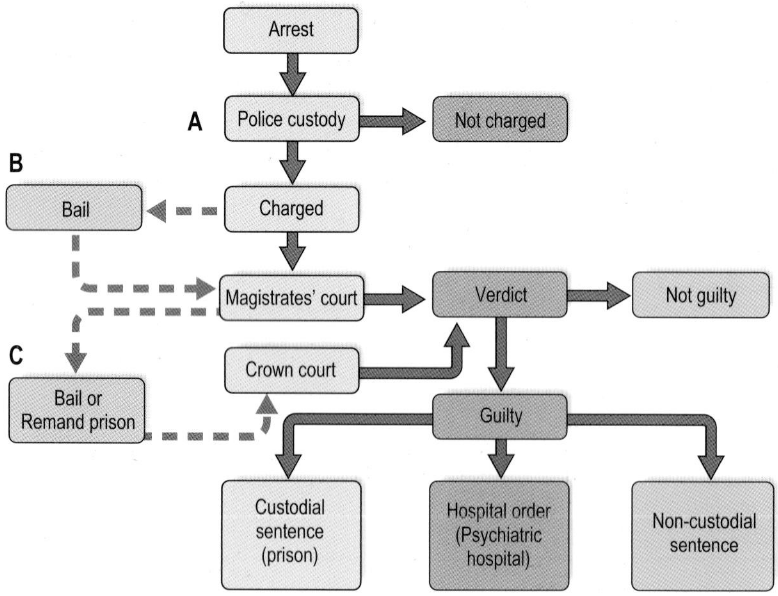

## Diversion of mentally disordered offenders

The need for forensic psychiatry is based on two important principles. The first is that if someone commits a crime because of a mental disorder, then treatment of the mental disorder is in the best interests of the individual and society. Table 1 summarises the common ways in which mental disorder leads to crime. Secondly, imprisonment usually exacerbates mental disorder and reduces the chance of rehabilitating the offender, and may result in unnecessary suffering. Therefore, it is often best for mentally disordered offenders to be dealt with by psychiatrists rather than remain within the criminal justice system. The process of getting them out of the criminal justice system is usually referred to as diversion of mentally disordered offenders.

Most crime is petty and this is true of crimes committed by people with mental disorder. Because of this, point **A** on Figure 1 is an important point of diversion. Most police officers now receive training in the recognition of mental disorder. They are encouraged to seek a psychiatric opinion if they suspect someone in their custody to have a mental disorder. For minor offences, they will often choose not to press charges if psychiatric treatment is to be offered. Alternatively, the magistrate hearing the case will take psychiatric recommendations into account when deciding on a sentence. This work is usually done by local psychiatric services, rather than forensic psychiatrists. In many areas, court diversion schemes operate in which psychiatrists, psychiatric nurses or social workers are available each day to carry out assessments at the request of the police or the magistrates' court.

Forensic psychiatrists are usually involved in the assessment of people who have committed more serious crimes that require trial by jury in a Crown court. These assessments usually take place at points **B** and **C** of Figure 1. The forensic psychiatrist will determine whether a mental disorder is present and whether treatment will reduce the risk of reoffending, or help the offender in other ways. If mental disorder is present, they will make recommendations about where treatment should be given based on their assessment of the level of risk the offender poses to the public. Often assessments will be made by more than one psychiatrist. If, after considering the psychiatric evidence, the judge believes that psychiatric treatment is required, then one of a number of options (Table 2) will be chosen, depending on the offence and the level of risk. These options for sentencing are also available to magistrates, except for restriction orders which can only be applied by a Crown court.

While the sentence in a criminal trial is influenced considerably by psychiatric evidence, the same is not usually true of the verdict. This is because psychiatric evidence does not usually help a jury decide whether the accused committed the act they are being tried for. The exception to this is in cases of homicide, where psychiatric evidence about the offender's state of mind at the time of the offence may result in a verdict of manslaughter on grounds of diminished responsibility rather than murder. This is an important distinction, as murder carries a mandatory life sentence whereas sentencing for other offences is at the discretion of the judge.

## Mental disorder and crime

The relationship between mental disorder and crime is complex. Sometimes they occur together by coincidence. Sometimes, mental disorder can lead to crime as shown in Table 1. There are also some offences which by their very nature suggest psychological problems. One of these is arson, which is sometimes committed in response to delu-

Fig. 1 **Pathways through the criminal justice system.**

Table 1 **Crimes associated with certain mental disorders**

| Disorder | Offence | Reasons |
|---|---|---|
| Schizophrenia | Low rate of violence and homicide, but more likely than in general population | Secondary to delusions and hallucinations<br>Frustration caused by negative symptoms<br>More likely to be caught |
| | Acquisitive offences | Difficulty shopping and organising finances caused by negative symptoms<br>Poverty due to social drift |
| Mania | Violence (usually minor), reckless driving, deception, inappropriate sexual behaviour | Disinhibition<br>Impaired judgement<br>Grandiosity |
| Depression | Homicide/infanticide, victims usually family members; often followed by suicide | As a result of guilt and hopelessness, may believe family need protecting or putting out of their misery<br>When depression caused by dysfunctional relationship, tension and frustration may lead to violence and homicide |
| | Shoplifting | Poor concentration and memory<br>Fear of being caught can lead to temporary alleviation of low mood |
| 'Cluster B' personality disorders | Increased rate of violence, arson, sexual offences and acquisitive offences | Disregard for feelings of others<br>Explosive outbursts of anger<br>Impulsivity and need for instant gratification |
| Paranoid personality disorder | Violence | Suspiciousness and jealousy |
| Drugs and alcohol | Violence | Disinhibition<br>Impaired judgement |
| | Acquisitive offences | To obtain money for alcohol/drugs |
| Dementia and brain damage | Violence and inappropriate sexual behaviour | Disinhibition<br>Impaired judgement |

Table 2 **Possible sentences for offenders requiring psychiatric treatment**

**Custodial sentence with treatment in prison**
- some prisons have hospital wings
- some prisons offer specific treatment programmes, e.g. for sex offenders, substance abuse

**Hospital order (Section 37 of Mental Health Act)**
- broadly similar to Section 3
- can be used in any case of mental illness or severe mental impairment
- can be used in cases of psychopathic disorder or mental impairment only if treatment will result in improvement or prevent deterioration
- requires recommendations from two doctors, one approved under Section 12
- treatment in Special Hospital, Regional Secure Unit or district psychiatric hospital, depending on level of risk
- renewable, so patient remains in hospital while still a risk to public or him/her self
- patient may appeal to Mental Health Review Tribunal which has the power to discharge them

**Restriction order (Section 41 of Mental Health Act)**
- added to Section 37, only if restrictions are necessary to protect the public from serious harm
- means the patient cannot be moved to less secure facilities or given leave from hospital without the permission of the Justice Minister

**Probation, conditional on attendance for treatment**
- requires patient's consent
- patient returned to court for resentencing if breaches conditions

sions and hallucinations, and sometimes as a 'cry for help' or as a genuine suicide attempt. Sexual offending also suggests psychological abnormalities although, as will be seen in the following description, mental illness is rarely a cause.

### *Sexual offences*

Child sexual abuse includes a variety of sexual offences against boys and girls under the age of 16 years. Intra-familial child sexual abuse is known as incest, extra-familial as paedophilia. There is a considerable overlap between these two groups, with up to half of incestuous fathers molesting children outside their own family. Some men are drawn to children because they are unable to form satisfactory relationships with adults, because of personality difficulties or low intelligence. Others have a sexual preference for children and may not believe that what they are doing is wrong. A significant proportion will have been sexually abused during their own childhood. Mental illness is uncommon.

Rape is defined as penetration by the penis of the vagina, anus or mouth of another person without consent. Perpetrators are often under the influence of alcohol and, sometimes, illegal drugs. As with child sexual abuse, they often have difficulty forming normal sexual relationships. Men may sometimes resort to violence, including rape, when stressed or facing a threat to their status. Some men rape in order to act out violent sexual fantasies. Mental illness is not common among rapists.

About 25% of rapists commit a further sexual assault and reoffending by child abusers is even more common. Because of this, various treatment approaches have been devised. Social skills training and education about why sexual offences are wrong are often used. Behavioural techniques may be used to try to alter sexual fantasies. Often it will not be possible to eliminate the desire to offend and so it will be necessary for the offender to learn to control these urges and avoid situations which exacerbate them. Antilibidinal drugs such as cyproterone acetate are sometimes used. Whether any of these treatments are effective is controversial.

Indecent exposure is committed when a woman or, nearly always, a man exposes their genitals to another person in a public place. The majority of cases are emotionally and sexually inhibited men who are more likely to offend during times of stress. A minority of offenders progress to more serious sexual offences. Rarely, indecent exposure may be a feature of mental retardation, dementia or other mental illnesses.

## *Case history 35*

A 28-year-old man with schizophrenia is arrested for shoplifting.

a. What should happen to him?
b. Would this be any different if he had commited a serious crime?

## Forensic psychiatry

- Most patients with mental disorders never commit an offence
- Mental disorder increases the likelihood of some offences
- Offenders with a mental illness should usually be diverted from the criminal justice system to psychiatric care

# Alcohol dependence I

## Introduction

Alcohol is the most popular of the psychoactive substances available for recreational use. In small quantities it has a stimulating effect, lifting the mood and causing disinhibition, but if larger amounts are taken sedation and depression result. Concentration, speech and movement are also affected. Behaviour after drinking large amounts of alcohol is often impulsive, ill-judged and may be aggressive. As a consequence alcohol can be an extremely damaging drug. Regular heavy drinkers can suffer devastating physical, mental and social damage, and their families are also profoundly affected. Alcohol is implicated in 40% of all road traffic accidents, 50% of murders and 80% of suicides. In very large quantities it can be fatal because it depresses brain centres controlling circulation and breathing.

About 90% of the adult population drinks alcohol at some time. There is a continuum between normal social drinking, problem drinking and dependence on alcohol, and it can be difficult to distinguish between these states (Fig. 1). Maximum 'safe' levels of consumption have been recommended, above which the risk of sustaining some social or physical damage rises considerably. These levels are 21 units per week for men, and 14 per week for women (Fig. 2). At least 25% of men and 15% of women exceed these quantities. About one in ten of these will experience some significant difficulties in their physical or mental health, relationships, ability to work or some other aspect of their lives. Twenty percent of all admissions to psychiatric units are for alcohol-related problems.

## Clinical features

The main characteristic of dependence on alcohol is that the drinking takes priority over all other aspects of life. The threat of a marital breakdown or unemployment is not enough to convince the dependent drinker to cut down or stop, instead they will continue to drown the sorrows that have been produced by the alcohol in the first place. Other typical features of dependence on alcohol include:

- **Feeling compelled to drink.** There is such a strong desire to drink that alcoholics often feel they have no control over their drinking behaviour, and if alcohol is not available it is craved for. Many dependent drinkers want to stop but feel they cannot.
- **Tolerance of the effects of alcohol.** Increasing quantities are required to produce the same effect.
- **Withdrawal symptoms which appear within 6 hours of the last drink.** Typically this occurs overnight, resulting in withdrawal symptoms first thing in the morning. The earliest symptom to occur is usually tremor. If alcohol is not drunk quickly other symptoms follow, including anxiety, agitation, nausea, vomiting and sweating. Generalised convulsions can occur, and one in 20 will develop delirium tremens (DTs). Withdrawal symptoms can continue for up to a week if untreated.
- **'Relief drinking' and a regular pattern of alcohol consumption.** Alcohol is consumed to relieve withdrawal symptoms. There is regular 'topping up', often beginning early in the morning and continuing throughout the day. A routine becomes established and all other aspects of life must fit around it.
- **Rapid reinstatement after abstinence.** The full dependence syndrome returns remarkably quickly, even after a long period off alcohol.

Some alcoholics present to medical services with a direct request for help with their drinking. More often the presentation will be with one of the physical, psychological or social consequences, and the underlying cause may not be immediately obvious. Sustained heavy drinking can have an impact on virtually every body system, as shown in Figure 3. Comorbidity with mental illness is common. A detailed history of alcohol use must therefore be included in all medical and psychiatric assessments.

## Aetiology

Social and cultural factors play an important role in the aetiology of alcoholism. Overall consumption of alcohol by the population depends upon its availability, which is determined by the number and type of outlets selling it, the legal restrictions on purchasing it and price. In the western world alcohol is widely available, relatively cheap, and its consumption is highly socially acceptable. The more it is consumed by the population as a whole, the greater the number of alcoholics. On an individual level, there is good evidence that dependence on alcohol runs in families, and this is likely to be due to both genetic and environmental factors.

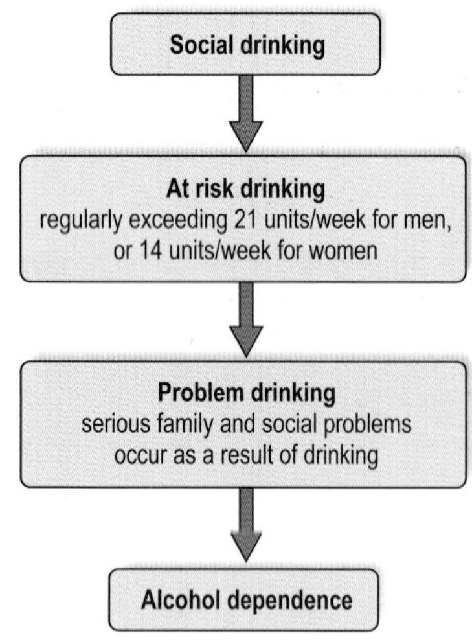


Fig. 1 **Continuum of alcohol consumption.**

1 Pint Beer
2 units
SPIRIT
30 units
1 unit
EXTRA STRONG LAGER
4 units
WINE
8 units
1 unit

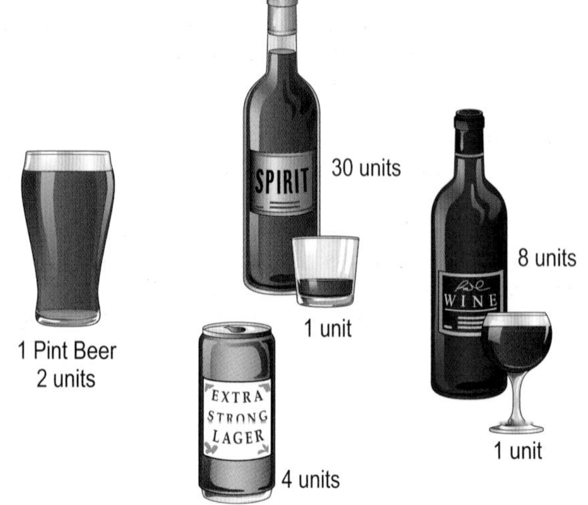

Fig. 2 **Units of alcohol.**

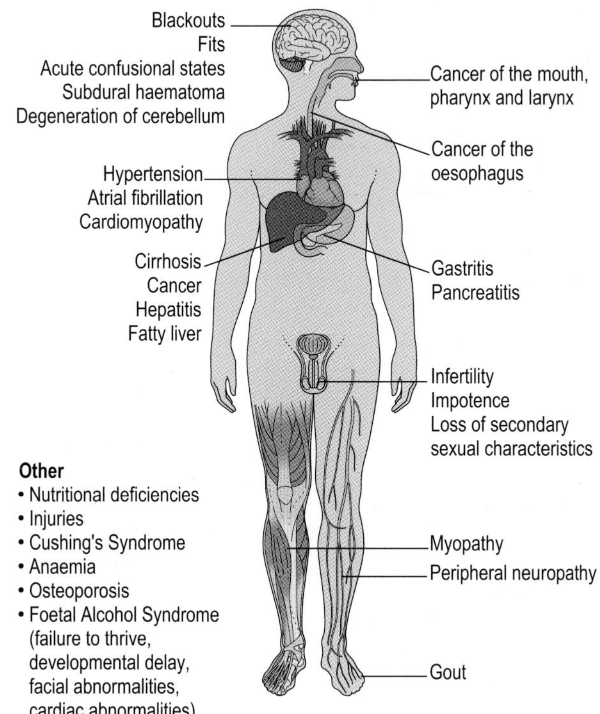


Fig. 3 **Physical effects of dependence on alcohol.**

## Psychiatric complications of alcohol dependence

### *Depression*

Alcohol dependence and depressed mood often go together, and it can be difficult to decide which came first. Both cause poor sleep, reduced appetite, feeling worse in the morning, loss of concentration, loss of interest in usual activities and low mood. Some patients with a primary depressive episode will begin to drink in an attempt to lift their mood or to blot out unbearable feelings. However, this does not usually result in problem drinking or dependence, and there is even some evidence that alcohol consumption overall is reduced during a depressive episode. Most commonly the depression is secondary to the alcohol dependence – 40% of alcoholics who present to psychiatrists for treatment meet the criteria for a diagnosis of depressive disorder. In at least three-quarters of these cases the depression resolves within two weeks of stopping drinking. It is only those patients who are still depressed when no longer drinking that will benefit from treatment with antidepressant medication.

### *Suicide*

Ten percent of alcoholics die by suicide due to a variable combination of the depressant and disinhibiting effects of alcohol, social problems and poor physical health.

### *Alcoholic hallucinosis*

This is an uncommon disorder in which auditory hallucinations occur in clear consciousness in an alcoholic who continues to drink. The hallucinations may be simple noises that last a few days only, or in more severe cases are of voices speaking in the second or third person, and persisting for many months or years. In contrast with schizophrenia there are no delusions, thought disorder or other first-rank symptoms. The aetiology is not known and treatment is with antipsychotic drugs.

### *Alcoholic dementia*

Chronic alcoholism may result in dementia, with cerebral atrophy that particularly affects the frontal lobes. The prevalence of dementia among alcoholics is not known, but about half have been shown to have some degree of cognitive impairment. In many of these cases the cognitive function returns to normal with abstinence from alcohol, but a proportion will have a continuing dementia.

### *Wernicke's encephalopathy and Korsakoff's psychosis*

These disorders are due to severe thiamine deficiency, and may occur for a number of reasons, most commonly alcohol dependence. Alcohol has high calorific content but no nutritional value, and alcoholics tend to replace their usual diet with alcohol. Dietary thiamine deficiency is made worse by the effects of alcohol on reducing absorption of thiamine from the gut and impairing its storage by the liver, while demand for thiamine is increased as it is required for the metabolism of alcohol. The encephalopathy has an acute onset, with confusion, ataxia, and ophthalmoplegia. Peripheral neuropathy is often found, but is not part of the acute syndrome. Urgent treatment with thiamine is needed as Wernicke's encephalopathy is potentially fatal and will progress to Korsakoff's psychosis if untreated. This is severe and permanent loss of memory, with an inability to lay down any new memories or retain information for longer than a few minutes, and in modern classifications is referred to as alcohol-induced amnesic syndrome.

### *Case history 36*

Edward is a 45-year-old businessman who presents to his GP with depression. He describes a 'disastrous' year in which he has separated from his wife, accumulated large debts and in the past week been notified that he is to be made redundant from his job. He has been consistently depressed for several months, with recurrent suicidal thoughts, loss of appetite, sleep disturbance and poor concentration. He says that he has been drinking alcohol in order to relieve his distress and forget his problems. His consumption has crept up to half to one bottle of whisky per day.

a. How would you establish whether he is dependent on alcohol?
b. What is the relationship between his depression and alcohol abuse?
c. How would you treat the depression?

### Alcohol dependence 1

Alcohol dependence is characterised by:

- priority of drinking over all other aspects of life
- tolerance of the effects of alcohol
- withdrawal symptoms on abstinence
- physical, psychiatric and social problems

# Alcohol dependence II

## Assessment

All patients should be asked about their alcohol consumption, and specific quantities recorded. Vague responses, such as 'I only drink socially', are not acceptable; many alcoholics consider themselves to be very sociable drinkers. As alcohol consumption varies for most people, it is usually easiest to enquire about a typical week and calculate the number of units consumed. Remember that measures poured at home are usually larger than the standard measures provided in bars. The pattern of alcohol consumption is important. Alcoholics typically have a rigid pattern, with regular consumption throughout the day, beginning with an early morning drink to alleviate withdrawal symptoms. The CAGE questionnaire is commonly used as a quick screening tool for alcohol dependence (Fig. 1).

If there is evidence of dependence, a detailed history of past and current drinking behaviour and its social, physical and psychological consequences should be obtained. It is important to ask about the patient's attitude to their drinking: do they consider it to be a problem and if so are they prepared to accept help to stop drinking? Motivation to stop is a vital prerequisite of any treatment package. Those who have no such motivation should be informed of the risks they are taking, and advised about the services available should they wish to seek help in the future.

Assessment of those with symptoms of alcohol dependence should include a full psychiatric history and mental state examination, looking particularly for depression, suicidal thoughts and cognitive impairment. A thorough physical examination will be necessary to search for the many medical complications of alcoholism, and this should be supported by investigations, including full blood count and liver function tests. The mean corpuscular volume (MCV) and serum gamma-glutamyl transpeptidase (GGT) are useful screening tests for alcohol abuse, as both are raised with chronic heavy alcohol consumption. A corroborative history may be useful to complete the assessment, but many alcoholics attempt to hide the full extent of their drinking from their families and may be unwilling to have them involved in the assessment.

## Treatment

Treatment of alcohol dependence consists of management of withdrawal from alcohol and prevention of relapse. It is relatively easy to persuade an alcoholic to stop drinking and treat the subsequent withdrawal symptoms; maintaining abstinence from alcohol is the real challenge.

### *Withdrawal from alcohol*

Management of withdrawal from alcohol, or detoxification, may be done in a planned, controlled way, with a patient who recognises that he has an alcohol problem and wishes to stop drinking. In these circumstances the withdrawal can often be managed at home with daily visits from the GP or Community Alcohol Team to monitor progress, and medication to control the symptoms. Hospital admission is only indicated if there is a history of serious problems during previous withdrawals, such as convulsions or delirium tremens.

Many withdrawals are not planned and happen after a period of enforced abstinence from alcohol. This may occur following admission to hospital and should always be considered in a patient who becomes tremulous or confused within a few days of admission. Symptoms of the withdrawal syndrome are summarised in Figure 2. They are usually treated with benzodiazepines (e.g. chlordiazepoxide) which, like alcohol, increase the activity of the neurotransmitter GABA. The drug is given in sufficient doses to control the symptoms, and the dose is then gradually reduced and stopped over the course of a week, by which time the symptoms will have resolved. Parenteral thiamine should be given to all patients to prevent Wernicke's encephalopathy. Detoxification should be offered to all alcoholics expressing a wish to stop drinking, including those who have been through this process many times in the past.

**Delirium tremens**, commonly known as DTs, is a serious condition that occurs within four days of stopping drinking. It usually begins suddenly with intense anxiety, agitation, tremulousness, confusion, a fluctuating level of consciousness and reduced awareness of the surroundings. Visual illusions and hallucinations are common and are typically fleeting visions of small animals but can be more complex. Dehydration occurs and autonomic disturbance causes sweating, a weak rapid pulse and often mild pyrexia. Without treatment the symptoms will settle within 3 days, but there is a mortality rate of 5% due to cardiovascular collapse, intercurrent infection, such as a pneumonia, or hyperthermia. DTs usually

**CAGE questionnaire**

If two or more of the following questions are answered positively, alcohol dependence is likely:

- Have you ever felt you should **c**ut down on your drinking?
- Do people **a**nnoy you by criticising your drinking?
- Do you feel **g**uilty about your drinking?
- Do you have an '**e**ye-opener' first thing in the morning to steady the nerves, or get rid of a hangover?

Fig. 1 **The CAGE questionnaire.**

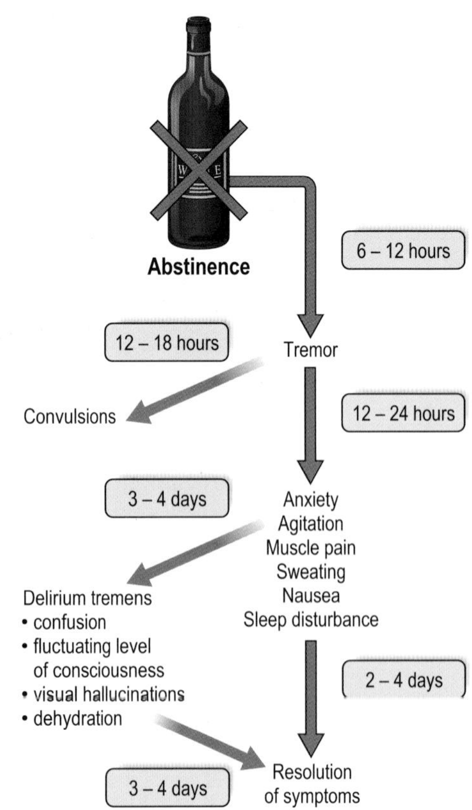


Fig. 2 **Withdrawal syndrome.**

require treatment in hospital and, in most circumstances, a general medical ward is better equipped to manage the disorder than a psychiatric ward. Close nursing observations are required and the patient should be examined for any evidence of infection, head injury or other physical disorder that may complicate the clinical picture. Relevant investigations should be performed, and appropriate treatment started quickly. The delirium should be treated with benzodiazepines, such as chlordiazepoxide, titrating the dose against the symptoms. Fluid replacement is important and may need to be provided intravenously. Parenteral thiamine should be given in every case.

### *Prevention of relapse*

A great variety of treatments are available for alcoholism, and it is best to tailor a package to suit the individual as far as is possible. Factors such as past experience of treatment, social supports and the amount of physical and psychological damage already sustained will influence the management plan (Fig 3). The goal of treatment for the majority of patients is lifelong abstinence from alcohol. A return to 'controlled' drinking is not a realistic possibility for most, as rapid reinstatement of the full dependence syndrome is characteristic of alcoholism.

Treatments are provided by the health service, private sector and voluntary organisations, and a combination of approaches is often helpful. Treatment options include:

1. **Pharmacological.** The drug disulfiram (Antabuse) is used to enhance patients' motivation to not drink. It works by interfering with the metabolism of alcohol, resulting in the build up of acetaldehyde if alcohol is drunk. This has extremely unpleasant effects, with flushing, headache, nausea, increased heart rate and hypotension. The patient will therefore have an additional reason to not drink after taking their medication each day and a powerfully reinforcing aversive effect if they do drink. However, there have been a few cases of people taking disulfiram who have died after consuming alcohol, so it should be prescribed with caution. Acamprosate is thought to reduce craving for alcohol through its effect on NMDA and GABA receptors in the brain, but has only been shown to be effective among people attending alcohol support groups.
2. **Residential rehabilitation programmes.** These are provided by the NHS and the private sector. Most use the Minnesota model of treatment, which consists of education, multiple group meetings and individual psychotherapy. Groups are important in the prevention of relapse and allow members to share their experiences and gain insight by seeing their own problems mirrored by others. They offer mutual support and work together to find strategies to cope without alcohol.
3. **Self-help organisations.** Alcoholics Anonymous (AA) is probably the best known of all self-help groups. It was founded in Akron, Ohio in 1935 and is now worldwide. AA relies on the principles of open self-scrutiny, help to others and fellowship, and the only membership requirement is a desire to stop drinking. Two parallel organisations, Al-Anon for the spouses of alcoholics and Al-Ateen for their children, are also available.
4. **Voluntary organisations.** Many organisations are available to provide advice and support either individually or in groups for alcoholics and their families. Some, such as the Salvation Army, also provide centres for detoxification and 'Dry Houses' for alcoholics to live in following detoxification.

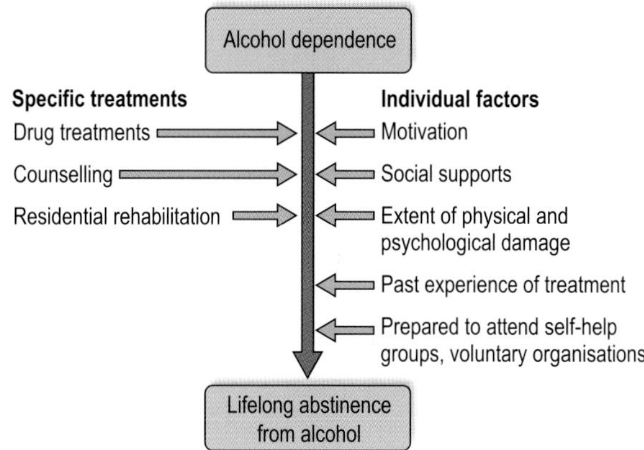


Fig. 3 **Prevention of relapse.**

## *Case history 37*

Mark is a 24-year-old man who was admitted to hospital following a fight in the street in which he was stabbed in the chest and sustained a pneumothorax. Three days after his admission he deteriorated suddenly. He did not appear to be aware of his surroundings, and had periods of drowsiness interspersed with extreme agitation. He was convinced that there were insects covering his bed, and was terrified by them.

a. What is the likely diagnosis?
b. What would be your short-term management plan?

## Alcohol dependence 2

- All patients should be asked about alcohol consumption
- The CAGE questions and MCV and GGT blood tests are useful screening tests
- Uncomplicated withdrawals from alcohol can be managed at home
- Delirium tremens is a serious condition that requires treatment in hospital
- A programme of care to prevent relapse is required following withdrawal

# Substance misuse

Psychoactive drug users come into contact with medical services when acutely intoxicated, dependent or mentally ill. Acute intoxication is a transient alteration in the level of consciousness, accompanied by changes in behaviour, mood, perceptions and cognition, occurring after taking the drug. Dependence on a psychoactive substance generally occurs after prolonged and regular use, and shares many of the characteristics of alcohol dependence, including primacy of drug taking over other activities, tolerance and withdrawal symptoms following abstinence.

The majority of adults in the developed world use psychoactive drugs at some time in their life. The legally available drugs, such as alcohol and tobacco, are the most widely used but a substantial proportion of young people regularly use illicit drugs such as cannabis and ecstasy, and up to a third of people will use an illicit drug at some time in their lives. The point at which 'use' of these drugs becomes 'misuse' or 'abuse' is unclear, and the various agencies involved apply different criteria. It is important to distinguish between unsanctioned drug use (use that is not approved of by society) and hazardous drug use that has harmful consequences for the user. It is the latter that mental health services are concerned with, in particular if the drug use impacts on the individual's psychological, social or occupational functioning.

Substance misuse occurs in all social classes, and there is little evidence that its onset is associated with social deprivation. There is though likely to be downward social drift as a consequence of dependence on drugs and those protected by social advantage are less likely to suffer adverse consequences. Most users of illegal drugs are young and a Merseyside study found that 92% of the opiate abusers were less than 30 years old. The middle-aged are more likely to be dependent on prescribed medication such as benzodiazepines. Men are twice as likely to use illicit drugs as women, and most are single and unemployed. Up to 50% of people attending drug treatment centres have a history of conviction, and the rate of criminal activity is inevitably much higher than this. The most commonly used drugs are described in Table 1.

## Assessment

Assessment of an individual seeking help for drug abuse or dependence begins with a thorough history, which must include a detailed account of current drug use. Quantities may be difficult to judge, but the amount of money spent on drugs will give some indication. Many drug users take a variety of drugs. They may have one preferred drug but supplement or replace this with others depending upon availability. Other aspects of the history to consider are previous treatment for drug abuse, social circumstances, legal issues including pending court cases and probation, and motivation for change. Physical examination should include a search for injection sites and investigations should include urinary drug screen, and, following counselling, blood tests for HIV and hepatitis B and C.

## Treatment of drug misuse

Drug services are provided by the health service, social services, probation service and voluntary sector. A number of different approaches are available, and packages of care should be designed to meet individual needs. Treatment options include the following.

### *Harm reduction measures*

In many cases it is not substance misuse itself that causes problems, but the lifestyle that accompanies it, in particular criminal activity to finance the drugs and other behaviour such as use of dirty needles to inject and unprotected sex. Prescribing a substitute for abused drugs reduces the need for users to fund their habit and the harm associated with use of street drugs and intravenous injection. Heroin addicts are prescribed the opiates methadone or buprenorphine, which

Table 1 **Drugs of abuse**

| Drug | Route | Effects |
|---|---|---|
| **Opiates**<br>Heroin, methadone, pethidine | Oral, sniffed, inhaled, smoked, injected | Intense, but brief euphoria. Tolerance and physical dependence occur.<br>Withdrawal symptoms include anxiety, depression, restlessness, insomnia, nasal secretion, musculoskeletal pains, anorexia, vomiting, diarrhoea, dilated pupils, yawning and gooseflesh ('cold turkey') |
| **Benzodiazepines**<br>Temazepam, Diazepam, Lorazepam, etc. | Oral, occasionally intravenous | Anxiolytic and sedative effects. Tolerance and physical dependence occur.<br>Withdrawal symptoms include anxiety, tremor and convulsions acutely, and over a longer period depression, fatigue, insomnia, sensitivity to light and sounds, visual distortions and muscle weakness |
| **Amphetamine** | Oral, sniffed, intravenous | Stimulant action, causing euphoria, increased energy, reduced need for sleep and reduced appetite. Tolerance and physical dependence may occur. Chronic use can result in an illness resembling schizophrenia |
| **Cocaine** | Oral, sniffed, smoked, intravenous | Causes a feeling of intense pleasure and excitement (the rush) lasting seconds, followed by less intense feelings for about 30 minutes, and then by depression, irritability, insomnia and craving for more. Repeated intoxication can result in hallucinations or persecutory delusions, and there may be violent behaviour. Tolerance develops |
| **Cannabis** | Oral, smoked | Causes mild euphoria and relaxation, sense of heightened perception and occasionally hallucinations. Physical effects include reddening of conjunctivae, dry mouth, and fast pulse |
| **LSD**<br>(Lysergic acid diethylamide) | Oral | Effects develop gradually over 2–4 hours, with mood changes, visual illusions and hallucinations and other perceptual changes. Flashbacks to these effects can occur weeks or months later |
| **Solvents**<br>Glue, lighter fluid, paint thinners, aerosol sprays, petrol | Sniffed | Causes mood swings, lack of judgement, disinhibition and visual hallucinations. The effects last about 30 minutes. Sudden death may occur due to direct cardiac toxicity |
| **Ecstasy (MDMA)** | Oral | Causes euphoria, a sense of heightened empathy and some perceptual changes. Tolerance may develop. Has been associated with a small number of sudden deaths |
| **Ketamine** | Oral, sniffed, inhaled, smoked, intramuscular, intravenous | Causes user to feel detached from their body and surroundings and to hallucinate. Intravenous injection dangerous. Long-term use associated with cognitive impairment |

has partial agonist and antagonist effects and can precipitate withdrawal if taken with other opiates. Amphetamine users can be prescribed dexamphetamine. Other measures include provision of clean needles and condoms, and education about safe practices.

### *Medical detoxification*

For many drugs no active medical intervention is needed during the period of withdrawal beyond reassurance and encouragement to persevere. Referral to the local drug advisory service for support and counselling is often helpful. Patients who are dependent may benefit from the prescription of medication to prevent the discomfort and risks of acute withdrawal. Methadone and buprenorphine are commonly used for withdrawal from opiates and diazepam for withdrawal from benzodiazepines. They are prescribed in sufficient dose to control symptoms and avoid the need for the patient to use any illicit drugs, and the dose is then reduced at a rate that is comfortable for the patient. For long-term addicts this may be a slow process over several months, and regular support and monitoring will be required throughout. A more rapid, managed withdrawal from opiates can be achieved using the alpha-2-adrenergic receptor agonists lofexidine or clonidine, which provide symptomatic relief.

### *Other forms of treatment*

Motivational techniques and individual support are used and without them many drug abusers would not engage with any of the treatments described above. Groups such as Narcotics Anonymous are often helpful. Social interventions, such as help with accommodation and financial problems, may help people who have given up hope of recovery back onto the right track. Residential rehabilitation is offered to people who are not helped by standard measures.

## Mental illness and substance misuse

There is a strong relationship between substance abuse and mental illness. The two occur together coincidentally, but more commonly there is a direct relationship, with the substance abuse causing mood disorders, anxiety disorders and psychotic illnesses. The social problems and adverse life events that frequently accompany substance abuse may also indirectly precipitate mental illness.

### *Drug-induced psychosis*

A psychotic illness with hallucinations and delusions can be precipitated by stimulants such as amphetamine, hallucinogens such as LSD, or cannabis. The symptoms may closely mimic schizophrenia, psychotic depression or mania, but resolve within a few weeks if no more of the drug is taken. It is not uncommon though for apparently drug-induced psychotic illness to persist despite cessation of the drug, most likely because the person affected has a predisposition to psychosis that is precipitated by the drug but probably would have occurred later anyway. Symptoms of drug-induced psychosis respond to antipsychotic drugs, which should be tapered off as the symptoms resolve and discontinued when the patient has recovered. This treatment will not be effective if the drug abuse continues.

### *Drug abuse in the severely mentally ill*

The severely mentally ill may take illicit drugs for a wide variety of reasons (Fig. 1). Drug abuse is a serious problem in the severely mentally ill because it is associated with a worse outcome, worse symptoms, more relapses, more medical and social complications, and a reduced response to medication. Compliance with all forms of treatment tends to be poorer. There is also an increased risk of violence and suicide. These patients need a comprehensive but flexible management plan, with good co-ordination between specialist drug and general psychiatric services, an emphasis on engaging them with the service and close monitoring.

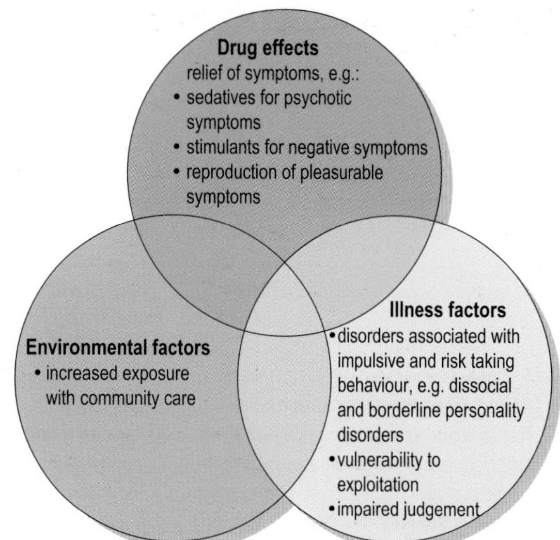


Fig. 1 **Causes of drug abuse in the severely mentally ill.**

### Case history 38

Nick is a 28-year-old man who has been diagnosed with paranoid schizophrenia. He abuses a variety of illicit drugs. He smokes cannabis every day, and uses amphetamines most days, usually intravenously. He also takes benzodiazepines, ecstasy and LSD intermittently. He is suspicious of mental health services because he has been admitted to hospital against his will in the past after attacking his mother because of auditory hallucinations of voices telling him that she was an impostor. He has no desire to address his drug use.

a. How should he be managed?

### Substance misuse

- Use of illicit drugs is very common, and the majority of drug users will not come into contact with psychiatric services
- Harm reduction measures form an important part of the management of drug users
- Drug abuse is a severe problem in the seriously mentally ill and requires a carefully co-ordinated management plan

# Psychosexual disorders

Psychosexual disorders fall into three main groups in ICD10: sexual dysfunction, gender identity disorders and disorders of sexual preference (Table 1). Sexual dysfunction is the most common of these groups, and so will be discussed in detail.

## Sexual dysfunction, not caused by organic disorder or disease

The title of this category in ICD10 is misleading. It implies that sexual dysfunction is caused either by organic illness and disease or by psychological factors when, in fact, it is often caused by a combination of the two. An example of this is given in Figure 1 which also demonstrates how sexual dysfunction is often the result of problems in both partners.

### *Clinical assessment*

The structure of a sexual history is similar to the history of other presenting complaints. It is important to help the patient describe their problems by asking open questions. Once you have clarified the nature of the problem, it is important to establish how long it has been going on and whether there have been any precipitating or maintaining factors. Sexual problems are often a manifestation of other problems in a relationship and so it is important to find out if there are any such problems. Enquiry should be made about sexual experience and beliefs and it is helpful to know whether the problem has occurred during other relationships. Clinical assessment should involve both partners if possible, as they may have different views about the problem and may both contribute to the problem. Treatment is more likely to be successful if both partners are involved.

A problem often encountered when taking a sexual history is that many people are not used to discussing sexual matters and feel embarrassed about doing so. If the person taking the history appears embarrassed, this will make matters worse. A particular problem is knowing what words to use and feeling comfortable in saying them. For example, terms such as ejaculation and orgasm are stilted and may not be familiar to some people. An alternative term like 'come' is more likely to be understood and using colloquial terms like this usually puts people at ease and encourages open discussion. Because of this, it is important to become confident in speaking about sexual matters using terms people understand.

| Table 1 **ICD10 classification of sexual disorders** |
|---|
| **Sexual dysfunction not caused by organic illness or disease** |
| Lack or loss of sexual desire |
| Sexual aversion and lack of sexual enjoyment |
| Failure of genital response |
| Orgasmic dysfunction |
| Premature ejaculation |
| Non-organic vaginismus |
| Non-organic dyspareunia |
| Excessive sexual drive |
| **Gender identity disorders** |
| Transsexualism. Desire to live and be accepted as a member of the opposite sex |
| Dual-role transvestism. Wearing clothes of the opposite sex in order to temporarily feel like a member of that sex |
| **Disorders of sexual preference** |
| Fetishism. Reliance on an inanimate object for sexual arousal |
| Fetishistic transvestism. Wearing clothes of the opposite sex to achieve sexual arousal |
| Exhibitionism. Recurrent exposure of genitals to strangers, usually leading to sexual arousal |
| Voyeurism. Recurrent, secretive observation of people involved in sexual or intimate behaviour such as undressing |
| Paedophilia. Sexual preference for children |
| Sadomasochism. Preference for sexual activity that involves bondage or infliction of pain or humiliation |
| Multiple disorders of sexual preference. Combinations of above disorders |

### *General principles of management*

It is important to investigate and treat any suspected organic illness or disease that may be contributing to the sexual problems. Common conditions to look for are summarised in Figure 2. It is also essential to check whether either partner has a mental illness, particularly depression – which is a common cause of loss of sexual desire. If sexual problems are just one aspect of more general relationship problems, these should be addressed through relationship counselling.



Fig. 1 **An example of the complexity of some sexual problems.**

## Sexual dysfunction in women

### *Lack or loss of sexual desire*

This has a number of psychological causes. It is common for sexual desire within a relationship to decrease over time. Women often have to fulfil a number of different roles such as worker, homemaker, parent, child and friend and as these roles expand it may be difficult to maintain the role of lover. Sexual desire is reduced by fatigue, stress, depression, relationship problems and previous adverse sexual experiences. These causes should be addressed during treatment. It is particularly helpful for couples to set aside time to spend together in surroundings that encourage them to relax and talk as this can often lead to a rejuvenation of sexual desire. It is important to help couples discuss what they like and don't like about their lovemaking as differences can lead to reduced sexual desire.

### *Failure of genital response*

In women this consists of vaginal dryness and failure of lubrication. By far the most common cause is postmenopausal oestrogen deficiency.

### *Orgasmic dysfunction*

This is more commonly known as anorgasmia. It is defined as failure to achieve orgasm despite adequate stimulation. While orgasm is central to many women's enjoyment of sexual intercourse, some women derive satisfaction from other parts of lovemaking. However, because most men cannot

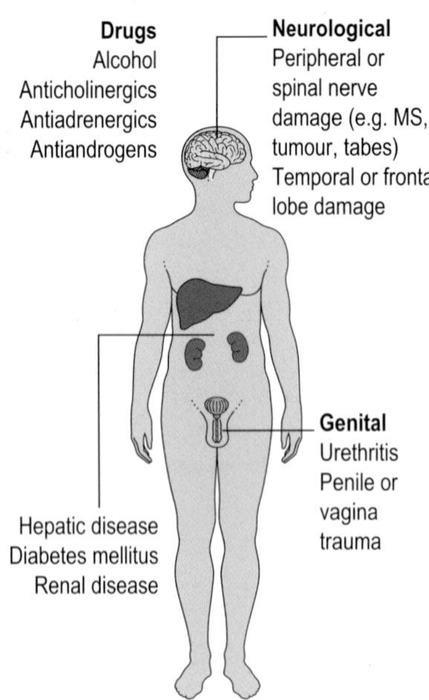


Fig. 2 **Organic disorders causing sexual problems.**

fully enjoy sexual activity without achieving orgasm, they assume that the same is true of a female partner. Therefore, even if a woman does not consider anorgasmia to be a problem, it may still cause problems in her sexual relationship. Encouraging partners to discuss these issues is a useful first step in treatment and behavioural therapy, in which intercourse is initially prohibited (sensate focus technique, Fig. 3), can be used to remove the pressure for a woman to achieve orgasm and allow couples to explore other sources of sexual pleasure. Encouraging masturbation and use of sexual fantasy may help women learn ways to heighten their sexual arousal and achieve orgasm.

### *Non-organic vaginismus*

This is an involuntary spasm of the muscles surrounding the lower third of the vagina. As well as causing sexual problems, it makes use of tampons difficult and may prevent women from attending for cervical smear tests. It is caused by a fear of vaginal penetration. In some cases this fear develops as a result of dyspareunia and continues even when pain is no longer a problem. In other cases, the fear develops in the absence of pain. Treatment has a high success rate. It starts with relaxation exercises that help the women learn to relax her vaginal muscles and reduce anxiety levels. The next step is to gently insert vaginal 'trainers' of increasing size while carrying out the relaxation exercises. 'Trainers' can be fingers or specially designed specula. The next step is insertion of a penis under the woman's control before finally transferring control to the partner.

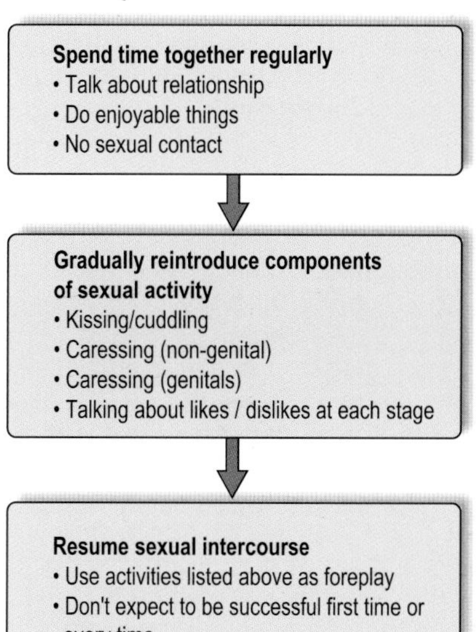


Fig. 3 **Sensate focus.**

### *Dyspareunia*

This is genital pain occurring during sexual activity. Non-organic dyspareunia is a misleading term as most cases are the result of both organic and psychological factors. Commonly, pain is caused initially by an organic problem and non-organic dyspareunia then develops because of fear of the pain recurring. Treatment should start with investigation and treatment of the organic causes. Often, no further treatment is required. If the problem persists, a programme similar to that used for vaginismus is likely to be successful.

## Sexual dysfunction in men

### *Lack or loss of sexual desire*

This is less common in men than women but its causes and treatment are similar to those described above.

### *Failure of genital response*

This is more commonly known as erectile dysfunction or erectile impotence. It refers to the failure to achieve or maintain an erection. It affects about 40% of men over 40 and 70% of men over 70. Up to 25% of cases are caused by psychological factors alone, 25% by physical factors alone and the rest by a combination of the two. Psychological factors are likely if a man is unable to achieve an erection during intercourse but does so at other times, such as on waking in the morning or when masturbating. Psychological aspects of the problem are often helped by the process of sensate focus which is outlined in Figure 3. Giving up smoking and reducing alcohol and illicit drug use can result in considerable improvement. The most commonly used physical treatment are phosphodiesterase inhibitors, which improve blood flow to the penis by reducing the breakdown of cyclic GMP in smooth muscle cells that line blood vessels in the corpus cavernosum.

### *Orgasmic dysfunction*

This takes the form of delayed or retrograde ejaculation. It can occur following prostatectomy and is a common side effect of antipsychotic drugs and antidepressants, particularly specific serotonin reuptake inhibitors. With SSRIs, the serotonergic antagonist cyproheptadine can be given prior to intercourse although this can precipitate a relapse of depression. Otherwise, treatment involves advice about increasing the amount of genital stimulation.

### *Premature ejaculation*

This can be defined in different ways. Ejaculation occurring before or shortly after penetration certainly constitutes premature ejaculation. A broader definition is that it is an inability to control ejaculation sufficiently for both partners to enjoy sexual intercourse. It occurs in about 20% of men. It is much more common in young men and usually improves with increased sexual experience. There are a variety of treatments. Performance anxiety has an important role in premature ejaculation and this can be reduced by advice and discussion, preferably involving both partners. The 'stop and squeeze technique' involves squeezing the base of the penis firmly just before ejaculation and then resuming intercourse once the sensation of being about to ejaculate has subsided. An alternative is for the man to work his way through a variety of masturbation exercises that teach him to recognise when ejaculation is imminent and develop techniques for delaying it.

### Psychosexual disorders

- Psychosexual disorders are classed into: sexual dysfunction, gender identity disorders and disorders of sexual preference
- Sexual dysfunction is the most common and is caused by physical, psychological and relationship problems, sometimes alone and sometimes in combination
- Gender identity disorders and disorders of sexual preference are uncommon and require specialist management

# Self-assessment

All the following statements are either true or false

1. Regarding mental health services:
   a) CMHTs are multidisciplinary teams
   b) Occupational therapists act as care co-ordinators
   c) Most cases of mental illness are seen by CMHTs
   d) CPA is a specific social care intervention
   e) Home treatment teams control hospital admissions
2. Early Intervention in Psychosis Teams:
   a) Work with recent onset cases, regardless of age
   b) Get involved once a diagnosis has been confirmed
   c) Avoid using medication in the early stages of illness
   d) Act as care co-ordinators for their patients
   e) Work with patients until psychosis has resolved
3. Assertive Outreach Teams:
   a) Work primarily with homeless patients
   b) Display a forceful attitude towards patients
   c) Work most with people with schizophrenia
   d) Do housework with patients to try to engage them
   e) Are ineffective when substance misuse is present
4. The following are examples of functional mental illnesses:
   a) Bipolar affective disorder
   b) Schizophrenia
   c) Borderline personality disorder
   d) Korsakoff's psychosis
   e) Somatisation disorder
5. The following demographic factors are associated with suicide:
   a) Female
   b) Older age
   c) Living in rural environment
   d) Working as an anaesthetist
   e) Unemployment
6. The following health and social factors are associated with suicide:
   a) Chronic arthritis
   b) Married
   c) Schizophrenia
   d) Alcohol dependence
   e) Bereavement
7. Neurotransmitters have the following characteristics:
   a) precursors are present in the synaptic cleft
   b) presynaptic excitation causes synthesis
   c) they bind to pre- and post-synaptic receptors
   d) receptor binding causes a biological effect
   e) they pass into the postsynaptic cell
8. The following are associated with an increased risk of violence:
   a) Male gender
   b) Past history of violence
   c) PTSD
   d) Substance misuse
   e) Cluster B personality disorders
9. In assessing the suicide risk of a patient following an overdose:
   a) impulsive overdoses suggest high suicide risk
   b) the number of tablets taken is a key factor
   c) writing a suicide note suggests higher risk of suicide
   d) if they called for help, the suicide risk must be low
   e) a history of previous self harm suggests a low risk
10. Third person auditory hallucinations:
    a) Are usually experienced as being inside the head
    b) By definition consist of three separate voices
    c) May suggest the patient should kill himself
    d) Are often associated with a diagnosis of schizophrenia
    e) May comment on the patient's actions
11. The following factors contribute to non-adherence with psychotropic drugs:
    a) Side effects of medication
    b) Good insight into the illness
    c) Stigma
    d) Financial concerns
    e) Complex drug regimes
12. The following concepts are typically used in Cognitive Therapy:
    a) Defence mechanisms
    b) Counter-transference
    c) ABC model
    d) Thinking errors
    e) Cognitive schemata
13. The following suggest a diagnosis of schizophrenia rather than psychotic depression:
    a) Second person auditory hallucinations
    b) Thought broadcasting
    c) Loosening of association
    d) Delusions of guilt
    e) Nihilistic delusions
14. Bipolar disorder:
    a) Is a form of cyclothymia
    b) Type 2 causes hypomanic and depressive episodes
    c) May present with a mixed affective state
    d) Can be made worse by antidepressants
    e) Is often treated with carbamazepine
15. The following interventions are recommended for the treatment of depressive episodes in primary care:
    a) Computerised CBT
    b) Problem solving
    c) Exercise programmes
    d) Guided reading
    e) Antidepressant medication
16. The following are features of manic episodes:
    a) Emotional lability
    b) Increased productivity at work
    c) Flight of ideas
    d) Persecutory delusions
    e) Irritability
17. SSRI antidepressants are commonly used in the following conditions:
    a) Hebephrenic schizophrenia
    b) Generalised anxiety disorder
    c) OCD
    d) PTSD
    e) Somatoform pain disorder
18. Mental state examination of a patient with obsessive–compulsive disorder will typically reveal:
    a) Dishevelled appearance
    b) Depressed affect
    c) Delusions of contamination
    d) Mood congruent auditory hallucinations
    e) Disorientation in time and place
19. The following are typical of bulimia nervosa:
    a) Disregard for calorific intake between binges
    b) Amenorrhoea
    c) Good response to treatment with SSRIs alone
    d) 40% of cases have onset after age 40 years
    e) Better prognosis in men
20. The following are correctly paired:
    a) Paranoid personality disorder: delusions of persecution
    b) Dissocial personality disorder: social withdrawal
    c) Borderline personality disorder: rejection sensitivity
    d) Histrionic personality disorder: shallow affect
    e) Anankastic personality disorder: feelings of ineptitude
21. In older people:
    a) Deliberate self-harm is often 'a cry for help'
    b) Early dementia is the condition most likely to cause suicide

c) Hearing impairment protects against auditory hallucinations
d) Alzheimer's disease is the most common form of dementia
e) Antipsychotic drugs are helpful in Lewy body dementia

22. The following suggest a diagnosis of delirium over dementia:
a) Acute onset
b) Hallucinations
c) Personality change
d) Varying impairment of attention
e) Evidence of acute physical illness

23. Dementia is a common feature of the following conditions:
a) Huntington's disease
b) HIV infection
c) Normal pressure hydrocephalus
d) Parkinson's disease
e) Multiple sclerosis

24. The following are usually of benefit in the management of acute alcohol withdrawal:
a) Antipsychotic drugs
b) Antidepressants
c) Benzodiazepines
d) Buprenorphine
e) Oral thiamine

25. The following processes maintain anxiety disorders:
a) Avoidance
b) Response prevention
c) Thinking biases
d) Extinction
e) Operant conditioning

26. The following conditions often present with physical symptoms:
a) Delirium
b) Depressive episodes
c) Somatisation disorder
d) Dissociative fugue
e) Factitious disorder

27. Obsessions:
a) Seem to the sufferer to be inserted in their head
b) Sometimes consist of images
c) If violent, suggest a high risk to others
d) Are usually resisted by the sufferer
e) Suggest a diagnosis of OCD rather than depression

28. The following are typical adverse effects of most antipsychotic drugs:
a) Dry mouth
b) Diarrhoea
c) Agitation
d) Tremor
e) Acute dystonia

29. The following are early signs of lithium toxicity:
a) Slurred speech
b) Fine tremor
c) Ataxia
d) Ophthalmoplegia
e) Nausea and vomiting

30. The following are often used to treat chronic (residual) schizophrenia:
a) Antidepressant medication
b) Family therapy
c) Psychiatric rehabilitation
d) Dynamic psychotherapy
e) Occupational therapy

31. The following are typical of alcohol dependence:
a) Intoxication early in the day
b) Able to maintain work and relationships
c) Opportunistic drinking of alcohol
d) Slow rate of relapse because of tolerance
e) Delirium tremens occurs within 24 hours of abstinence

32. The following increase the likelihood of recognising depression in primary care:
a) Ask open questions
b) Respond to emotional cues
c) Save time with closed questions
d) Ask directly about emotions
e) Maintain eye contact for around 50% of time

33. The following are features of mental incapacity:
a) Mental retardation
b) Decisions most people would consider foolish
c) Not weighing evidence in the balance
d) Decision not supported by the nearest relative
e) Unable to communicate decision

34. Autism:
a) Causes narrow repetitive patterns of behaviour
b) Is often associated with learning disability
c) Is a specific developmental disorder
d) Is characterised by excessive 'make believe' play
e) Typically features language problems

35. The following are true of ADHD:
a) Also known as hyperkinetic disorder
b) Persistence into adulthood in most cases
c) Good response to mild tranquillisers
d) Impulsivity is typical of the condition
e) Helped by behavioural interventions

36. Regarding conduct disorder:
a) It is usually diagnosed in primary school
b) Genetic factors are the main cause
c) Having friends makes the diagnosis unlikely
d) Many go on to exhibit dissocial behaviour as adults
e) School refusal is a common manifestation

37. The following conditions are likely to be made worse by tricyclic antidepressants:
a) Glaucoma
b) Prostatic hypertrophy
c) Ischaemic heart disease
d) COPD
e) Myaesthenia gravis

38. The Mental Health Act can be used:
a) To detain a patient in a general hospital
b) By a police officer
c) To force a patient to accept medication at home
d) As an alternative to a prison sentence
e) To give antibiotics to an incapacitous patient

39. The following conditions are psychotic in nature:
a) Schizotypal disorder
b) Schizoaffective disorder
c) PTSD
d) Body dysmorphic disorder
e) Anorexia nervosa

40. The following are correctly paired:
a) Phobias: Anticipatory anxiety
b) Generalised anxiety disorder: Fear of illness
c) Social phobia: Worse in shops
d) Panic attacks: Metabolic acidosis
e) Depressive episodes: High rate of anxiety symptoms

## Answers

1. TTFFT. CMHTs are multidisciplinary teams in which all qualified staff act as care coordinators, using the CPA process to review and plan care. Most cases of mental illness are seen in primary care. Home treatment teams are best placed to decide whether admission is needed.
2. FFFTF. EIP teams work with people aged 14–35 years, for up to 3 years, assessing suspected psychosis and coordinating care for established cases, and starting antipsychotic medication at an early stage.
3. FFTFF. Assertive outreach teams work in a highly patient-centred manner with people who would otherwise disengage from treatment, typically people with schizophrenia, often with comorbid alcohol or substance misuse. Homelessness is an issue for some of their patients.
4. TTFFT. Mental disorders are either organic, i.e. have a demonstrated physical cause, or functional. Korsakoff's psychosis results from brain lesions caused by thiamine

deficiency. Personality disorders are mental disorders, not illnesses.

5. FTFTT. Middle aged and older men living in cities are at greatest risk. Employment is a protective factor, except for a few high risk professions, usually those that provide easy access to methods of suicide.
6. TFTTT. Mood disorders and alcohol and substance misuse carry the highest risk, but rates are raised in most forms of mental disorder. Marriage is protective, separation and bereavement increase the risk.
7. FFTTF. Neurotransmitters are synthesised in the presynaptic neurone, stimulation of which causes their release into the synaptic cleft, where they exert their biological effects by binding to pre- and post-synaptic receptors.
8. TTFTT. Risk factors for violence are male gender, alcohol and substance misuse and, as is often found in cluster B personality disorders, a history of violence and impulsivity. Once these factors are taken into account, the effect of mental illness on rates of violence is small.
9. FFTFF. Planned overdoses, with evidence of suicidal intent, that the person thought would kill them are the most concerning. Calling for help suggests ambivalence but this is not the only factor that determines subsequent risk. Previous DSH suggests a high risk of repetition and a raised risk of suicide.
10. FFTTT. Hallucinations are heard from external space. Third person hallucinations refer to the patient as he or she, e.g. 'He should kill himself' and are a first rank symptom of schizophrenia, as are voices giving a running commentary on the patient's actions, usually in the third person.
11. TFTTT. People are less likely to take medication if they don't believe they need to take it or feel stigmatised by doing so, have side effects, have to pay for it, or have to deal with complex regimes.
12. FFTTT. Defence mechanisms and transference are concepts used in dynamic psychotherapy. CBT teaches people that cognitive schemata lead to thinking errors, so that ***A***ntecedents result in unhelpful ***B***eliefs and ***C***onsequences.
13. FTTFF. Second person auditory hallucinations occur in both schizophrenia and depression. Thought broadcasting is a first rank symptom and loosening of association is the thought disorder typical of schizophrenia. Delusions of guilt and nihilistic delusions are typical of psychotic depression.
14. FTTTF. Cyclothymia involves less severe mood changes. Bipolar disorder, type 1 is diagnosed if mania or mixed affective states occur, with or without depression; type 2 if only hypomania and depression occur. Antidepressants may cause conversion to hypomania and rapid cycling. Carbamazepine is used less often than lithium, valproate and antipsychotics.
15. TTTTT. These are all available in primary care, as part of the stepped care of depression.
16. TFTTT. Emotional lability and flight of ideas are typical of mania, as are grandiose delusions, but persecutory delusions also occur. Patients are often irritable as well as elated. Mania is only diagnosed if the patient is too unwell to function normally.
17. FTTTF. SSRIs should be offered to patients with GAD, OCD and PTSD, but psychological treatment is often more effective. Hebephrenic schizophrenia is treated with antipsychotic drugs, somatoform disorders with psychological treatment.
18. FFFFF. Poor self care and depression occur in OCD but are not typical. Some patients fear contamination but recognise their concerns are misfounded, so are not deluded. Hallucinations and cognitive impairment are not a feature.
19. FFFFF. Most restrict calories between binges. Most cases are not underweight so amenorrhoea is not typical. SSRIs can reduce the urge to binge but should be used to augment psychological treatments. Onset is in adolescence or early adulthood in the vast majority of cases. Male cases are less common but have a worse prognosis.
20. FFTTF. Mistrust and suspiciousness are typical of paranoid PD, but delusions are not a feature of personality disorders. People with dissocial PD engage with the world, but in an abrasive way. Rejection sensitivity is typical of borderline PD, as is a shallow affect of histrionic PD. Feelings of ineptitude are typical of anxious PD.
21. FFFTF. DSH in older people is usually a failed suicide attempt. Dementia is not usually a cause of suicide. Auditory hallucinations are more likely with hearing impairment. Alzheimer's disease is the most common form of dementia, followed by vascular dementia. Antipsychotic drugs make Lewy body dementia worse and are associated with an increased risk of stroke in all forms of dementia.
22. TTFTT. Delirium is caused by the toxic effects of physical illness on the brain. It typically has an acute onset and causes fluctuating levels of confusion and perceptual disturbance, including hallucinations. Personality change is typical of dementia.
23. TTTTT. These five conditions can all present with dementia, in addition to their other manifestations. In the case of HIV and normal pressure hydrocephalus, the dementia will improve with treatment of the underlying condition.
24. FFTFF. Benzodiazepines and alcohol both activate GABA receptors and each reduces withdrawal from the other. Antipsychotic drugs are occasionally needed for rapid tranquillisation, but can reduce the seizure threshold, as can antidepressants. Buprenorphine is an opiate agonist used in opiate dependence. Oral thiamine takes too long to restore levels to be helpful acutely.
25. TFTFT. Operant conditioning maintains anxiety disorders by causing avoidance. Thinking errors can cause anxiety. Response prevention is a form of treatment and extinction is the abatement of anxiety that occurs if a person manages to stay in a feared situation.
26. FTTFT. Delirium is a psychiatric presentation of a physical condition. Physical symptoms are common in depression. Medically unexplained physical symptoms are typical of somatisation disorder and symptoms are fabricated in factitious disorder. Dissociative fugue presents with amnesia.
27. FTFTF. Obsessions are recognised by the sufferer as a product of their own mind and can be thoughts, images or impulses. The sufferer finds them unpleasant and often repugnant, and resists them and doesn't act on them, unlike compulsions. They occur in depressive episodes as well as OCD.
28. FFTTT. Antimuscarinic effects such as dry mouth are caused by some antipsychotics, but are more typical of tricyclic antidepressants. Diarrhoea is typical of SSRIs.

Akathisia, Parkinsonism, dystonia and tardive dyskinesia are typical of antipsychotics and can occur even with atypicals other than clozapine.

29. FFFFT. Nausea, vomiting and coarse tremor are the early signs, slurred speech and ataxia occur later. Fine tremor is a benign effect that occurs at therapeutic levels. Ophthalmoplegia is typical of Wernicke's encephalopathy.
30. FTTFT. Antipsychotic drugs are still needed, but antidepressants are seldom required. Family therapy to educate carers and reduce expressed emotion is helpful and rehabilitation and occupational therapy can improve function. Dynamic psychotherapy would not help.
31. FFFFF. Early morning drinking is typical, but not intoxication because of tolerance. The person continues to drink despite damage to work and relationships. There is a regular pattern of drinking, not an opportunistic one and rapid relapse is typical. Withdrawal symptoms occur within hours but DTs usually after 2–3 days.
32. TTFTF. Best practice is to be empathic, maintain good levels of eye contact, respond to emotional cues, ask open questions that directly address the patient's emotional state.
33. FFTFT. Mental capacity involves understanding and retaining information, weighing it in the balance and communicating the decision. It should not be assessed on the basis of a diagnosis, such as learning disability (mental retardation), or the decision that is made.
34. TTFFT. Autism is a pervasive developmental disorder, characterised by restricted and repetitive behaviour and impaired social interaction and communication. Learning disability occurs in 75% of cases.
35. TFFTT. ADHD is classified as hyperkinetic disorder in ICD10. It is characterised by hyperactivity, inattention and impulsivity. Most cases remit by adulthood. Stimulant drugs and behavioural and family interventions are effective.
36. FFFTF. It is usually diagnosed in secondary school. Genes play a part but family and environmental factors are more important. Friendships with similar children are typical of the socialised form. Truancy occurs, not school refusal. 50% exhibit dissocial personality disorder as adults.
37. TTTFF. TCAs have antimuscarinic effect that exacerbate glaucoma and prostatism and, in addition, affect the cardiovascular system because of anti-adrenergic and membrane stabilising properties.
38. TTFTF. The MHA can be used to detain a person in any hospital but only to enforce the treatment in hospital of mental disorder and its manifestations. The MHA can be applied to people at all stages of the Criminal Justice System. Section 136 allows a police officer to take a person to a place of safety if they pose a risk to themselves or others as a result of mental disorder.
39. FTFFF. Brief periods of psychosis can occur in schizotypal disorder but the core features are not psychotic in nature. Schizoaffective disorder is only diagnosed if psychotic symptoms typical of schizophrenia and mood disturbance occur simultaneously. Flashbacks in PTSD are not considered psychotic in nature and distorted body image in anorexia nervosa is thought to be caused by culturally determined views of thinness and the effects of starvation on self-perception. Delusional disorder and not body dysmorphic disorder should be diagnosed if concerns about appearance are of delusional intensity.
40. TTFFT. Anxiety about being exposed to the feared situation is typical of phobias, as are health concerns in GAD. Social phobia will only be worse in crowded places if it is likely the sufferer will have to interact with others. Metabolic alkalosis occurs in panic attacks. Depression and anxiety commonly coexist.

# Case history comments

## Case history 1

a. John will need to have regular contact with a psychiatrist, who will prescribe his antipsychotic drugs, and monitor his mental state. The psychiatrist may also need to arrange inpatient treatment, and consider the use of the Mental Health Act if necessary. In view of John's poor compliance with medication it would be worth considering use of injected depot antipsychotic medication. If this were used it would be administered by a community psychiatric nurse (CPN). The CPN could also investigate the possibilities of alternative accommodation for John, help him engage in appropriate activities and social contact, and provide support to his parents. An assessment of his independent living skills by an occupational therapist would help in deciding what sort of accommodation would suit him best. A social worker may also be involved in finding the accommodation.

b. The CPN would probably be the most appropriate care co-ordinator, because John's treatment will need to include long-term medication, but other members of the team may be competent to monitor medication, even if they are from a different professional background.

## Case history 2

a. The care co-ordinator from the community mental health team and representatives of the home treatment and assertive outreach teams should be invited to the CPA, along with any friends or family Jess wants to attend.

b. The home treatment team could work with Jess regarding adherence to medication and could monitor her mental state. The assertive outreach team may be able to engage with her more effectively than the CMHT, so could take over her care co-ordination.

## Case history 3

a. Emily has experienced the following psychiatric disorders:
- dependent personality disorder
- panic disorder
- depressive disorder with secondary obsessional symptoms
- organic depressive episode due to steroids.

## Case history 4

a. The history suggests she will be unable to retain the information needed to make a decision, or to weigh it in the balance, but test this formally. She is unlikely to regain capacity without treatment for pneumonia, so you need to decide whether she would have wanted you to start her on antibiotics. Find out if she has made an advance directive that covers these circumstances or if she has granted a LPA for personal welfare. If she hasn't, talk to relatives and other people who know her well and if necessary involve an IMCA.

## Case history 5

a. There is evidence of mental illness, the patient is not accepting treatment in the community and she is neglecting herself and therefore risking her own health and safety. She will not accept voluntary hospital admission, so compulsory admission should certainly be considered.

b. If she is relatively new to mental health services, Section 2 of the Mental Health Act should be considered. If she is well known, and the diagnosis established, then Section 3 would be more appropriate. In either case she should be assessed by two doctors, ideally a consultant psychiatrist and a GP who knows her, and by an approved mental health practitioner (AMHP). If possible these assessments should take place at the same time, and would probably take place in the patient's home. The AMHP has responsibility for co-ordinating the section assessment, and arranging for the patient to go into hospital.

## Case history 6

a. Antidepressant treatment is likely to help Nilanjan, but so will psychological and social treatments. He has cardiovascular risk factors so amitriptyline is not a good choice, but the modified tricyclic lofepramine is an alternative. Citalopram could be tried again, starting at a low dose and increasing slowly.

## Case history 7

a. Cognitive behavioural therapy would target Mary's depression and anxiety and schema work could help her understand how her childhood contributed to any thinking errors. Dynamic psychotherapy would help Mary understand how her relationship with her parents affects her response to the problems she faces in the present. The final decision about what form the therapy should take would depend on factors such as Mary's preference, her willingness and ability to work within a therapeutic framework, and local availability of resources.

## Case history 8

a. It is unlikely that Rose will be able to live independently immediately, although this may be an appropriate longer term goal. Possible options include:
- group home
- hostel providing lower levels of support.

b. An occupational therapy assessment would help to establish her current abilities in performing activities of daily living (e.g. road safety, ability to handle money, cooking skills, etc.). This would then contribute to the decision-making process which should also involve Rose, her family (if she wishes them to be involved), the hostel staff, care co-ordinator and psychiatrist. The least restrictive environment that meets her needs should be selected.

## Case history 9

a. The most likely diagnosis is paranoid schizophrenia, given the age of onset, delusions of thought control, possible auditory hallucinations, thought disorder (demonstrated by the family's difficulty following his speech) and social withdrawal. Other diagnoses to consider include drug-induced psychosis, and depressive episode with psychotic symptoms.

## Case history 10

a. His parents should be reassured that they are in no way to blame for his illness. Schizophrenia is caused by a number of biological and environmental factors, but there is no evidence that style of parenting or stressful events can cause schizophrenia. However, the family and home environment can have an effect on the course of schizophrenia, and it may be possible to help the family reduce the level of expressed emotion in the home.

### Case history 11

a. The three symptoms described are common positive symptoms of schizophrenia.
b. The course of schizophrenia is very variable; however, it is likely that he will experience further acute episodes of illness and he may develop negative symptoms.
c. His prognosis is likely to be much worse if he fails to comply with antipsychotic medication, abuses illicit drugs, has little social support or lives in an environment with high levels of expressed emotion.

### Case history 12

a. Antipsychotic treatment should be changed to a drug with less antimuscarinic and sedative effects. If he doesn't respond to this, consider switching to clozapine. Cognitive therapy targeting delusions and hallucinations should be considered, especially if there is only a partial response to medication. His daily living skills should be assessed to determine whether he needs rehabilitation, supported accommodation or other community support. His financial situation should be reviewed and optimised. He should be helped to establish meaningful activity and to stay involved with his local community. It is important to explain the nature of his illness and treatment to him and his family and let them know how to obtain help if needed in the future. His mental state and treatment should be monitored by his care co-ordinator from the CMHT and by outpatient appointments with a psychiatrist. His care should be co-ordinated through regular CPA meetings.

### Case history 13

a. Tell Sarah she is correct in her view that her depressive episodes have been a response to life events and explain that it was the symptoms she developed at the time, their duration and the extent to which they affected her life that led to the diagnosis. She describes what sounds like hypomanic episodes, but check that she didn't experience the disruption of normal function or the psychotic symptoms that occur during manic episodes. Her diagnosis is probably bipolar affective disorder, type 2, and this should help her by identifying the treatments most likely to be of benefit.

### Case history 14

a. Kwame's children are at raised risk of bipolar and unipolar mood disorders, but are more likely than not to remain free of either condition. If they do develop a mood disorder, effective treatment is available. There is no evidence of measures that can be taken to prevent the onset of mood disorders, but most people feel better for maintaining regular sleep patterns and find it helpful to read self-help books based on the principles of CBT. It would be important to bear the family history in mind if one of his children developed any persistent mood disturbance, and if he has a daughter who becomes pregnant, she should mention it to the antenatal team.

### Case history 15

a. The diagnoses to consider are:
   - manic episode of bipolar disorder
   - intoxication with alcohol or illicit drugs (such as amphetamines or cocaine)
   - normal variation in mood (she may be excited about going to the very important meetings).
b. Further evidence of mania should be sought, such as difficulty sleeping, racing thoughts, poor judgement (e.g. spending too much money) and psychotic symptoms. The GP should also ask about alcohol and illicit drug use. A history from an informant (e.g. parent, friend) may be useful. Risks associated with disinhibited behaviour, such as overspending, sexual disinhibition and dangerous driving must be considered.

### Case history 16

a. Sharon is low in mood with tearfulness. She has psychological symptoms of depression, as she is taking a pessimistic view of things and has lost confidence. Biological symptoms are also present with sleep disturbance, loss of energy and forgetfulness and difficulty coping at work probably due to poor concentration.
b. You would need to know how long the symptoms had been present, and what had precipitated them. You should also look for other symptoms of depression such as suicidal ideas, changes in appetite and diurnal variation in mood. A past history and family history of depression would help confirm the diagnosis. It is also important to exclude common differential diagnoses by asking about alcohol consumption, physical health and use of both prescribed and illicit drugs.

### Case history 17

a. Janet is likely to be helped by interventions from step 2 and step 3 of the stepped care model for depression. CBT and antidepressants should be offered. Problem solving may be relevant if the end of her relationship has led to practical problems. An exercise programme may be of benefit.
b. The treatment options should be explained to Janet and she should decide, with advice if necessary, what are the best options for her.

### Case history 18

a. It is important to exclude physical causes for his symptoms by taking a full medical history, and performing a physical examination and relevant investigations. You should ask about psychological symptoms of anxiety, such as feelings of fear, dread or panic. Physical symptoms of anxiety include dry mouth, sweating, tremor and diarrhoea in addition to the shortness of breath and chest pain that he complains of. If the shortness of breath is due to anxiety it is likely that he is hyperventilating. And this would resolve if he breathed into a paper bag.
b. Social phobia is most likely because the symptoms were precipitated by the prospect of a public performance.

### Case history 19

a. Management of Anton's social phobia should start with reassurance and explanation of the symptoms he is experiencing. CBT is the treatment of choice. His specific fears about public speaking could be addressed by a programme of systematic desensitisation, combined with anxiety management and challenges of any thinking errors underlying his anxiety. There may be a limited role for drug treatments. SSRIs are effective in some cases of social phobia and taking beta-blockers prior to doing a presentation may be helpful.

### Case history 20

a. Mary's differential diagnosis should include:
   - obsessive–compulsive disorder
   - depressive disorder with secondary obsessional symptoms
   - schizophrenia.
   - In addition, it is likely that she

has an obsessional personality disorder.

b. Treatment:
   - *Drug treatment* – antidepressants with predominantly serotonergic action, such as SSRIs, or the tricyclic clomipramine.
   - *Psychological treatment* – may be delivered individually or in a group. Behavioural therapy would be appropriate, such as exposure and response prevention.
   - *Social treatment* – it may be helpful to look at Mary's sources of social contact and support to see if these can be enhanced. Her mother's needs should also be considered.

## Case history 21

a. Post-traumatic stress disorder is most likely, although it would be important to exclude depressive disorder and to enquire about any psychiatric disorders present prior to the incident in the lift.

b. In the first instance he will require some reassurance and advice about managing the panic attacks. Cognitive behavioural therapy would be an appropriate treatment option. Antidepressant medication may be helpful if he is depressed, and to relieve some of the anxiety symptoms. Tricyclic antidepressants should be avoided as he has a history of ischaemic heart disease.

## Case history 22

a. Mike experienced a strong impulse to hit someone. In normal circumstances he would have acted on the impulse, but in this case was unable to because of his desire to maintain his new relationship. This resulted in an emotional conflict that he found difficult to resolve.

b. Conversion – his psychological conflict was 'converted' into a physical symptom and thereby resolved.

c. Primary gain was relief of the anxiety and discomfort aroused by being unable to act on his impulse. Secondary gain was the concern and attention of his girlfriend and her family.

## Case history 23

a. Somatisation disorder is most likely. She may have a concurrent depressive disorder

b. There are a number of things that may help:
   - Book regular appointments with her in advance, possibly weekly at first with a view to extending the interval between appointments in time. Make it clear that the expectation is that she will not be seen outside these appointments except in an emergency.
   - Tell her she has somatisation disorder, which is a real condition but not life threatening.
   - Avoid unnecessary investigations, referrals or interventions.
   - Treat depression if present and deal with social and interpersonal problems.
   - Enlist support from her husband.

## Case history 24

a. The first step should be to confirm the diagnosis. In order to do this the focus must shift from the children to Jane. She may be reluctant for this to happen, and it will require tact and sensitivity. The diagnosis can be confirmed by enquiring about psychological and biological symptoms of depression, past history of depression and family history of mental illness. Other diagnoses should be excluded by enquiring about alcohol and illicit drug use, and physical health. Investigations might include blood tests to look for anaemia and thyroid dysfunction. When the diagnosis is confirmed, treatment should be offered including antidepressant drugs, counselling and support in addressing social problems (e.g. financial advice, help with child care).

b. The health visitor may have a role in monitoring the children's wellbeing, and giving Jane support in her maternal role. The practice counsellor may be able to offer psychotherapy to treat the depression.

## Case history 25

a. The possible causes are:
   - MS may be the direct cause of depression and anxiety
   - drug treatment of MS with steroids may cause depression
   - depression and anxiety may be an emotional response to the stress of a deterioration in the MS and admission to hospital
   - coincidental occurrence of the depression, anxiety and MS.

b. Management depends to some extent on the cause, but in all cases it is reasonable to consider the following:
   - active treatment of the MS relapse
   - limit prescription of steroids, if used, to minimum dose and duration
   - antidepressant medication
   - psychological treatment, such as supportive psychotherapy or cognitive behavioural therapy
   - consider any social problems that may prevent recovery.

## Case history 26

a. $\text{BMI} = \dfrac{\text{weight (kg)}}{\text{height (m)}^2} = \dfrac{48}{1.7^2} = 16.6.$

b. Normal BMI is 20 or over. Therefore if ideal weight is $x$:
   $20 = \dfrac{x}{1.7^2}.$
   Ideal weight = at least 57.8kg.

c. Anorexia nervosa, because her weight is more than 15% below normal. She is deliberately losing weight by keeping to a low calorie diet, and has a distorted body image.

d. She is likely to have amenorrhoea, bradycardia, hypotension, constipation and muscle weakness.

## Case history 27

a. It is important to establish whether Bronwyn has suicidal thoughts and whether there are any social or family factors involved in causing her depression. How severe have her previous episodes of depression been, including the one that occurred postnatally? Has she had treatment for depression other than sertraline and was any of this helpful? Is she planning to breast-feed?

b. In collaboration with Bronwyn, and bearing in mind the issues mentioned above, come to a decision whether intervention is needed and whether family, social and psychological treatments should be tried. If she decides medication is needed, imipramine would be the safest drug. The risks with SSRIs like sertraline are low, particularly after the first trimester. She could breast-feed when taking imipramine or sertraline.

## Case history 28

a. Further information would be needed from David and others to confirm a diagnosis of personality disorder, but the most likely diagnosis is of anxious personality disorder. Other possibilities to be considered are emotionally unstable personality disorder, and dissocial personality disorder.

## Case history 29

a. An assessment should be completed, looking for evidence of mental illness, drug or alcohol abuse, or other factors which may have contributed to the current crisis. If present these should be treated in the usual way. The intervention should aim to diffuse the crisis in a practical way. For example, a low-dose antipsychotic drug may help with the feelings of tension. It may help to give him an opportunity to discuss the problems with his girlfriend, and if necessary he could be given advice about where to seek help with rehousing. A sick note allowing him to take a period of leave from work may allow the problem with his boss to be resolved. The GP should arrange to see him at regular intervals to offer support throughout the crisis period.

## Case history 30

a. She is grieving for her mother. This is, of course, a normal and appropriate reaction, although not expressed in an entirely normal way because of her mental retardation.
b. At this stage no formal treatment is required, but the staff may be able to help her grieve by giving her opportunities to talk about her mother, look at photographs and have access to some of her personal possessions as mementoes. If things do not settle over the following months, or if her behaviour escalates (for example, with self harm), then treatment needs to be considered, including antidepressant medication and referral to a therapist who is skilled at working with people with learning disability.

## Case history 31

a. Hyperkinetic disorder is the most likely diagnosis, but unsocialised conduct disorder should also be considered.
b. Difficulties in family relationships may well be contributing to Liam's difficult behaviour. His parents divorced when he was 3 years old, and he has a new step-father. There is clearly inconsistency between his mother and step-father in their parenting styles, and his step-father may be overly strict. He has a new baby sister, with whom he will be competing for his mother's attention. It is also possible that his mother may be feeling unable to cope because she has postnatal depression.
c. It is important that the mother and step-father are united and consistent in their approach to Liam. Wherever possible any good behaviour (or even absence of 'bad' behaviour) should be rewarded, and undesirable behaviour ignored. Having some one-to-one time with Liam each day may help address some of the frustration and jealousy he may feel following the birth of his sister. The mother should also be advised to liaise closely with the school.

## Case history 32

a. Secondary nocturnal enuresis – bedwetting occurring after a period of being dry. It is most likely to be due to the stress and worry of her parents separating.
b. Urinary tract infection is the commonest differential diagnosis.
c. The mother should be reassured that this is a common problem, due to stress, and cannot possibly be deliberate as it is occurring in Charlotte's sleep. Mother has clearly also been through a stressful time, and may find it easier to deal with Charlotte calmly if she has an opportunity to express her feelings of anger and distress elsewhere. Charlotte should not be punished for the bedwetting; instead the mother should work with her gently to sort the problem out. A star chart is likely to be effective. Charlotte would earn one star for each dry night, possibly with the added inducement of a present of her choice after one full week of being dry.

## Case history 33

a. Frank probably has dementia. The gradual onset and global nature of his presentation is suggestive of Alzheimer's disease, but his vascular risk factors and abnormal gait raise the possibility of vascular dementia. Normal pressure hydrocephalus causes dementia, ataxia and urinary incontinence and must be excluded.
b. If psychometric testing and neuroimaging support a diagnosis of Alzheimer's disease, then a cholinesterase inhibitor may help. Normal pressure hydrocephalus, if present, is treatable. Check there is no prescribed medication, alcohol use or physical illnesses that may be exacerbating his condition. Person-centred non-drug interventions are most likely to be of benefit.

## Case history 34

a. Depressive disorder with nihilistic delusions (also known as Cotard's syndrome).
b. As she has stopped eating and drinking, urgent treatment is necessary, under the Mental Health Act if necessary. ECT should be considered, because of the rapid onset of action.

## Case history 35

a. The police should request a psychiatric opinion before pressing charges, ideally from the psychiatrist who has been treating the man. If the psychiatric opinion is that the crime was committed because of the schizophrenia, and treatment is offered, the police will usually decide not to press charges, and he will be diverted out of the criminal justice system at this stage.
b. If a serious crime has been committed then the police will usually press charges, and a forensic psychiatry opinion will be sought prior to trial by jury in a crown court. If found guilty the judge may decide that the patient should receive psychiatric treatment under a hospital order.

## Case history 36

a. If he is dependent on alcohol he would feel compelled to drink, and have a regular pattern of consumption. He would also experience withdrawal symptoms, usually in the mornings, and may drink to relieve them. He would also be increasingly tolerant to the effects of the alcohol.
b. It is not clear whether the depression or alcohol abuse came first, but each is likely to make the other worse. It is possible that the social problems he describes (marital breakdown, debts and loss of employment) could all be a direct result of his alcohol abuse. This accumulation of problems in addition to the alcohol could then precipitate a depressive episode.
c. It is not advisable to treat a depressive episode in the usual way (with antidepressant drugs and/or psychotherapy) in the face of this considerable alcohol consumption. The first step in treatment should be to address the alcohol abuse. If he remains depressed after several weeks of abstinence from alcohol, then specific treatment should be started.

## Case history 37

a. The timing and presentation is suggestive of delirium tremens. Other causes of delirium should also be considered.
b. The following should be considered:
   - medication to reduce his distress and agitation and allow him to be nursed safely; a benzodiazepine such as chlordiazepoxide would be most appropriate for treatment of DTs
   - nurse in separate room that is well lit and quiet
   - physical examination and investigations to confirm the cause of the delirium
   - give parenteral thiamine to prevent Wernicke's encephalopathy.

## Case history 38

a. Active treatment is desirable for this man, as he poses a risk of violence when unwell. Both the schizophrenia and drug abuse will need to be managed, ideally with involvement of specialist services. In some areas there are 'dual diagnosis' services aimed specifically at treating individuals with a combination of severe mental illness and drug misuse. An assertive outreach approach is likely to be necessary, i.e. services will have to go to him rather than wait for him to attend clinics. The emphasis should be on building a relationship with him that will encourage him to engage with treatment. Harm minimisation measures such as provision of clean needles and advice about sexual behaviour may be helpful. Depot antipsychotic medication should be considered, as he is unlikely to take prescribed oral medication consistently.

# Index



Page numbers followed by f indicate figures; t, tables; b, boxes